Contemporary Issues in Breast Cancer

Jones and Bartlett Series in Oncology

Contemporary Issues in Breast Cancer

Edited by

Karen Hassey Dow, PhD, RN, FAAN
Associate Professor
School of Nursing
University of Central Florida
Orlando, Florida

JONES AND BARTLETT PUBLISHERS
Sudbury, Massachusetts
Boston   London   Singapore

Editorial, Sales, and Customer Service Offices
Jones and Bartlett Publishers
40 Tall Pine Drive
Sudbury, MA 01776
(508) 443-5000
(800) 832-0034

Jones and Bartlett Publishers International
Barb House, Barb Mews
London W6 7PA
UK

Library of Congress Cataloging-in-Publication Data
Contemporary issues in breast cancer/edited by Karen Hassey Dow.
      p.   cm. — (Jones and Bartlett series in oncology)
   Includes bibliographical references and index.
   ISBN 0-86720-713-2
   1. Breast—Cancer.   I. Dow, Karen Hassey.   II. Series.
  RC280.B8C639 1996   96-14427
  616.99'449—dc20   CIP

The selection and dosage of drugs presented in this book are in accord with standards accepted at the time of
publication. The authors, editor, and publisher have made every effort to provide accurate information.
However, research, clinical practice, and government regulations often change the accepted standard in this
field. Before administering any drug, the reader is advised to check the manufacturer's product information
sheet for the most up-to-date recommendations on dosage, precautions, and contraindications. This is
especially important in the case of drugs that are new or seldom used.

P06081

Printed in the United States of America
00 99 98 97 96   10 9 8 7 6 5 4 3 2 1

*For women with breast cancer
and their families, and the nurses who have cared for them.*

Contents

Preface

There are many medical textbooks devoted specifically to breast cancer, so why a book on *contemporary issues* in breast cancer? Other texts carefully describe the pathology, natural history, treatment, and progression from the perspective of the disease. Many fine oncology nursing reference texts contain chapters on breast cancer that provide a comprehensive and excellent description of breast cancer and associated symptom management from the perspective of active treatment. There are also books written specifically for the lay audience. Witness the several first-person accounts of women surviving treatment and living with breast cancer. These books are written from the perspective of the individual woman. Yet, there was no text available for nurses and other health care professionals that brought together the issues in medical management, nursing concerns beyond symptom management and support, and the larger family and community experiences in living with the disease. Thus, *Contemporary Issues in Breast Cancer* is contemporary in its attempt to examine the issues of breast cancer with the backdrop of one's family, community, and culture.

This book is divided into eight parts: prevention, screening, and early detection of breast cancer; issues in the treatment of breast cancer, including concerns about tamoxifen and choices in newer breast cancer treatment modalities; survivorship issues such as menopausal symptoms, exercise, depression, and social support; first-person accounts of living with breast cancer; breast cancer as a family issue; innovative community models or interventions; ethnicity and culture in breast cancer; and, finally, activism, health policy, and research. Each chapter is comprehensive in its scope of the history of the topic and suggests areas of future research.

Contemporary Issues in Breast Cancer is the result of many individual talents, gifts, and skills, as well as a great deal of patience. First and foremost, a special tribute to the women with breast cancer and their families who shared their lives, fears, hopes, and dreams. They have helped to focus our concerns in surviving breast cancer and in living with the disease. They have armed the public with more information and have greatly challenged the prevailing thinking about breast cancer. Second, an enormous thanks to the book's contributors who have given their time and talent in writing about their clinical experiences and presenting their research on breast cancer. They represent a wide range of clinical specialists, researchers, educators, activists, and advocates. They live in geographically and ethnically diverse parts of the country and give us insights into the unique aspects of their practices. Third, a special appreciation for our families, friends, and significant others who have supported us in our writing and editing endeavors. They have sacrificed valuable family time so that we could write our chapters and get them published in due time. I would like to especially thank my husband, Norman Dow, and my daughter, Lauren Hassey. Finally, wholehearted thanks to the staff at Jones and Bartlett— to Jan Wall, RN, for her foresight and patience and to Suzanne Crane for her humor and patience.

Contributors

Jennifer L. Aikin, RN, MSN, OCN
Clinical Nurse Specialist
National Surgical Adjuvant Breast
and Bowel Projects
Pittsburgh, Pennsylvania

Madeline M. Barnicle, RN, MS, OCN
Oncology Clinical Nurse Specialist
Rush Cancer Institute
Rush Presbyterian St. Luke's Medical Center
Chicago, Illinois

Beverly Brandt, RN, MSN
Clinical Nurse Specialist
Allegheny General Hospital; and
Adjunct Faculty
University of Pittsburgh, Graduate School
of Nursing
Pittsburgh, Pennsylvania

Jeannine M. Brant, RN, MS, AOCN
Oncology Clinical Nurse Specialist/
Pain Consultant
Saint Vincent Hospital and Health Center
Billings, Montana

Barbara J. Carter, DNSc, RN, CS
Associate Professor
Division of Nursing
Massachusetts College of Pharmacy and
Allied Health Sciences
Boston, Massachusetts

Patricia M. Clark, RN, MSN, CS, AOCN
Nurse Practitioner
Breast Evaluation Center
Dana-Farber Cancer Institute
Boston, Massachusetts

Elizabeth Ann Coleman, PhD, RNP, AOCN
Associate Professor
College of Nursing
University of Arkansas for Medical Science
Cancer Prevention and Control Research
Program; and
Program Leader
Arkansas Cancer Research Center
Little Rock, Arkansas

Karen Hassey Dow, PhD, RN, FAAN
Associate Professor
School of Nursing
University of Central Florida
Orlando, Florida

Johanna Lombardo Ehmann, RN, AAS, OCN
President/Founder
Johanna's of Albany, Ltd.
Cancer Rehabilitation Nurse Consultants
Albany, New York

Barbara A. Given, PhD, RN, FAAN
Professor and Director
Research Center
College of Nursing
Michigan State University
East Lansing, Michigan; and
Associate Director
Cancer Prevention and Control
The Cancer Center at Michigan State University
East Lansing, Michigan

Judith Hirshfield-Bartek, RN, MS, OCN
Clinical Nurse Specialist
Beth Israel Hospital
Boston, Massachusetts

Lizbeth A. Hoke, PhD
Clinical Psychologist
Department of Psychiatry
Beth Israel Hospital
Boston, Massachusetts

Marjorie Kagawa-Singer, PhD, RN, MN
Associate Researcher
National Research Center on Asian American
Mental Health
UCLA
Los Angeles, California

M. Tish Knobf, RN, MSN, FAAN
Associate Professor
Yale University School of Nursing;
Oncology Clinical Nurse Specialist
Ambulatory Service
Yale New Haven Hospital
New Haven, Connecticut

Kathy LaTour, MFA
Journalist and Instructor
Southern Methodist University
Dallas, Texas

Susan A. Leigh, RN, BSN
Cancer Survivorship Consultant
Tucson, Arizona

Deborah K. Mayer, RN, MSN, AOCN, FAAN
Oncology Consultant
Portland, Oregon

Victoria Mock, DNSc, RN, OCN
Director of Oncology Nursing Research
The Johns Hopkins Oncology Center
Baltimore, Maryland

Laurel L. Northouse, PhD, RN, FAAN
Associate Professor
College of Nursing
Wayne State University
Detroit, Michigan

Nancy O'Rourke, RN, MSN
Clinical Nurse Specialist
Radiation Oncology
Beth Israel Hospital
Boston, Massachusetts

Janice Mitchell Phillips, PhD, RN
*Assistant Professor and ACS Professor
of Oncology*
School of Nursing
University of Maryland
Baltimore, Maryland

Lucette M. P. Robinson, RN, BSN
Clinical Nurse III
Radiation Oncology
Beth Israel Hospital
Boston, Massachusetts

Nelda Samarel, EdD, RN
Associate Professor
Department of Nursing
William Patterson College of New Jersey
Wayne, New Jersey

Amy Strauss Tranin, RN, MS, OCN
Genetic Cancer Risk Counselor
Trinity Lutheran Hospital
Kansas City, Missouri

Sandra Millon Underwood, PhD, RN
Associate Professor
University of Wisconsin
Milwaukee, Wisconsin

Nancy J. White, RN, MS, OCN
Clinical Nurse Coordinator
Rural Cancer Care Project
Michigan State University
Kalamazoo, Michigan

Contemporary Issues
in Breast Cancer

PART 1 | Prevention, Screening, and Early Detection of Breast Cancer

CHAPTER 1 | Genetics and Breast Cancer Risk

Amy Strauss Tranin, RN, MS, OCN

INTRODUCTION TO MOLECULAR GENETICS

The health-care professional's present understanding and practice of oncology relies on a sophisticated knowledge of human anatomy, physiology, biochemistry, and pathology. Dealing with disease in the future will require a detailed understanding of the molecular anatomy, physiology, and biochemistry of the human genome. It will be necessary for health-care practitioners to intimately understand molecular anatomy and physiology of chromosomes and genes.

Cancer, in its various forms, is a genetic disease (Sandberg, 1994). It involves deviations in the normal genetic mechanisms that regulate cell growth. A malignancy is the result of genetic mutations in somatic cells and its progression involves a series of genetic changes. The mutations that lead to cancer affect the genes responsible for cell proliferation and development, as well as other fundamental cellular activities.

Currently, the treatment of breast cancer begins only after the patient's diagnosis, that is, after initiation and progression have taken place (Caskey, 1993). The time is fast approaching when technology will make it possible to predict the development of breast cancer through a simple blood test involving DNA analysis. The prediction of these events, based on our knowledge of gene function and pathogenic progression, will provide us with an entirely new approach to the diagnosis and treatment of breast cancer.

Keeping up with the continuing advances in molecular genetics will be essential for nursing practice in the future. Nurses must begin to understand this information as well as they currently understand anatomy, physiology, and disease pathology because the advances in molecular genetics will affect all aspects of health care. Many of the genetic changes that underlie

Figure 1-1   Human Karyotype Form

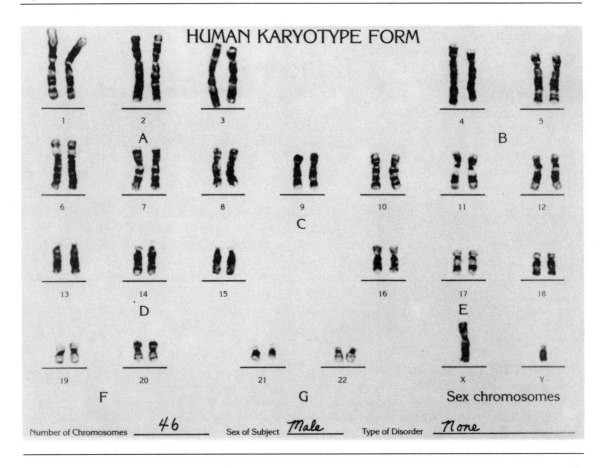

malignant transformation of cells and/or distinguish malignant clones are used as markers to diagnose, monitor, or characterize breast cancer (Gilchrist et al., 1993; Lonn, Lonn, Nilsson, & Stenkvist, 1994; Normanno, Ciardiello, Brandt, & Salomon, 1994; Wenger et al., 1993).

This chapter provides an overview of molecular genetics to help nurses caring for women with breast cancer better comprehend preventive, diagnostic, and treatment methods currently being used and those that will be forthcoming. The patients and clients that nurses work with will also need to know and understand much of this information to make decisions for themselves. In order to provide ac-

curate risk information, the nurse must be able to evaluate an individual's risk based on inheritance and sporadic (multifactorial) factors.

STRUCTURE OF HUMAN CHROMOSOMES

The 46 chromosomes of the human genome, which contains approximately 50,000 to 100,000 genes, are illustrated in Figure 1-1. These genes control all aspects of embryogenesis, development, growth, reproduction, and metabolism—essentially all aspects that make a human being a functional organism (Thompson, McInnes, & Willard, 1991).

Approximately 5% to 10% of the total number of genes have been identified—about 4,000 genes in all (Hoffman, 1994). It is predicted that by the year 2005, every one of the estimated 100,000 human genes will have been identified (Nowak, 1994). When that work has been completed, it is generally assumed that it will be possible to characterize and understand the genes and their organization in the genome. This will have an enormous impact on the understanding of physiological processes in humans, in both healthy and disease states, and consequently on the practice of health care in general.

Each of the numbered structures in Figure 1-1 is a pair of chromosomes. The 46 chromosomes of human somatic cells constitute 23 pairs (Thompson et al., 1991). Of those 23 pairs, 22 are alike in both males and females. The remaining pair comprises the sex chromosomes: two XX's in females and an X and Y in males. One member of each pair of chromosomes is inherited from the father, the other from the mother. Members of a pair of chromosomes usually carry matching genetic information. Each human chromosome is believed to consist of a single, continuous DNA double helix; that is, each chromosome is a long, linear double-stranded DNA molecule, as illustrated in Figure 1-2 (McLendon, 1993).

The anatomic structure of DNA carries the chemical information that allows the exact transmission of genetic information from one cell to its daughter cells, and from one generation to the next (Thompson et al., 1991). DNA is a macromolecule composed of three types of units:

1. A 5-carbon sugar—deoxyribose
2. A nitrogen-containing base—which can be one of two types:
   • purine bases—adenine and guanine
   • pyrimidine bases—thymine and cytosine
3. A phosphate group

These units are illustrated in Figure 1-3.

The sequence of bases in a DNA molecule represents the information content of the gene, and is critical in determining its function. In

Figure 1-2   DNA Double Helix

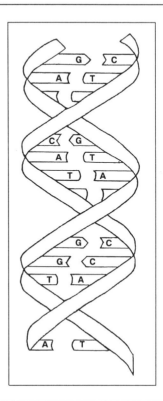

the human genome, these linear molecules range in size from approximately 50 million base pairs (for the shortest chromosome, chromosome 21) to 250 million base pairs (for the longest chromosome, chromosome 1). The human genome consists of approximately 6 to 7 billion base pairs (or 6 to 7 million kilobase pairs (kb)) of DNA organized linearly into the 23 pairs of chromosomes. Some genes are less than 1 million bases (1 kb) in length, while others, such as the factor VIII gene, stretch on for hundreds of million bases.

FUNCTION OF CHROMOSOMES AND GENES

Genetic information is contained in DNA in the chromosomes within the cell nucleus; however, protein synthesis, during which the

Figure 1–3   DNA Double Helix

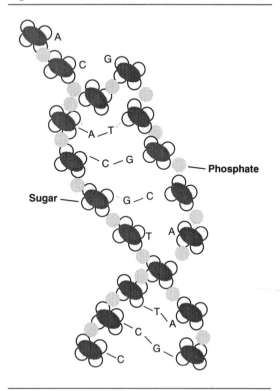

of information from gene to polypeptide involves many steps. These steps are transcription, translation, and protein synthesis. At each step in this complex pathway an error can occur. Mutations that interfere with the individual steps have been implicated in a number of inherited genetic disorders, including cancer.

PATTERNS OF MENDELIAN (SINGLE-GENE) INHERITANCE

There are three main categories of genetic disorders—single-gene, chromosomal, and multifactorial. This chapter focuses on single-gene and multifactorial disorders because they have been implicated in the etiology of cancer.

A single-gene disorder is one that is determined by a specific piece of genetic information at a particular locus on one or both members of a chromosome pair. Single-gene traits are often called Mendelian because, like the characteristics of garden peas studied by Gregor Mendel, they segregate within families and usually occur in fixed proportions among the offspring of specific types of matings (Brock, 1993).

Single-gene disorders are characterized by their patterns of transmission in families. To establish a pattern of transmission, a usual first step is to obtain information about the family history of the patient. In order to summarize the details of the family history, a pedigree is constructed, using standard symbols. A family pedigree, indicating a history of cancer, is illustrated in Figure 1-5. The legend at the bottom of the figure explains the meaning of each symbol.

Disorders carried by mutant genes at a single genetic locus show one of three patterns of inheritance: autosomal dominant, autosomal recessive, or x-linked. The distinction between autosomal and x-linked inheritance depends solely on the chromosomal location of the gene. The distinction between dominant and recessive inheritance is not absolute; rather, it is an arbitrary designation, based on clinical features, that may be without significance at the level of gene action.

information encoded in the DNA is used, takes place in the cytoplasm (Brock, 1993). The molecular link between these two related types of information (the DNA code of genes and the amino acid code of proteins) is RNA.

The informational relationships among DNA, RNA, and protein are circular: DNA directs the synthesis and sequence of RNA; RNA directs the synthesis and sequence of polypeptides; and specific proteins are involved in the synthesis and metabolism of DNA and RNA. This is represented in Figure 1-4.

Genetic information is stored in DNA by means of a specific code (the genetic code), in which the sequence of adjacent bases determines the sequence of amino acids in the encoded polypeptide (Thompson et al., 1991). One switch of the purine or pyrimidine bases can cause a noticeable phenotypic change. The flow

Figure 1-4   The Genetic Code

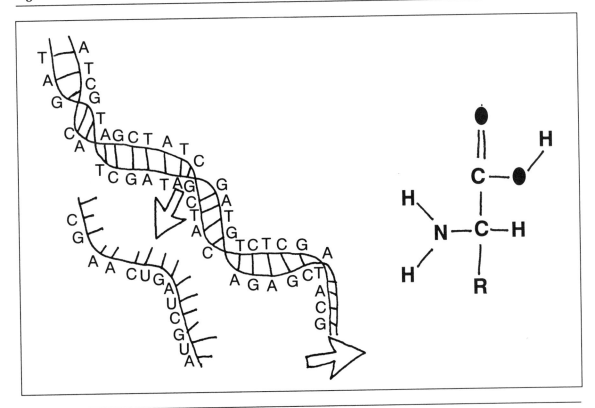

Establishing differences between a dominant and a recessive mutant gene is based on a relatively simple question. If in one chromosome pair the gene is normal and in the other the gene is abnormal or mutant, can the one normal gene perform the function of two? If the answer is yes, then the mutant gene is recessive, because both genes on each chromosome would have to be mutant to cause changes in the function of the gene. If the answer is no, then the mutant gene is dominant. Figure 1-6 illustrates autosomal dominant transmission. A carrier is an individual who "carries" a mutant gene, but is currently unaffected by the trait.

CANCER ETIOLOGY

The concept of cancer as a genetic disease is relatively new. Perhaps 15% of all cancers appear to follow a familial pattern (Schneider, Diller, & Garber, 1994). Most cancers are not inherited, but occur as sporadic events in people who have little relevant family history. Cancers appear most often to be caused by acquired genetic alterations within a mature cell (somatic) at a specific tissue site. Since cancer involves changes in the genetic material, all cancer could be considered genetic in origin.

A tumor can arise either from an initial precipitating event in a single precursor cell (unicellular origin) or from a series of such events in a population of susceptible cells (multicellular origin) (Brock, 1993). Most cancers are thought to arise from a single-cell defect that leads to uncontrolled growth. In other words, one cell undergoes the necessary changes, and as that cells divides and multiplies, a malignancy is initiated. The clonal na-

Figure 1-5   Family Pedigree

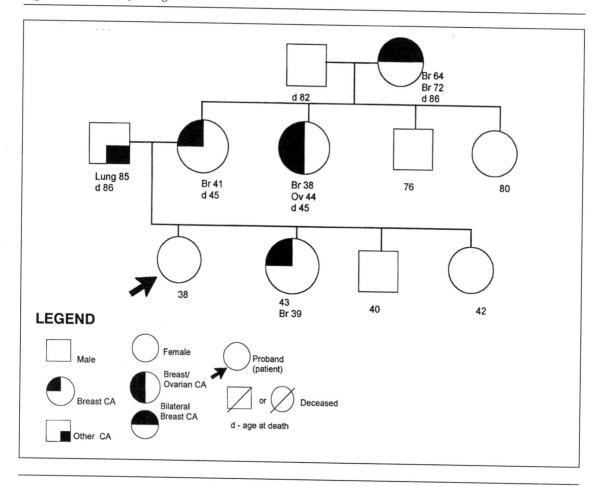

Figure 1-6   Autosomal Dominant Heritance

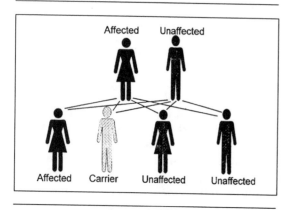

ture of most tumors suggests that mutation at a specific genetic locus might be an early event in the development of malignancy. Major exceptions to the unicellular, or clonal, origin of tumors are to be found in colon carcinoma, hereditary neurofibromatosis, and hereditary trichoepitheliomas (Brock, 1993).

Oncogenes and Tumor-Suppressor Genes

There are two distinct types of genes that cause cancer: *oncogenes* and *tumor-suppressor genes* (Weinberg, 1994). These two genes have

Table 1-1 Selected Examples of Proto-oncogene Abnormalities in Human Tumors

Proto-oncogenes	Tumor
abl	CML
erbB1	Squamous cell carcinoma, astrocytoma
erbB2	Adenocarcinoma of breast, ovary, and stomach
myc	Burkitt's lymphoma, carcinoma of lung, breast, and cervix
H-ras	Carcinoma of colon, lung, and pancreas, melanoma
sis	Astrocytoma
src	Colon carcinoma

opposite effects in carcinogenesis. Oncogenes are the genes that affect normal cell growth and development by facilitating malignant transformation. Tumor-suppressor genes, on the other hand, block tumor development by regulating genes involved in cell growth.

Most oncogenes are mutated ("activated") forms of normal genes. These normal genes are called proto-oncogenes and are found in normal cells. When proto-oncogenes are disrupted, they can promote abnormal cell proliferation. The protein products of proto-oncogenes have key roles in the cellular signalling network and may be seen as relays in the biochemical circuitry that governs the behavior of normal cells. Proto-oncogenes can be altered as a result of a mutation in the gene itself or by an external control. The different mechanisms for proto-oncogene activation are thought to lead to gain-of-function changes that enhance the positive signals for cell growth.

Oncogenes have a dominant effect at the cellular level, that is, when activated, a single mutant area on one chromosome is sufficient to change the function of the cell from normal to malignant. Over 50 different proto-oncogenes are now known, and of these, about 20 have actually been found in mutant form in human tumors (Weinberg, 1994). A representative list of proto-oncogenes consistently shown to be

mutated in human cancer is shown in Table 1-1 (Hodgson & Maher, 1993).

The largest group of cancers in humans involves the epithelial cells (breast, colon, lung, prostate), where the problem of carcinogenesis appears to be one of unrestrained growth of an already specialized cell type. The normal role of a tumor-suppressor gene is to restrict undue cell proliferation. Tumor-suppressor genes are a built-in braking system against runaway cell proliferation. A mutation in a tumor-suppressor gene leads to a loss of function of this role.

Some chromosomes carry tumor-suppressor genes, and either chromosome loss or loss-of-function mutations can lead to the emergence of malignancy. Tumor-suppressor genes have been implicated in several Mendelian forms of cancer, including retinoblastoma; Wilms tumor; familial polyposis coli; neurofibromatosis, type 1; and the rare form of inherited cancer known as Li-Fraumeni syndrome (Brock, 1993). Although in each of these cancers autosomal dominant inheritance is either the rule or at least seen in a proportion of cases, loss or alteration of *both* copies of the responsible tumor-suppressor gene is required for tumor development. Tumor-suppressor genes are also involved in the progression of several common, nonheritable forms of cancer, such as breast and colorectal cancer. The number of tumor-suppressor genes discovered to date is less than a dozen (Weinberg, 1994). Some examples of tumor-suppressor genes are listed in Table 1-2.

DNA Mismatch Repair Genes

A third type of gene that can cause cancer is one involved in DNA repair during cell growth. This newly discovered type of cancer gene has been linked to hereditary nonpolyposis colorectal cancer and sporadic colon cancers (Leach et al., 1993; Papadopoulos et al., 1994). The result of this type of cancer gene is an intrinsic genetic instability (Cleaver, 1994). DNA repair processes are indispensable for protection from spontaneous and environmentally induced cancers. A

> absolutely necessary.

Table 1-2   Selected Examples of Tumor-Suppressor Genes

| Tumor-Suppressor Genes | Disorders in Which Gene Affected | |
	Familial	Sporadic
RB1	Retinoblastoma	Lung cancer
WT1	Wilms tumor	Lung cancer
p53	Li-Fraumeni syndrome	Many epithelial carcinomas
NF1	Neurofibromatosis, type 1	Unknown
DCC	Unknown	Colorectal cancer

defect in DNA repair is a major contributor to this observed genetic instability.

Mutations in the two recently uncovered genes, hMLH1 and hMSH2, have a central role in a process known as DNA mismatch repair. Mismatched nucleotides signal a genetic error. In their normal roles, DNA mismatch repair genes, like genetic proofreaders, seem able to spot mismatches and orchestrate the necessary repairs (Cleaver, 1994). If these repair genes don't work, errors accumulate in the course of many generations of cell division and eventually a cancerous mutation occurs. These genes have been described as being like the spell-check in a word processing computer program (Service, 1994). One gene, hMSH2, is said to be primarily a replication editor and the other gene, hMLH1, a recombination editor (Radman & Wagner, 1993). When working right, DNA mismatch repair genes find the errors.

It is interesting to note that in clinical practice, none of the known dominant oncogenes has been implicated in an inherited human cancer, but both recessive tumor-suppressor genes and DNA mismatch repair gene defects have been demonstrated to account for inherited predisposition to cancer.

Recessive Mutations Leading to Cancer

Some tumors appear to occur in an inherited form and others occur sporadically. Understanding the mechanisms involved is important in understanding cancer etiology. Knudson's "two-hit" hypothesis proposed that forms of cancer such as retinoblastoma, which occur in both hereditary and sporadic forms, could be explained on the basis that in the hereditary form the first gene mutation is carried in the germline, whereas in the sporadic form both mutations are somatic, occurring in the same somatic cell (Knudson, 1989). The normal genes referred to are now known as tumor-suppressor genes. A single functional copy of a tumor-suppressor gene is enough to provide a normal functioning cell; however, a cell in which one copy is already altered or lost, by either germline or somatic mutation, will lose its ability to suppress tumor development if by chance it acquires a somatic mutation at the remaining gene. Because of the clonal nature of tumors, this event can cause a tumor even if it occurs in only one of the numerous cells of a tissue.

Sporadic (Multifactorial) Cancer Development

The development of a malignancy requiring only the activation of a proto-oncogene, or the loss of function of a DNA repair gene, or both copies of a tumor-suppressor gene, is grossly oversimplified. Instead, tumor formation is a multistep process involving a succession of genetic changes in the evolving tumor cell population. Loss or inactivation of the same gene may contribute to the development of several different common cancers.

It must be emphasized that most common cancers, even when showing familial aggregations, are not inherited. A large number of genes may be involved in tumorigenesis. Several different cancer genes may be involved in the same tumor. The same genes may be lost

Table 1-3   Familial Cancers Associated with Breast Cancer

Syndrome	Clinical Manifestation	Genetic Mutation	Mode of Inheritance
Breast/ovarian cancer syndrome[a]	Breast cancer, ovarian cancer prostate cancer, colon cancer	BRCA1	Autosomal dominant
Site-specific breast cancer[a, b]	Breast cancer (male and female), ovarian cancer	BRCA2	Autosomal dominant
Li-Fraumeni syndrome[a]	Breast cancer, sarcoma, brain tumors, leukemia, adrenocortical carcinoma	p53	Autosomal dominant
Muir-Torre syndrome[c]	GI and GU cancers, skin cancer, breast cancer, benign breast tumors, uterine and ovarian cancer	MSH2, MLH1	Autosomal dominant
Cowden's disease[c]	Multiple mucocutaneous lesions, vitiligo, angiomas, benign proliferative disease of multiple organ systems, breast cancer, thyroid cancer, GI neoplasms, GU lesions	Unknown	Autosomal dominant
Peutz-Jeghers syndrome[c]	Abnormal melanin deposits, GI polyposis, GI cancer, breast cancer, cancer of uterus, ovarian cancer, cancer of testis	Unkown	Autosomal dominant
Ataxia-telangiectasia[c]	Cerebral ataxia, oculocutaneous telangiectasias, radiation hypersensitivity, leukemia, lymphoma, breast cancer and other solid tumors	Linked to chromosome 11q21	Autosomal recessive

a Inherited cancer syndrome.
b Cancers that cluster in families.
c Genetic syndromes.

or mutated in different types of cancer. It is also possible that there may be an ordered or sequential loss of tumor-suppressor genes as a cell progresses from predisposed to overtly cancerous. Finally, several chromosomal regions also harbor oncogenes.

FAMILIAL CANCERS

There are three main categories of familial cancers: 1) inherited cancer syndromes; 2) genetic disorders; and 3) familial clusters of cancer (Schneider et al., 1994). It is estimated that 15% of all cancer cases are thought to be familial cancers. Familial cancers are defined as cancers that occur in families at greater than expected rates. Since cancer is a common dis-

ease, separating familial from nonfamilial cancers is not always simple. Table 1-3 organizes the different familial cancers associated with breast cancer. For each familial cancer, there is a noninherited or sporadic form that is currently clinically indistinguishable.

Inherited Cancer Syndromes

Malignancy is the central (and sometimes only) feature of inherited cancer syndromes, which tend to be autosomal dominant (Schneider et al., 1994). The underlying genetic error can be a germline mutation in a growth regulatory gene or a DNA repair gene. Epidemiologic studies have indicated that 5% to 10% of breast cancer cases are due to inheritance of highly penetrant dominant genes (King, Rowell, & Love, 1993).

Inherited cancer syndromes often have an earlier age of onset and may be associated with multiple primary tumors. These cancer syndromes are complicated by variable penetrance, expressivity, and age of onset, which may make it difficult to distinguish between inherited and sporadic forms. The genes involved in dominantly inherited cancers may be many in number and heterogeneous in function. Examples of dominantly inherited cancers related to breast cancer are briefly described.

Li-Fraumeni Syndrome. The Li-Fraumeni syndrome is a rare disorder associated with increased risk of several tumors, including soft tissue sarcomas, carcinoma of the breast, osteosarcoma, adrenocortical carcinoma, brain tumors, acute leukemia, and possibly other cancers (Li & Fraumeni, 1992). Clinically, the range of cancers in the syndrome remains to be clarified (Li et al., 1992). Approximately half of patients with this disorder have been shown to have germline mutations that fall within a single small region on the *p53* tumor-suppressor gene (Malkin et al., 1990). About 50% of women with the Li-Fraumeni syndrome may develop breast cancer; however, this disorder probably affects less than 1% of all breast cancer cases (Evans et al., 1994).

Breast/Ovarian Cancer Syndrome. Linkage studies have established that a gene predisposing to breast and ovarian cancer, called the *BRCA1* gene, is located on chromosome 17 (Hall et al., 1990). The gene itself was isolated in the fall of 1994 (Miki et al., 1994). It is estimated that 45% of families with apparent autosomal dominant transmission of breast cancer susceptibility and approximately 90% of families with dominant inheritance of both breast and ovarian cancer possess *BRCA1* germline mutations (Hoskins et al., 1995).

Inheritance in these families follows the classic autosomal dominant transmission, with each child of mutation carriers having a 50% chance of inheriting *BRCA1* mutations

(Hoskins et al., 1995). Female carriers are estimated to have an 87% cumulative risk by age 70 of developing breast cancer and a 62% cumulative risk by age 70 of developing ovarian cancer (Ford et al., 1994). There is also evidence of significant excesses of colon and prostate cancer in *BRCA1* carriers (Ford et al., 1994). Carriers with one cancer have an additionally high risk of developing a second breast or ovarian cancer.

Cancers That Cluster

In some families, it is clear that the increased incidence of cancer is due to some type of underlying hereditary predisposition, but the genetic factors have not yet been elucidated (Schneider et al., 1994). It may be discovered that some of these families have a single-gene inherited cancer syndrome. In other families the etiology may be polygenic or complex multifactorial disorders. Breast cancer is one of the common familial cancers that cluster in families.

Site-Specific Breast Cancer. In a number of families with familial breast cancer, possibly representing 50% or more of all genetic breast cancer patients, no linkage to the *BRCA1* gene has been found (van de Vijver, 1993). In these cases, it remains to be discovered to which chromosomal region, and eventually to which gene, breast cancer development should be attributed. A second breast cancer susceptibility gene was localized to chromosome 13 and is called *BRCA2* (Wooster et al., 1994). Like *BRCA1*, *BRCA2* appears to confer a high risk of early onset breast cancer, but differs in that the risk of ovarian cancer may be lower and the risk of male breast cancer may be higher than for *BRCA1* carriers.

Genetic Syndromes

Genetic syndromes have three features in common: a predisposition to malignant disease, increased sensitivity to an environmental agent, and some form of spontaneous or induced chromosome abnormality (Brock,

1993). There are many genetic syndromes that have primarily nonmalignant features but are also associated with the development of cancer (Schneider et al., 1994). In these syndromes, there is an increased occurrence of somatic mutations that can lead to cancer development. The increased susceptibility to cancer is a secondary effect and although cancer risk is elevated it is not as high as in the inherited cancer syndromes.

Ataxia-telangiectasia.   One genetic syndrome associated with breast cancer is ataxia-telangiectasia (van de Vijver, 1993). This is an autosomal recessive disorder characterized by the development of cerebellar ataxia in the first decade, along with choreoathetosis, dysarthria, and abnormalities of ocular movements (Hodgson & Maher, 1993). Affected individuals have a 10% to 20% risk of developing cancer, especially lymphomas and lymphocytic leukemias, but also epithelial tumors, including breast cancer. Relatives of individuals with ataxia-telangiectasia appear to have an increased risk of breast cancer (Swift, Morrell, Massey, & Chase, 1991).

Muir-Torre Syndrome.   This is a rare autosomal dominant condition that includes multiple benign sebaceous adenomas and carcinomas, basal and squamous cell carcinomas, and keratoacanthomas of the skin, as well as multiple internal malignancies (Hodgson & Maher, 1993). The internal cancers include tumors of the colon, stomach, esophagus, breast, uterus, ovaries, bladder, and larynx, as well as squamous cell carcinoma of the mucous membranes.

Cowden's Disease.   This is also an autosomal dominant trait characterized by multiple hamartomatous lesions of skin, mucous membranes, breast, and thyroid (Hodgson & Maher, 1993). Approximately 50% of affected females have fibrocystic disease of the breast as well as breast cancer. Thirty-three percent of breast cancers are bilateral. There is also increased incidence of cancers of the thyroid,

colon, uterus, cervix, lung, bladder, skin, and lymphoreticular system.

Peutz-Jegher Syndrome.   This autosomal dominant disorder is characterized by the association of black or bluish melanin spots on the lips, perioral region, buccal mucosa, hands, arms, feet, and legs, with gastrointestinal polyposis (Hodgson & Maher, 1993). Individuals with this syndrome also have an increased risk of cancers of the breast, uterus, and ovarian sex cord.

GENETIC MUTATIONS AS PROGNOSTIC INDICATORS IN BREAST CANCER

In an effort to improve prognosis, markers that detect molecular alterations are being studied (Institute of Medicine, 1992). These markers include alterations in proto-oncogenes, growth factors, growth factor receptors, tumor-suppressor genes, and genes believed to be associated with metastasis. In breast cancer, the genes that have received the greatest attention include two proto-oncogenes / growth factor receptors, *HER-2/neu* and epidermal growth factor receptor (EGFR), and the *NM23* tumor-suppressor gene. EGFR and *HER-2/neu* overexpression has been shown to correlate with a poor prognosis in both node-negative and node-positive breast cancer (Fox et al., 1994; van de Vijver, 1993). Tumors expressing little or no *NM23* were more likely to relapse (Institute of Medicine, 1992). Many other genetic markers are being investigated.

Another tumor-suppressor gene defect seen frequently in breast cancer is the *p53* gene (van de Vijver, 1993). This gene has been found on the short arm of chromosome 17. Deletions of this area of the chromosome have been seen in over 50% of breast cancers (van de Vijver, 1993). Four different changes in *p53* gene configuration may be present in breast cancers. Little information is available concerning the association of *p53* gene defects and clinicopathological parameters.

Table 1-4   Situations That May Warrant a Breast Cancer Risk Counseling Referral

- Cancer within the family is recognized to have familial components (i.e., bilaterality, multiple primaries, young age at onset).
- Cancer in the family occurs at young ages (<45 years).
- Family members, themselves, are concerned about their cancer risk, regardless of risk factors.
- Families have a known genetic condition that predisposes them to breast cancer.
- Individuals are interested in predictive testing research.

Table 1-5   Indications for Breast Cancer Risk Counseling

- Breast and/or ovarian cancer in relatives
- Any cancer in two or more close relatives
- Two or more generations of cancer
- Bilateral breast cancer
- Early age of onset (<45 years)
- Li-Fraumeni syndrome in a relative
- Multiple childhood sarcomas in relatives
- Ataxia-telangiectasia in a relative
- Signs of proliferative breast on own biopsy
- Inheritance of known tumor-suppressor gene mutations

Note. Adapted from "Familial Cancer Risk, Part II: Breast Cancer Risk Counseling and Genetic Susceptibility Testing" by J.A. Peters, 1994, *Journal of Oncology Management*, November/December, 18–26.

Most of the studies performed on chromosomal mutations in breast cancer have been either from relatively small heterogeneous populations or with short follow-up times (van de Vijver, 1993). It will be important to validate study results using prospective study design and homogenous groups, allowing enough time for sufficient follow-up before clinical standards can be established. No genetic markers are used clinically at this time.

BREAST CANCER RISK COUNSELING

Cancer risk counseling is a communication process concerning an individual's risk of developing specific forms of cancer. The risk may stem from lifestyle choices, exposures to carcinogens, precursor diseases such as carcinoma in situ of the breast, or inherited susceptibilities. Many women perceive themselves to be at high risk, yet possess no significant risk factors. A wide variety of activities may fall under the cancer risk counselor's umbrella:

identifying families with increased risk; obtaining detailed family, medical, and lifestyle histories; documenting cancer-related diagnoses; constructing and analyzing risk pedigree; providing counseling; recognizing familial cancers; and discussing the options for early detection and prevention (Peters, 1994). Table 1-4 identifies situations that may warrant a breast cancer risk counseling referral. Table 1-5 identifies indications for breast cancer risk counseling.

An assessment of an individual's family is the first step in providing cancer risk counseling. The nurse should construct a family pedigree, including both the maternal and paternal sides, going back at least two generations. When possible, medical records should be reviewed to verify diagnosis. Medical records can also be used to determine whether the early demise of a relative may have been due to the late stage of cancer at diagnosis. The counselor can then reinforce the importance of early detection by showing the client that these days a diagnosis can be made much ear-

Table 1-6   Elements of Cancer Risk Counseling

- Ascertain beliefs, concerns, and experiences
- Construct a framework of understanding risk information
- Present background information
- Analyze risk and convey risk information
- Present clinically relevant information tailored to the individual

Note. Adapted from: "Cancer Risk Counseling for Individuals and Families at Increased Cancer Risk." by P. T. Kelly, 1994, *The Cancer Bulletin, 46,* pp. 275–276.

lier and lives can be saved. Table 1-6 outlines the elements of cancer risk counseling.

Exploring the family history is only the beginning in providing comprehensive breast cancer risk counseling (Kelly, 1991). It is also important to assess beliefs, past experiences, feelings regarding the medical community, lifestyle habits, and lifestyle risk factors. A more complete understanding of the individual will allow the counselor to use a framework of information more appropriate for that particular individual. The cancer risk counselor's goal should be to provide important information, but it must be presented in a manner that is meaningful to the individual.

Conveying risk information to individuals is challenging. Discussion of risk frequently includes relating how risk estimates are derived, the limitation of epidemiologic methods and evaluation of specific studies, the multi-step process of carcinogenesis, and the patterns of inheritance associated with hereditary cancers. Recent molecular characterization of well-defined hereditary cancer syndromes, as described earlier, offers the potential for more accurate estimates of inherited cancer risk (Offit & Brown, 1994). In selected cases, this analysis of risk includes DNA linkage to cancer susceptibility genes or direct gene mutation analysis, i.e., predictive testing. Predictive testing issues in the cancer risk counseling environment are described below.

For families that do not meet the criteria for hereditary syndromes, a growing amount of population-derived information is available to estimate familial cancer risk. There are a number of risk assessment models currently

in use. These can be broken down into two categories: 1) mathematical computer models weighing combinations of risk factors; and 2) empiric data collected from population studies, registries, or oncology clinics with long-term follow-up of relatives (Peters, 1994). Offit and Brown (1994) and Hoskins et al. (1995) provide excellent resources for review of the various risk assessment models.

Breast cancer risk counseling provides an individual with a framework for understanding risk estimates and may allow the individual to make informed and thoughtful decisions. Cancer risk counseling provides an opportunity to devise appropriate surveillance plans as well as lifestyle changes that may improve an individual's health and well-being. Education about current prevention and early detection methods is essential to developing this plan. Individuals can be empowered to care for themselves by using state-of-the-art knowledge of prevention and early detection methods and can make decisions that are appropriate for themselves.

PREDICTIVE TESTING

Presymptomatic detection of individuals at risk of developing cancer as a result of susceptibility genes is an important aim of current research, both in familial cases and in the larger number of sporadic cases. The human genome project has already resulted in the discovery of genes localized to specific chromosomal regions that demonstrate a predisposition to common cancers such as breast and colon, as well as other diseases like hypertension, diabetes, and Alzheimer's disease (Collins & Galas, 1993) Knowing which genes cause or contribute to the occurrence of disease enables scientists to develop tests to detect which people might suffer from a disease, *before they experience symptoms,* so they can benefit from early intervention.

Predictive or presymptomatic testing and screening can provide clues about genetic susceptibility or predisposition to genetic disorders. For some diseases, like the single-gene inherited cancers referred to earlier, these tests will most likely be highly predictive. However, for many common diseases, like most cancers that have multifactorial or complex causation, including both multiple genetic factors and environmental effects, prediction will be less certain (Scanlon & Fibison, 1995). Even when an individual is known to be a carrier of a cancer susceptibility gene, considerable uncertainty remains. When or if a cancer will ever manifest itself cannot be forecast with any certainty. Genetic testing for cancer does not provide definitive information about whether an individual will ever be diagnosed with cancer, the age at which a cancer will be diagnosed, or even (in some cases) the type of cancer that might develop (Kelly, 1994).

The issues surrounding predictive testing are numerous (Biesecker et al., 1993). Tests for predisposition to common disorders will be of great commercial interest. They could have substantial potential for harm to individuals and families in terms of insurability and employability, as well as substantial benefit from the potential of early preventive and therapeutic interventions (Institute of Medicine, 1994). Many genetic tests, when they are available, will be ordered and interpreted by primary-care health practitioners, not only by geneticists or genetic counselors. The ethical principles of voluntariness, informed consent, and confidentiality must be the guiding force in presymptomatic testing and risk counseling. Predictive testing for inherited susceptibility to breast cancer can be obtained through research and clinical laboratories that are accepting samples as part of research protocols.

SUMMARY

An understanding of molecular genetics will be necessary for future practitioners to help women and their families understand its relationship to breast cancer. The role of the cancer risk counselor, likewise, will continue to develop and expand given the growing needs of women at risk for breast cancer. These are challenging and exciting times.

GENETIC TERMINOLOGY

DNA—Deoxyribonucleic Acid—A molecule that encodes the genes responsible for the structure and function of living organisms. DNA assists in the transmission of genetic information from generation to generation.

Gene—Most simply, a gene is a hereditary unit. In molecular terms, a gene is a sequence of chromosomal DNA that is required for production of a functional product. Inherited characteristics are determined by genes.

Chromosomes—Chromosomes are composed of DNA and therefore genes. The normal human chromosome number is 46.

Human Genome—The human genome is the complete DNA sequence. The human genome contains the entire genetic information of human beings.

References

Biesecker, B. B., Bohnke, M., Calzone, K., Markel, D. S., Garber, J. E., Collins, F. S., & Weber, B. L. (1993). Genetic counseling for families with inherited susceptibility to breast and ovarian cancer. *Journal of the American Medical Association, 269,* 170–174.

Brock, D. J. H. (1993). *Molecular genetics for the clinician.* Cambridge, Great Britain: Cambridge University Press.

Caskey, C. T. (1993). Presymptomatic diagnosis: A first step toward genetic health care. *Science, 262,* 48–49.

Cleaver, J. E. (1994). It was a very good year for DNA repair. *Cell, 76,* 1–4.

Collins, F., & Galas, D. (1993). A new five-year plan for the U.S. human genome project. *Science, 262,* 43–46.

Evans, D. G. R., Fentiman, I. S., McPherson, K., Asbury, D., Ponder, B. A. J., & Howell, A. (1994). Familial breast cancer. *British Medical Journal, 308,* 183–187.

Ford, D., Easton, D. F., Bishop, D. T., Narod, S. A., Godgar, D. E., & the Breast Cancer Linkage Consortium. (1994). Risks of cancer in *BRCA1*-mutation carriers. *Lancet, 343,* 692–695.

Fox, S. B., Smith, K., Hollyer, J., Greenall, M., Hastrich, D., & Harris, A. L. (1994). The epidermal growth factor receptor as a prognostic marker: Results of 370 patients and review of 3009 patients. *Breast Cancer Research and Treatment, 29,* 41–49.

Gilchrist, K. W., Gray, R., van Driel-Kuller, A. M. J., Mesker, W. E., Ploem-Zaaijer, J. J., Taylor, S. G., & Tormey, D. C . (1993). High DNA content and prognosis in lymph node positive breast cancer: A case control study by the University of Leiden and EGOG. *Breast Cancer Research and Treatment, 28,* 1–8.

Hall, J. M., Lee, M. K., Newman, B., Morrow, J. E., Anderson, L. A., Huey, B., & King, M-C. (1990). Linkage of early-onset familial breast cancer to chromosome 17q21. *Science, 250,* 1684–1689.

Hodgson, S. V., & Maher, E. R. (1993), *A practical guide to human cancer genetics.* Cambridge, Great Britain: Cambridge University Press.

Hoffman, E. P. (1994). The evolving genome project: Current and future impact. *American Journal of Human Genetics, 54,* 129–136.

Hoskins, K. F., Stopfer, J. E., Calzone, K. A., Merajver, S. D., Rebbeck, T. R., Garber, J. E., & Weber, B. L. (1995). Assessment and counseling for women with a family history of breast cancer: A guide for clinicians. *Journal of the American Medical Association, 273,* 577–585.

Institute of Medicine. (1992). *Advances in understanding genetic changes in cancer.* Washington, DC: National Academy Press.

Institute of Medicine. (1994). *Assessing genetic risks: Implications for health and social policy.* Washington, DC: National Academy Press.

Kelly, P. T. (1991). *Understanding breast cancer risk.* Philadelphia: Temple University Press.

Kelly, P. T. (1994). Cancer risk counseling for individuals and families at increased cancer risk. *Cancer Bulletin, 46,* 275–276.

King, M-C., Rowell, S., & Love, S. (1993). Inherited breast and ovarian cancer: What are the risks? What are the choices? *Journal of the American Medical Association, 269,* 1975–1980.

Knudson, A. G. (1989). Hereditary cancers disclose a class of cancer genes. *Cancer, 63,* 1888–1891.

Leach, F. S., Nicolaaides, N. C., Papadopoulos, N., Liu, B., Jen, J., Parsons, R., Peltomäki, P., Sistonen, P., Aaltonen, L. A., Nyström-Lahti, M., Guan, X.-Y., Zhang, J., Meltzer, P. S., Yu, J.-W., Kai, F.-T., Chen, D. J., Cerosaletti, K. M., Fournier, R. E. K., Todd, S., Lewis, T., Leach, R. J., Naylor, S. L., Weissenbach, J., Mecklin, J.-P., Järvinen, H., Petersen, G. M., Hamilton, S. R., Green, J., Jass, J., Watson, P., Lynch, H. T., Trent, J. M., Chapelle, A., Kinzler, K. W., & Vogelstein, B. (1993). Mutations of a *mutS* homolog in hereditary nonpolyposis colorectal cancer. *Cell, 75,* 1215–1225.

Li, F. P., & Fraumeni, J. F. (1992). Predictive testing for inherited mutations in cancer-susceptibility genes. *Journal of Clinical Oncology, 10,* 1203–1204.

Li, F. P., Garber, J. E., Friend, S. H., Strong, L. C., Patenaude, A. F., Juengst, E. T., Reilly, P. R., Correa, P., & Fraumeni, J. F. (1992). Recommendation on predictive testing for germ line *p53* mutations among cancer-prone individuals. *Journal of the National Cancer Institute, 84,* 1156–1160.

Lonn, U., Lonn, S., Nilsson, B., & Stenkvist, B. (1994). Breast cancer: Prognostic significance of c-*erb-B2* and *int-2* amplification compared with DNA ploidy, S-phase fraction, and conventional clinicopathological features. *Breast Cancer Research and Treatment, 29,* 237–245.

Malkin, D., Li, F. P., Strong, L. C., Fraumeni, J. F., Nelson, C. E., Kim, D. H., Kassel, J., Gryka, M. A., Bischoff, F. Z., Tainsky, M. A., & Friend, S. H. (1990). Germ line *p53* mutations in a familial syndrome of breast cancer, sarcomas, and other neoplasms. *Science, 250,* 1233–1238.

McLendon, W. W. (1993). Celebrating 40 years of the double helix: From a theory of biology to the care of patients. *Journal of the American Medical Association, 269,* 1993–1994.

Miki, Y., Swenson, J., Shattuck-Eidens, D., Futreal, P. A., Harshman, K., Tavtigian, S., Liu, Q., Cochran, C., Bennett, L. M., Ding, W., Hussey, C., Tran, T., McClure, M., Frye, C., Hattier, T., Phelps, R., Haugen-Trano, A., Katcher, H., Yakumo, K., Gholami, Z., Shaffer, D., Stone, S., Bayer, S., Wray, C., Bogden, R., Dayananth, P., Ward, J., Tonin, P., Narod, S., Bristow, P. K., Norris, F. H., Helvering, L., Morrison, P., Rosteck, P., Lai, M., Barrett, C., Lewis, C. M., Neuhausen, S. L., Cannon-Albright, L. A., Goldgar, D. E., Wiseman, R., Kamb, A., Skolnick, M. H. (1994). A strong candidate for the breast and ovarian cancer susceptibility gene BRCA1. *Science, 266,* 66–71.

Normanno, N., Ciardiello, F., Brandt, R., & Salomon, D. S. (1994). Epidermal growth factor-related peptides in the pathogenesis of human breast cancer. *Breast Cancer Research and Treatment, 29,* 11–28.

Nowak, R. (1994). Mining treasures from 'junk DNA'. *Science, 263,* 608-610.

Offit, K., & Brown, K. (1994). Quantitating familial cancer risk: A resource for clinical oncologists. *Journal of Clinical Oncology, 12,* 1724–1736.

Papadopoulos, N., Nicolaides, N. C., Wei, Y.-F., Ruben, S. M., Carter, K. C., Rosen, C. A., Haseltine, W. A., Fleischmann, R. D., Fraser, C. M., Adams, M. D., Venter, J. C., Hamilton, S. R., Petersen, G. M., Watson, P., Lynch, H. T., Peltomäki, P., Mecklin, J.-P., Chapelle, A., Kinzler, K. W., & Vogelstein, B. (1994). Mutation of a *mutL* homolog in hereditary colon cancer. *Science, 263,* 1625–1629.

Peters, J. (1994). Breast cancer risk counseling. *Genetic Resource, 8*(1), 20–25.

Radman, M., & Wagner, R. (1993). Missing mismatch repair. *Nature, 366,* 722.

Sandberg, A. A. (1994). Cancer cytogenetics for clinicians. *CA: A Cancer Journal for Clinicians, 44,* 136–159.

Scanlon, C., & Fibison, W. (1995). *Managing genetic information: Implications for nursing practice.* Washington, DC: American Nurses Association.

Schneider, K. A., Diller, L. R., & Garber, J. C. (1994). Overview of familial cancers. *Genetic Resource, 8*(1), 12–18.

Service, R. F. (1994). Stalking the start of colon cancer. *Science, 263,* 1559–1560.

Swift, M., Morrell, D., Massey, R. B., & Chase, C. L. (1991). Incidence of cancer in 161 families affected by ataxia-telangiectasia. *New England Journal of Medicine, 325,* 1831–1836.

Thompson, M. W., McInnes, R. R., & Willard, H. F. (Eds.). (1991). *Genetics in medicine* (5th ed.). Philadelphia: W. B. Saunders.

van de Vijver, M.J. (1993). Molecular genetic changes in human breast cancer. *Advances in Cancer Research, 61,* 25–56.

Weinberg, R. A. (1994). Oncogenes and tumor suppressor genes. *CA: A Cancer Journal for Clinicians, 44,* 160–170.

Wenger, C. R., Beardslee, S., Owens, M. A., Pounds, G., Oldaker, T., Vendely, P., Pandian, M. R., Harrington, D., Clark, G. M., McGuire, W. L. (1993). DNA ploidy, S-phase, and steroid receptors in more than 127,000 breast cancer patients. *Breast Cancer Research and Treatment, 28,* 9-20.

Wooster, R., Neuhausen, S. L., Mangion, J., Quirk, Y., Ford, D., Collins, N., Nguyen, K., Seal, S., Tran, T., Averill, D., Fields, P., Marshall, G., Narod, S., Lenoir, G. M., Lynch, H., Feunteun, J., Devilee, P., Cornelisse, C. J., Menko, F. H., Daly, P. A., Ormistron, W., McManus, R., Pye, C., Lewis, C. M., Cannon-Albright, L. A., Peto, J., Ponder, B. A. J., Skolnick, M. H., Easton, D. F., Goldgar, D. E., & Stratton, M. R. (1994). Localization of a breast cancer susceptibility gene, BRCA2, to chromosome 13q12–13. *Science, 265,* 2088–2090.

CHAPTER 2 | Screening Women for Breast Cancer

Elizabeth Ann Coleman, PhD, RNP, AOCN

This chapter was written to assist nurses in dealing with the current issues involved in screening women for breast cancer. Specifically, this chapter focuses on 1) helping women understand the risk of breast cancer; 2) helping women understand the need for and limitations of screening mammography, clinical breast examinations (CBE), and breast self-examination (BSE); and 3) teaching women about current screening issues. The latter helps women to be aware of recommended guidelines for breast cancer screening, to choose a mammography facility that provides optimum screening at low cost, and to take responsibility for their own breast health through breast cancer screening.

HELPING WOMEN UNDERSTAND THE RISK OF BREAST CANCER

As the most common non-skin cancer in women in the United States, breast cancer causes more deaths among women than any other cancer, except lung cancer (Miller et al., 1993). During 1995, approximately 182,000 women in the United States were diagnosed with breast cancer; 46,000 were expected to die from the disease (Wingo, Tong, & Bolden, 1995). As these facts indicate, all women are at risk for breast cancer.

The risk for breast cancer increases greatly with age. For example, an analysis of data for 1987 through 1991 from the National Cancer Institute's (NCI) Surveillance, Epidemiology, and End Results Program (SEER) shows that for women aged 35 to 39 years, the rate of breast cancer was 32 per 100,000, while for women aged 65 to 69 years, the breast cancer incidence rate was 228 per 100,000 (Barbara Lyles, personal communication, NCI Cancer Statistics Branch, June 15, 1994). Table 2-1 shows the incidence rate specified by each 5-year age group.

The risk of breast cancer increases for a woman who has had breast cancer in one breast, has a history of breast cancer in her

Table 2-I Breast Cancer (Invasive) Age-Specific Rates, 1987–1991

Age at Diagnosis	Rates per 100,000
0–4	0.0
5–9	0.0
10–14	0.0
15–19	0.0
20–24	0.5
25–29	3.9
30–34	12.9
35–39	32.2
40–44	64.5
45–49	100.7
50–54	117.5
55–59	143.5
60–64	186.0
65–69	227.5
70–74	259.2
75–79	293.7
80–84	312.6
85+	310.1

Note. Data from National Cancer Institute Cancer Statistics Branch SEER Program.

Table 2-2 Risk of a 40-Year-Old Woman Being Diagnosed with Breast Cancer in the Next 10 Years with Specified Risk Factors

Risk Factor	Risk
Age at menarche—under 12	1.5%
One prior breast biopsy	2.1%
Age at first live birth over 30	2.4%
One first-degree relative (mother or sister) with breast cancer	2.6%

Note. From "Projecting Individualized Probabilities of Developing Breast Cancer for White Females Who are Being Examined Annually," by M. H. Gail, L. A. Brinton, D. P. Byar, D. K. Corle, S. B. Green, C. Schairer, and J. J. Mulvihill, 1989, *Journal of the National Cancer Institute, 81,* pp.1879–1886.

The probability of her developing breast cancer over the next 10 years is 1.2%. Next, consider a 40-year-old woman with no risk factors except for menarche at 11 years of age. Her risk of developing breast cancer over the next 10 years is 1.5%. Table 2-2 shows the probability of developing breast cancer for other risk factors. Now, reconsider the 40-year-old woman who has no major risk factors when she is 50. Her risk of developing breast cancer over the next 10 years increases from 1.2% to 1.6%; and at age 60, her risk increases to 18%. Thus, age has a strong effect on breast cancer risk, and the effect of other risk factors strengthens with increasing age (Gail et al., 1989).

family, has had breast biopsies, has never had children, had her first child after age 30, began menstruating before age 12, or completed menopause after age 55. While these factors are associated with an increased breast cancer risk, they do not imply causation. With the exception of approximately 5% of women who carry the breast cancer gene, the cause of breast cancer remains unknown. Furthermore, the majority of women with breast cancer has none of the associated risk factors.

How does age compare with other risk factors for breast cancer? First, consider a 40-year-old woman with no major risk factors.

HELPING WOMEN UNDERSTAND THE NEED FOR AND LIMITATIONS OF CURRENT SCREENING MAMMOGRAPHY, CBE, AND BSE

Need for Mammography

Mammography is currently the most sensitive method for detecting early-stage breast cancer (U.S. Preventive Services Task Force, 1989). A mammogram can detect a tumor as small as ¼" in diameter; in comparison, a CBE or BSE can detect a tumor about ½" in diameter. The major benefit of screening mammography is the ability to detect nonpalpable or small tumors. Detecting a smaller tumor is correlated with a better prognosis.

Limitations of Mammography

Mammography does not detect breast cancer 100% of the time. High-quality mammography is most important. The competence of the radiologist who reads the mammogram probably affects the quality of mammography more than any other factor. Traditionally, radiology residency programs have provided inadequate training in mammography. In addition, the American Board of Radiology has not provided a satisfactory mammography examination for radiologists (McLelland, 1989).

Mammography facilities accredited by the American College of Radiology (ACR) usually offer high-quality mammograms. The ACR requires that radiologists read 480 mammograms a year and take continuing education courses. In addition, the facility must maintain records of outcome data that correlate positive mammograms to biopsies done and the number of detected cancers. Since the 1992 Mammography Quality Standards Act (MQSA), and interim regulations issued to implement MQSA, facilities that accept Medicare payment have even stricter requirements for quality assurance (Federal Register, 1993).

Need for CBE

A health professional who is well trained in performing a breast examination can detect very small breast tumors. It is recommended that women have a CBE with every general physical examination and should continue to do so annually when they reach the age of 40. Women should also have a CBE with each mammography because a small percentage of tumors are palpable even though they are not visible with mammography (U.S. Preventive Services Task Force, 1989).

Limitations of CBE

The accuracy of the CBE depends to a great extent on the experience and skill of the examiner. The National Strategic Plan for the Early Detection and Control of Breast and Cervical Cancer identifies the need for improved CBE training and makes this a priority area of focus (U.S. Dept. of Health & Human Services, Public Health Service, 1992)

Need for BSE

It is recommended that women should perform a self-examination on a monthly basis beginning at adolescence, and should continue BSE in conjunction with CBE and mammography.

Limitations of BSE

Similar to the clinical examination, the accuracy of BSE depends in large measure on the skill and experience of the examiner. The preferred method is to teach BSE to an individual on her own breasts at a young age (Coleman, 1991; Coleman, Riley, Fields, & Prior, 1991). Neither BSE nor CBE should replace mammography because mammography is effective in detecting nonpalpable breast lesions.

TEACHING WOMEN ABOUT CURRENT SCREENING ISSUES

Women are concerned about breast cancer and want to learn more about the disease, including the following current breast cancer screening issues: screening guidelines and choosing a mammography facility.

Guidelines for Screening

The International Workshop on Screening for Breast Cancer, which met February 24–25, 1993, in Bethesda, MD, reiterated the following guidelines:

1. For asymptomatic women aged 50 to 69 years, scientific data from eight randomized controlled trials provide evidence that mammography alone or mammography combined with CBE can reduce mortality from breast cancer by approximately 30% to 35% (Fletcher, Black, Harris, Rimer, & Shapiro, 1993).

2. For asymptomatic women aged 40 to 49 years, screening mammography found no reduction in mortality from breast cancer in the first 5 to 7 years.

Elwood, Cox, and Richardson (1993) performed a meta-analysis using the breast cancer death rates for each year of follow-up in each of the published randomized trials. They found similar death rates in screened and unscreened groups at 7 to 10 years and found no basis for the promotion of mammographic screening in women younger than 50 years.

Younger women in the general population need to be more aware of the current information regarding breast cancer and screenings. Even though more research is needed, it would be extremely difficult, if not impossible, to conduct a prospective randomized trial in the United States because many women 40 to 50 years of age already use mammographic screening. The United Kingdom is conducting a study of mammographic screening in younger women. The differences in the effectiveness of screening women younger and older than 50 years may result from the greater difficulty in distinguishing normal from abnormal tissue in younger women. The differences in the biological characteristics of tumors (e.g., the faster tumor growth in younger women) would also affect the results.

Researchers need to address screening for women at high risk for breast cancer, the impact of improved and more frequent screening for younger women, and the age when effectiveness of mammographic screening changes, rather than considering younger age as a decade group of 40 to 49 years. Perhaps, a significant decrease in mortality may occur with

mammographic screening for women 45 to 49 years of age.

If a prospective randomized trial of breast cancer screening in younger women is impossible in the United States, researchers need to link data from mammography screening facilities with data from pathology laboratories with population-based, quality-controlled cancer registries to determine the effectiveness of screening (National Cancer Institute [NCI], 1992). Also, this would determine the quality of screening facilities.

Currently, the NCI recommends that women aged 50 years and older have a screening mammogram every 1 to 2 years and receive an annual CBE. The NCI recommends that women ages 40 to 49 discuss with a health professional whether they should have a screening mammogram. This discussion should include family history of breast cancer and other risk factors. The NCI recommends that women 40 to 49 years of age have an annual CBE and that women of all ages practice monthly BSE and consult with a health care professional on BSE.

Choosing a Mammography Facility

The reports of an over-supply of mammography equipment (Brown, Kessler, & Rueter, 1990) and an under-supply of trained personnel to make (Dodd & McLelland, 1990) and read (McLelland, 1990) the mammograms are of great concern to both health care professionals and women. If facilities perform mammography infrequently, they are more likely to charge more for each mammogram to defray the cost of the expensive mammography equipment. Thus, the higher priced mammogram does not necessarily mean a better quality mammogram (NCI, 1989).

A woman should choose a mammography facility that uses machines specifically designed for mammography (called "dedicated mammography machines") that a qualified medical physicist calibrates at least once a year. The facility should employ a registered mammography technologist and a radiologist specially trained to read mammograms. The ACR suggests choosing a facility that performs at least 10 mammograms per week. Mammography facilities accredited by the ACR meet standards in the following quality assurance areas: radiation exposure, equipment specifications, facility quality control program, and personnel qualifications. The MQSA mandates that all facilities receiving payment for services through Medicare meet standards in these same areas. Thus, if a woman approaches a facility and asks if they accept Medicare reimbursement for screening mammograms, she will be more likely to find an accredited ACR facility.

HOW TO ENCOURAGE WOMEN TO TAKE RESPONSIBILITY FOR THEIR OWN BREAST HEALTH IN BREAST CANCER SCREENING

Goals for the year 2000 from the U.S. Public Health Service for Healthy People include having 80% of women in the United States in compliance with breast cancer screening guidelines (NCI, 1990). An analysis of data from the National Health Interview Survey in 1993 reveals a gulf between the goal and actual practice. This survey indicated that during the previous year approximately 33% of American women had a mammogram, 65% a BCE, and 38% had practiced monthly BSE.

Often, women say they do not have mammograms because, "I did not need it because I haven't had a problem," "never knew I should have one," and "doctor never recommended it" (Coleman, Feuer, & the NCI Breast Cancer Screening Consortium, 1992; the NCI Breast Cancer Screening Consortium, 1990). Women need to know that they should have a mammogram even when they do not have a problem with their breasts, and that they can request that their physician order a mammogram or go on their own to a screening mammography facility.

Among women with low income, particularly below $10,000 annually, the price of mammography represents a deterrent (Kiefe,

Siripoom, Halevy, & Brody, 1994). The average cost of a screening mammogram is about $90, but can range from $0 to $225 (Houn & Brown, 1994). Insurance coverage for mammography is becoming more prevalent, and Medicare and many state Medicaid programs pay 80% of the mammography cost after the insured has met the required deductible. The CDC Breast and Cervical Cancer Control state projects provide vouchers for screening mammography for the medically underserved below the 200% poverty level (slightly less than $15,000 annual household income for one-person households). The health departments in participating states administer these projects.

Nurses need to teach women how to perform a BSE on their own and use a checklist for evaluating BSE proficiency (Coleman & Pennypacker, 1991). While teaching BSE, nurses can inform women that they need an annual breast examination by a health care professional who uses these same techniques. With an understanding of the current developments in screening techniques and early detection of breast cancer, nurses can help women facing breast cancer understand the issues before them. Current issues include the risk for breast cancer, the need for and limitations of breast cancer screening, the current recommended screening guidelines, and how to choose a mammography facility. When nurses help women gain an understanding of these issues, they help them take responsibility for their own breast health.

References

Brown, M. L., Kessler, L. G., & Rueter, F. G. (1990). Is the supply of mammography machines outstripping need and demand? *Annals of Internal Medicine, 113*, 547–552.

Coleman, E. A. (1991). Practice and effectiveness of breast self examination: A selective review of the literature (1977–1989). *Journal of Cancer Education, 6*(2), 83–92.

Coleman, E. A., & Pennypacker, H. (1991). Measuring breast self-examination proficiency. A scoring system developed from a paired comparison study. *Cancer Nursing, 14*(4), 211–217.

Coleman, E. A., Riley, M. B., Fields, F., & Prior, B. (1991). Efficacy of breast self-examination teaching methods among older women. *Oncology Nursing Forum, 18*(3), 561–566.

Coleman, E. A., Feuer, E. J., & the NCI Breast Cancer Screening Consortium. (1992). Breast cancer screening among women from 65 to 74 years of age in 1987–88 and 1991. *Annals of Internal Medicine, 117,* 961–966.

Dodd, G. D., & McLelland, R. (1990). Breast disease programs and mammography training. *American Journal of Obstetrics and Gynecology, 163,* 689–691.

Elwood, J. M., Cox B., & Richardson, A. K. (1993, Febuary 25). The effectiveness of breast cancer screening by mammography in younger women. *The Online Journal of Current Clinical Trials* [on-line serial]. Available: Doc. No. 32

Federal Register (Tuesday, December 21, 1993).Vol. 58, No. 234 (21 CFR Part 900). *Mammography Facilities—Requirements for Accrediting Bodies and Quality Standards and Certification Requirements: Interim Rules.*

Fletcher, S. W., Black, W., Harris, R., Rimer, B. K., & Shapiro, S. (1993). *Report of the International Workshop on Screening for Breast Cancer.* Bethesda, MD: National Cancer Institute.

Gail, M. H., Brinton, L. A., Byar, D. P., Corle, D. K., Green, S. B., Schairer, C., Mulvihill, J. J. (1989). Projecting individualized probabilities of developing breast cancer for white females who are being examined annually. *Journal of the National Cancer Institute, 81,* 1879-1886.

Houn, F., & Brown, M. L. (1994). Current practice of screening mammography in the US: Data from the National Survey of Mammography Facilities. *Radiology, 190,* 209–215.

Kiefe, C. I., Siripoom, V. M., Halevy, A., & Brody, B. A. (1994). Is cost a barrier to screening mammography for low-income women receiving Medicare benefits? *Archives of Internal Medicine, 154,* 1217–1223.

McLelland, R. (1989). Challenges and progress with mammography. *Cancer, 64,* 2662–2666.

McLelland, R. (1990). Supply and quality of screening mammography: A radiologist's view. *Annals of Internal Medicine, 113,* 490–491.

Miller, B. A., Ries, L. A., Hankey, B. F., Kosary, C. L., Harras, A., Devesa, S. S., & Edwards, B. K. (Eds.) (1993). *SEER Cancer Statistics Review: 1973–1990.* (NIH Publication No. 93-2789.) Washington, DC: U.S. Department of Health and Human Services, National Cancer Institute.

National Cancer Institute. (1989). Latest facts about mammography. *Primary Care & Cancer, Oct. 1989,* 23–27.

National Cancer Institute. (1990). *90 Annual Report: Division of Cancer Prevention and Control.*

National Cancer Institute. (1992). *Surveillance Research: Breast cancer screening, performance, diagnosis, biological characteristics, treatment and outcomes. RFA-CA-93-13.* Bethesda, MD: National Cancer Institute.

NCI Breast Cancer Screening Consortium. (1990). Screening mammography: A missed clinical opportunity? Results of the NCI Breast Cancer Screening Consortium and National Health Interview Survey Studies. *Journal of the American Medical Association, 264,* 54–58.

U.S. Dept. of Health & Human Services, Public Health Service. (1992). *National Strategic Plan for the Early Detection and Control of Breast and Cervical Cancer.*

U.S. Preventive Services Task Force. (1989). Screening for breast cancer. In *Guide to clinical preventive services: An assessment of the effectiveness of 169 interventions* (chap. 6, pp. 39–45). Baltimore, MD: Williams & Wilkins.

Wingo, P. A., Tong, T., & Bolden, S. (1995). Cancer statistics, 1995. *CA: Cancer Journal for Clinicians, 45,* 8–30.

PART 2 | Issues in the Treatment of Breast Cancer

CHAPTER 3 | Managing Symptoms Related to Chemotherapy

Madeline M. Barnicle, RN, MS, OCN

The prospects of chemotherapy are fraught with fear and uncertainty. Women requiring chemotherapy due to breast cancer fear the devastating realities of hair loss, as well as the nausea and vomiting; however, they are more willing to endure the side effects when the goal is cure. For those whose cancer recurs following chemotherapy, the fact that they face an uncertain future dependent on effective chemotherapy is more than some can imagine.

Managing side effects from chemotherapy is a multifaceted challenge. Patients are primarily treated in outpatient settings illustrating the need for patient and family awareness of toxicities and methods to maximize coping. The advances in symptom management over the past decade have significantly improved patient outcomes. The nurse, in providing information, empowers the patient and decreases her vulnerability, thus enabling her to make decisions and participate in the treatment plan. The purpose of this chapter is to review side effects related to chemotherapy and to discuss innovative management. The most frequent physical symptoms experienced by women receiving chemotherapy for breast cancer are nausea and vomiting, mucositis, alopecia, menopausal symptoms, weight gain, and fatigue. Less common effects include hemorrhagic cystitis and neurotoxicity.

PRIOR TO CHEMOTHERAPY

Many patients experience intense anticipatory anxiety. Jacobsen, Bovbjerg, and Redd (1993) examined the prevalence and course of anxiety in 53 women receiving adjuvant chemotherapy for breast cancer. Findings indicated 91% reported feeling anxious with their first course of treatment; however, this declined to 64% between the first and second infusions. Patients experiencing side effects were more likely to report persistent anxiety.

The intense anticipatory anxiety experienced by patients on the first day of therapy can be diffused by meeting with the oncology nurse on a day prior to the treatment day. This gives the patient an opportunity to discuss apprehensions, clarify information, and tour the treatment facility at a less threatening time. Through assessment, the nurse can identify medical and psychological factors that predispose certain women to heightened anxiety. The anxious patient will benefit from a benzodiazepine such as lorazepam or alprazolam (Holland & Swain, 1991; Razavi et al., 1993). Patients also benefit from frequent, consistent communication with their oncology nurse. Information can help shift patients' reactions toward treatment compliance resulting in lower risks and improved treatment outcomes (Given & Given, 1989).

NAUSEA AND VOMITING

Nausea and vomiting are two of the most common and dreaded side effects of chemotherapy in breast cancer (Coates et al., 1983). New insight into the pathophysiology and standardization of antiemetic trial methodology, and the discovery of a new class of antiemetics (serotonin antagonists), have significantly improved control of chemotherapy-induced nausea and vomiting. In fact, for most patients receiving moderate to highly emetogenic therapy, complete control of nausea and vomiting is a realistic goal.

Predictions can be made relevant to the emetogenicity of various breast cancer protocols. To accurately establish risk, consideration needs to be given to patient characteristics. Variation in responses among women receiving same-dose therapy emphasizes the impact of individual factors. Jacobsen et al. (1988) interviewed women receiving adjuvant chemotherapy for breast cancer to evaluate non-pharmacologic factors contributing to the development of posttreatment nausea. Results identified patients with a poor Karnofsky score, increased anxiety, history of nausea and vomiting, and expectation of posttreatment side effects contributed to development of nausea. Other characteristics enhancing risk are gender, age, history of motion sickness,

(Morrow, 1985; Tonato, Roila, & Del Favera, 1991), or previous exposure to chemotherapy.

Nausea and vomiting can be divided into three categories: acute, delayed (beginning greater than 24 hours after therapy), and anticipatory, a classic conditioned response from inadequate antiemetic therapy. Antiemetic regimens must ensure sufficient control from the onset of therapy as well as quick responses to failures; anticipatory vomiting is high unless complete control is achieved. A posttreatment phone call can evaluate the patient's control of acute nausea and allow for expedient rescue if needed. Ongoing evaluation of recommended therapy is essential.

Drugs with well-established activity in the management of chemotherapy-induced nausea and vomiting include the phenothiazines, metoclopramide, haloperidol, cannabinoids, dexamethasone, and more recently, the serotonin antagonists (see Table 3-1). Improved efficacy and decreased side effects are demonstrated when active agents are used in combination (Kris, 1994). For example, dexamethasone increases the efficacy of the serotonin antagonists (Roila et al., 1991). The information available detailing the central and peripheral neurological pathways of chemotherapy-induced emesis provides rationale for effective antiemetic combinations. These anatonomic pathways include areas activated by chemical stimuli as well as psychological factors (Morrow, 1985). Although the specific mechanisms underlying nausea and vomiting are not completely understood, the most widely favored is that cytotoxic drugs cause cellular damage in the intestinal mucosa, which elicits the release of chemical mediators including serotonin (5-HT3) from the enterochromaffin cells. This was first observed with high doses of metoclopramide, which demonstrated 5-HT3 antagonist activity. These neurotransmittors are thought either to depolarize the vagal and splenic afferent neurons or to sensitize them to other stimuli. This, in turn, initiates the vomiting reflex by stimulating receptors in the nervous system. The drugs discussed below have significantly reduced the incidence of posttreatment nausea and vomiting (PTNV) (Perez, 1994)

Currently the most commonly used chemotherapy regimens for breast cancer include cyclophosphamide, doxorubicin, fluorouracil (CAF); cyclophosphamide, methotrexate, fluorouracil (CMF); and methotrexate, fluorouracil with leucovorin rescue. Other drugs used alone or in combination include paclitaxel, thiotepa, vinblastine, novantrone, and navelbine (Burroughs Wellcome Co.). Table 3-2 details emetogenic potential of these agents and recommendations for pharmacologic management. Serotonin antagonists have been compared with metoclopramide with superior results seen in the breast cancer population (LeBonniec et al., 1990; Marschner, 1991; Soukop et al., 1992).

In one study granisetron was compared with compazine and dexamethasone primarily in the breast cancer population, with results favoring granisetron for alleviating emesis 70% to 34% (Warr et al., 1991). The serotonin antagonists with their specificity have no doubt improved the acute phase of nausea and vomiting in patients receiving doxorubicin and cyclophosphamide, with minimal side effects. In fact, most patients receiving this combination experience no emesis.

With the acute phase becoming more manageable, delayed nausea is the greater challenge. Although not as severe as acute nausea and vomiting, delayed nausea and vomiting can be more debilitating. Patients report that these symptoms interfere with their ability to care for family and decrease their ability to engage in routine activities of daily living (Lindley, Bernard, & Fields, 1989). In cases of delayed nausea and vomiting, metoclopramide or dexamethasone have a better established efficacy.

Current recommended actions for emetogenic therapy include combining a neurotransmittor blocking agent, corticosteroid, and benzodiazepine or antihistamine, which offers the best results (Pisters & Kris, 1992). Another alternative is to combine a serotonin antagonist and corticosteroid for the same benefit with less sedation (Bonneterre et al., 1990). Not all regimens will require a serotonin antagonist. Patients considered to be low risk should be reassured that nausea and vomiting are unlikely to occur. They should be given a prescription for metoclopramide or prochlorperazine to be used as needed. Consideration needs to be given to cost since many patients lack insurance for oral prescriptions.

Anticipatory nausea and vomiting (ANV) appears in 25% to 67% of patients within approximately four courses of treatment (Wickham, 1989). Patients receiving short-term therapy are at less risk; however, 33% of patients receiving standard doses of CMF experience ANV. Patients who have already experienced posttreatment nausea and vomiting during the first four cycles are at greatest risk (Wilcox, Fetting, Nettesheim, & Abeloff, 1982).

Patients frequently describe an unrelenting nausea while taking oral cyclophosphamide. Symptoms are reported to be similar to morning sickness, or a burning, gnawing, hunger-like feeling that is relieved by eating. Strategies to minimize this sensation are outlined in Table 3-3.

HEMORRHAGIC CYSTITIS

Hemorrhagic cystitis develops in 2% to 40% of patients who receive cyclophosphamide (Levine & Richie, 1989). Symptoms can range from microscopic hematuria to frank bleeding. Patients are at low risk if they are receiving oral therapy and maintain a fluid intake of at least 80 ounces daily. High-risk patients on dose-intensive therapy will require hyperhydration, frequent voiding, and diuresis. Complaints such as dysuria, irritation, or suprapubic pain are evaluated through urine culture. Reinstating therapy after the development of hemorrhagic cystitis should be done cautiously as the patient is at risk of recurrent problems. Cyclophosphamide is a major player in adjuvant therapy; education and early communication of symptoms makes it

Table 3-1 Common Antiemetic Regimens

Classification/Action	Drugs	Dose/Schedule	Schedule	Side Effects	Comments
A. Benzodiazepines CNS depressant Interferes with afferent nerves from cerebral cortex Sedative Anxiolytic	Lorazepam (Ativan)	Tablets: 0.5, 1, 2 mg Parenteral 2-4 mg/ml	Every 3 to 4 hr prn	Sedation Amnesia Confusion	Effective for anticipatory nausea and vomiting Use with caution with hepatic or renal dysfunction
B. Phenothiazines Dopamine antagonist	Prochlorperazine (Compazine)	Tablets: 5, 10, 25 mg SR: 10, 15 mg Rectal supp: 25 mg IV: 20–40 mg	Every 4 to 6 hr Every 10 to 12 hr Every 4 to 6 hr Every 3 to 4 hr	Sedation (less common with SR) Orthostatic hypotension	Extrapyramidal SE more common <30 age Side effects can be cumulative in elderly
Inhibits vomiting center by blocking afferent impulses via vagus nerve	Triethylperazine (Torecan)	Tablets: 10 mg Supp: 10 mg	Every 4 to 6 hr Every 6 hr	Dizziness Drowsiness	Diphenhydramine combats EPS or dystonic reactions
C. Substituted benzamides Accelerates gastric emptying 5-HT$_3$ antagonist	Metoclopramide (Reglan)	Tablet: 5–10 mg IV: 1–3 mg/kg	tid: 30 min before meals Every 2 to 3 hr	Sedation Diarrhea Anxiety Fatigue	EPS common Use with caution in patients with renal dysfunction
D. Steroids Antiprostaglandin synthesis Exact mechanism is unknown Mild epigastric burning	Dexamethasone (Decadron)	PO: 4 mg IV: 10–20 mg	tid × 2 days bid × 2 days daily × 2 days	Insomnia Euphoria Anxiety Hypertension Edema	Rapid infusion causes perineal itching compatible with and enhances efficacy of ondansetron and granisetron
	Prednisone	PO: 20 mg	tid × 2 days bid × 2 days daily × 2 days		

E. Antihistamines				
Histamine H-1 receptor antagonist	Diphenhydramine (Benadryl)	PO: 25-50 mg IV: 12.5-50 mg	Every 6 hr Every 4 to 6 hr	Sedation Hypotension	Prevent extrapyramidal side effects Use cautiously in the elderly
F. Serotonin antagonists				
Seritonin receptor (5-HT$_3$) antagonist	Ondansetron (Zofran)	PO: 4-8 mg IV: 32 mg x 1 IV: 0.15 mg/kg x 3 doses	Twice daily Every 24 hr	Headache Hypotension Constipation Sedation	Most effective in acute phase of nausea Lightheadedness less common
	Granisetron (Kytril)	IV: 10 mg/kg	Every 24 hr		

SE, side effects; SR, sustained release.

Note. From "Nursing Care in Patient Management and Quality of Life" by K. Hassey Dow & M. Barnicle, 1996, *Diseases of the Breast,* Harris, Lippman, Morrow, & Hellman (Eds.). Philadelphia: Lippincott-Raven, pp. 954–955.

Table 3-2 Combination Antiemetic Options

Chemotherapy Combinations	Antiemetic Combinations

1. Low emetogenic potential (patient at low risk)
• Paclitaxel (taxol)
• Novantrone-thiotepa
• Navelbine
	A. Prochlorperazine 15 mg
	    sig: 1–2 q 12 hours pm or
	B. Thiethylperazine 10 mg
	    sig: 1 q 6 hours prn or
	    with leucovorin rescue
	C. Metoclopramide 10 mg
	    sig: 1 tid
	D. Lorazepam[a] 1 mg
	    sig: 1–2 q 3–4 hours prn

2. Moderate emetogenic potential (patient at risk)
• Cyclophosphamide, methotrexate, fluorouracil (CMF)[b]
• Cyclophosphamide, doxorubicin, fluorouracil (CAF) (low dose)
	A. Prochlorperazine SR 15 mg
	    sig: 1q 12 hours scheduled
	    Lorazepam 1 mg
	    sig: 1–2 q 4 hours prn
	B. Ondansetron 15 mg/kg combined
	    with dexamethasone 20 mg or
	    Granisetron .1 µg/kg combined with dexamethasone[c] 20 mg
	    At HS:
	        Lorazepam 1 mg
	        Diphenhydramine 25–50 mg
	        Prochlorperazine 15 mg
	    Take home prescriptions:
	    Prochlorperazine 15 mg 1–2 q 12 hours
	    Lorazepam 1 mg q 4 hours prn

Delayed nausea
• patients will require emetics on a scheduled basis
	A. Prochlorperazine 15 mg bid day 2 and 3 or
	B. Zofran 8 mg bid day 2 and 3 or
	C. Dexamethasone 8 mg PO bid × 2 days followed by 4 mg
	    bid × 2 days
	D. Dexamethasone 4 mg tid × 2 days bid × 2 days
	    followed by 1 daily for 2 days

3. Severely emetogenic potential (patient at high risk)
   - Doxorubicin, cyclophosphamide (AC)
   - CAF (high dose)

   A. Ondansetron .15 mg/kg or 32 mg total daily dose / combined with dexamethasone 20 mg IV or granisetron .1 μg/kg or 1 mg total daily dose combined with dexamethasone 20 mg IV

   At HS:

   Lorazepam 1–2 mg
   Diphenhydramine 50 mg
   Prochlorperazine 15–30 mg

Delayed nausea

   - patients will require antiemetics on a scheduled basis

   A. Prochlorperazine 15–30 mg q 12 hours days 2 and 3

   Lorazepam 1 mg q 4 hours prn

   B. Ondansetron 8 mg bid

   Lorazepam 1 mg PO q 4 hours prn
   Prochlorperazine 15–30 mg SR q 12 hours for days 2 and 3

   C. Dexamethasone 8 mg bid x 2 days
   Dexamethasone 4 mg bid x 2 days

   D. Prednisone 20 mg tid x 2 days
   Prednisone 20 mg bid x 2 days
   Prednisone 20 mg q day x 2 days

Anticipatory nausea

   A. Lorazepam 1 mg PO 30 minutes prior to treatment

   B. Lorazepam 0.5–2 mg IV prior to treatment (avoid before vesicant chemotherapy)

   C. Consider behavioral therapy options

---

a Lorazepam is best used in combination with the drugs listed above it. "Ativan" dissolves sublingually and is useful for "waves" of nausea.

b Patients with no risk factors generally tolerate adjuvant CMF requiring only prn low-dose antiemetics.

c Dexamathasone improves efficacy of serotonin antagonists.

Note. Pretreatment considerations include: having patients meet with an oncology nurse; establishing the level of risk (patient treatment characteristics); possibility of treatment on an outpatient basis.

TABLE 3-3   Strategies to Minimize Nausea
Related to Oral Cyclophosphamide

- Take long-acting antiemetic
- Eat small amounts of low-calorie food frequently
- Consider taking one-time daily dose
    Confirm with MD
    Preferably in the AM
- Take antacid

possible to treat those symptoms rather than
simply discontinue this drug, which can be a
potentially curing therapy.

MUCOSITIS

Chemotherapy-induced mucositis occurs in
less than 20% of breast cancer patients and is
highest in those receiving antitumor antibiotics or intense treatment modalities such as
bone marrow transplant. Breast cancer is the
most common neoplasm treated with chemotherapy, yet literature specific to oral complications is lacking.

Maintaining the integrity of the oral cavity
during chemotherapy is essential and can best
be accomplished through prevention, application of interceptive guidelines, and aggressive
maintenance of oral and dental hygiene (Toth,
Martin, & Fleming, 1991). Pretreatment strategies to prevent or decrease the incidence of
oral complications include a baseline oral assessment, treatment of pre-existing dental disease, and patient education (JNIH, 1989).
Patients who have pre-existing dental problems corrected and incorporate an oral care
regimen consistently have a significant decrease in oral complications (Beck, 1992).

Chemotherapy directly affects the integrity
of the oral cavity at the basement membrane
where susceptible stem cells are rapidly divid-
ing. The destruction of epithelial cells initiates
the inflammatory response. Chemotherapy
treatments are indirectly stomatotoxic with
their effect on the bone marrow. The degree of
mucositis and risk of infection is directly correlated with the extent of pancytopenia (Beck,

1992). Patients with metastatic disease may
have a slower bone marrow recovery, placing
them at greater risk. Distinguishing between
the types of oral complications is not simple.
For example, infectious processes, whether viral, fungal, or bacterial, may mimic or accompany stomatitis or mucositis (Poland, 1991).
Although there is no way to predict whether a
patient will develop stomatitis, one can expect
those who develop symptoms within the first
cycle will most assuredly develop recurrence
with continued therapy.

McCarthy and Skillings (1992) investigated the incidence of orofacial complications
in 34 women receiving cyclophosphamide,
methotrexate, fluorouracil, vincristine, and
prednisone. Patients were interviewed bi-
weekly and received orofacial exams weekly.
Mucositis occurred in 21% of the women studied. Characteristics common among affected
patients were oral lesions at baseline, age over
50, poor oral hygiene, restricted performance
status, anemia, or denture wearer. Additional
factors adding to mucosal vulnerability include tobacco, alcohol, and compromised organ function. Patients with compromised renal
function receiving moderate doses of methotrexate can experience a delayed elimination of
the drug, increasing their risk for mucositis.

The ultimate goal of any oral care protocol is a clean, smooth, pink, moist, and intact
oral cavity (Beck, 1992). Table 3-4 outlines an
oral care program. Brushing and flossing are
the most effective cleansing techniques. Rinsing with normal saline or sodium bicarbonate
enhances the removal of debris. The effectiveness of hydrogen peroxide rinses is inconsis-
tent; they break down granulating tissue and
have an unpleasant taste. Chlorhexadine has
demonstrated significant reductions in oral
infections and mucositis in patients receiving
bone marrow transplants (Ferretti et al., 1990).
Treatment of chemotherapy-induced stomatitis is primarily palliative, with emphasis on
maintaining hydration and nutritional status.
Monitoring a patient's condition on an outpatient basis requires diligence both in the nurse
and the patient.

Identification and early treatment of infectious processes avoids potential complications of sepsis. *Candida albicans* is the most common fungal infection, which presents with a classic raised cottage cheese-like plaque. Treatment is either topical with Nystatin rinses or clotrimazole troches, or oral with fluconazol. *Herpes simplex* is the most commonly seen viral infection; immunosuppression increases the risk of reactivating these infections. Acyclovir can be used in patients who test seropositive to prevent reactivation (Seral, 1990). Bacterial infections such as *pseudomonas* and *streptococcus* require broad spectrum antibiotics as well as aggressive oral hygiene. Vitamin E can be used topically in patients with stomatitis (Wadleigh et al., 1992).

Cryotherapy can reduce the incidence and severity of stomatitis. This intervention decreases oral toxicities in patients receiving leucovorin and fluorouracil and has been reported to be effective for mucositis induced by doxorubicin (Mahood et al., 1991; Twelves & Seymour, 1991). Of interest is that colony stimulating factors decreased the incidence and severity of oral complications through rapid restoration of neutrophil counts (Gabrilove et al., 1988).

MYELOSUPPRESSION

Myelosuppression is the most common dose-limiting toxicity of chemotherapy. Factors contributing to a patient's risk are age, prior radiation therapy, presence of bone metastasis (Goodman, 1989), prescribed therapy, and long-term therapy. Commonly used drugs in breast cancer with myelosuppressive risks are doxorubicin, cyclophosphamide, and paclitaxel. This risk is enhanced when these drugs are used in combination. There is no doubt that the discovery of colony stimulating factors has significantly decreased the severity and duration of neutropenic episodes. Currently, their role in the adjuvant setting is reserved for dose intensification protocols and recovery from neutropenic fevers. In the patient with metastatic disease, it is not uncommon for patients to receive more intense therapy with colony stimulating factors for bone marrow rescue.

Teaching patients about myelosuppression and their level of risk is imperative. The nadir and recovery of leukocytes and granulocytes can be predicted depending on the prescribed therapy. Patients receiving oral cyclophosphamide experience mild neutropenia, often requiring delays or dose reductions. Patients receiving doxorubicin, intravenous cyclophosphamide, and/or paclitaxel experience more intense nadirs with more rapid recovery. Myelosuppression and its morbidity can be successfully treated when recognized and treated early.

ALOPECIA

Hair contributes significantly to a women's body image and sexuality. Patients have described hair loss as one of the most distressing side effects of chemotherapy (Coates et al., 1983). However, patients are more able to adapt when they have a realistic appraisal of the situation and know that it is temporary. Surgical scars are devastating; however, hair loss can be publicly stigmatizing.

Chemotherapy causes partial or complete atrophy of the hair root bulb, with constriction of the hair shaft. On the average, 85% of hair follicles are in a proliferative phase; the majority of other body hair follicles are in a resting phase. However, with repeated doses, pubic, axillary, and facial hair may be lost. Fortunately, this effect is temporary and hair will regrow. With regrowth, changes in hair pigment, texture, and type may be evident. Hair will generally return to its pretreatment state within a year.

Drug combinations at low risk from hair loss are methotrexate-fluorouracil with leucovorin rescue, novantrone, thiotepa, and vinblastine. Oral cyclophosphamide weakens the hair shaft and causes generalized hair thinning, especially at the crown. Forty-one percent of patients receiving standard 6-month therapy lose greater than 50% of their hair (Fischer et al., 1990). Patients with thicker hair

Table 3-4   Stomatitis Oral Care Guide

- Consider pretreatment evaluation by dentist
- Goal: Prevention/reporting symptoms early

    I.   Potential Stomatitis
        A. Assess oral cavity daily
        B. Promote oral hygiene:
            - perform PC and HS
            - use soft toothbrush
            - floss daily (unwaxed)
            - apply lip lubricant
        C. Mouth rinse options:
            - Sodium bicarbonate solution:
              1 tsp baking soda, 8 oz water
            - ½ tsp salt in 8 oz water
            - warm water and saline
            - nonalcohol commercial mouthwashes
        D. Maintain adequate nutrition/hydration
    II. Mild or moderate stomatitis
        A. Assess oral cavity twice daily
        B. Continue oral hygiene
            - increase frequency
            - omit flossing with gum tenderness or bleeding
            - avoid dry mouth and lips
        C. Remove dentures
            - replace for meals only
        D. Culture suspicious lesions
        E. Topical anesthetics prn/ac options
            - Lidocaine 2% or 5%
            - Cetacaine or Hurricane spray sig: 1–2 sprays as needed
            - Stomatitis cocktail (equal parts viscous lidocaine, diphenhydramine HCL elixir and Maalox)
              sig: 15–30 cc q 4hours—may swish, spit, or swallow
            - Zilactin–hydroxypropyl cellulose sig: apply directly to lesion
            - Oratech gel sig: apply directly to lesion
            - Dyclonine hydrochloride 0.5–1% sig: 15 cc, swish and spit—also available in extra-strength
              Sucrets lozenges or spray
        F. Oral analgesics as needed, i.e., Tylenol #3
        G. Adapt diet to enhance nutrition and hydration needs
            - eat soft, bland, non-irritating foods
            - increase protein intake
            - ensure > 2,000 cc/day fluids
        H. Communicate with doctor or nurse as needed
    III. Severe stomatitis
        A. Assess oral cavity q 4 hours
        B. Oral hygiene
            - alternate warm saline rinses with antifungal or antibacterial oral suspensions
            - rinse with oxidizing agent, i.e., diluted hydrogen peroxidase (1.5%) for mucolytic areas
        C. Culture any lesions
            - patient may require antifungal, antiviral, and antibacterial agents
        D. Continue topical/systemic analgesics

Table 3-4 *Continued*

    E. Nutrition/hydration status
- may require intravenous hydration
- continue high protein intake
- ensure > 2,000 cc/day fluids

    F. Communication
- evaluate progress daily

Table 3-5 Strategies to Minimize Hair Loss

- Cut hair to a manageable and easy-to-maintain style prior to chemotherapy
- Use mild, protein-based shampoo and conditioner
- Use electric hair dryer on lowest setting
- Avoid electric curlers, curling irons, hair spray, and dyes that may increase fragility of hair
- Avoid excessive brushing or combing
- Purchase wig to fit normal hair color and style
- Send prescription for "therapeutic cranial prosthesis; medically indicated for alopecia from cancer chemotherapy"
- Consider referral to Look Good . . . Feel Better program
- Consider hair preservation techniques for patients receiving low-dose palliative chemotherapy

may not require a wig. Women with fine, sparse hair generally need a wig following the fourth cycle of treatment. Certain measures can minimize or delay hair loss; for examples, see Table 3-5.

Patients receiving higher doses of doxorubicin and cyclophosphamide, or paclitaxel, can expect complete hair loss. Patients should be advised to purchase a wig (cranial prosthesis) prior to hair loss. Wigs can be shaped and thinned to one's natural hair style. Patients receiving adjuvant therapy are devastated by the prospects of alopecia; however, they are often willing to accept it as a trade-off for curative intent. Patients with metastatic disease facing indeterminant chemotherapy may be less willing to accept these side effects.

Hair preservation techniques, such as scalp hypothermia, are controversial and ineffective with higher doses of doxorubicin and cyclophosphamide. Opponents believe that it creates a drug sanctuary, protecting cells from cytotoxic therapy. Although this risk is mini-

mal, it warrants consideration when treating patients with curative intent. When oral cyclophosphamide is given, hair preservation techniques are not practical, because the drug is taken orally. Hypothermia applied 15 to 20 minutes before and 20 to 30 minutes after can be effective for patients receiving less than 30 mg/m^2 doxorubicin and contributes to the patient's quality of life.

Dealing with appearance changes has become a recognized part of the healing process for many patients. Programs such as the Look Good . . . Feel Better program have been designed to help women restore their appearance and self-esteem.

WEIGHT GAIN

Increased body weight occurs in 50% to 90% of women receiving adjuvant chemotherapy (Foltz, 1985; Knobf, Mullen, Xistris, & Moritz, 1983; Goodwin, Panzarella, & Boyd, 1988; Heasman, Sutherland, Campbell, Elhakim, &

Boyd, 1985; Knobf, 1983; Knobf, 1986). In one study patients not receiving adjuvant therapy also demonstrated weight gain (Goodwin et al., 1988). Weight gains up to 22 pounds are particularly problematic for premenopausal women on longer combination therapy (Camoriano et al., 1990). In addition, results of one study indicated that weight gain was still evident at 2 years of follow-up (Levine, Raczynski, & Carpenter, 1991). This contributes to body image problems as well as health risks, including risk of disease recurrence. Camoriano et al. (1990) in their review of 646 women treated with adjuvant chemotherapy reported that women gaining more than the median weight at 1 year on chemotherapy were 1.5 times more likely to have relapsed, and 1.7 times more likely to have died compared with women gaining less.

The underlying mechanism of energy imbalance among women is unknown. Several theories have been postulated to explain this phenomenon: nutritional theory, hormonal changes, and depression (Demark-Wahnefried, Winer, & Rimer, 1993; Camoriono et al., 1990; Chlebowski et al., 1991). Other researchers found a high incidence of fatigue in their breast cancer patients, suggesting a relationship between weight gain and exercise/fatigue levels (Huntington, 1985).

Foltz (1985) investigated factors influencing weight gain in 34 women receiving 6 months of adjuvant chemotherapy with CMF. Weight gain was significant for 70%, with a mean gain of 10 pounds. Pre- and peri-menopausal patients experienced more gain than post-menopausal patients. Interestingly, in comparing weight gaining and non-weight gaining women, no significant difference was observed in activity, resting metabolic rate, and oral intake. In addition, activity, depression, metabolic rate, estradiol, and intake were not predictive of weight gain. Depression and resulting compensatory eating has been explored as a potential cause of weight gain (Demark-Wahnefried et al., 1993).

Patients can avoid weight gain through a regular exercise program and decreased fat in-take. Research reports that women who exercised routinely had stable body weight, reduced fat deposition, increased functional capacity (MacVicar, Winningham, & Nickel, 1989; Winningham, MacVicar, Bondoc, Anderson, & Minton, 1989), and a higher quality of life (Young-McCaughan & Sexton, 1991). Educating patients of their risk and establishing goals toward good nutrition and safe exercise provide a preventive direction for patients.

INTIMACY ISSUES

Theoretically, estrogen deficiency due to natural menopause or prematurely due to adjuvant chemotherapy is considered favorable due to the biology of breast tumors; however, it can have a negative impact on a woman's sexuality. Knobf (1986) studied 78 women receiving adjuvant chemotherapy to establish the degree of physical and psychological distress as well as life-style changes experienced. Fifty-six percent of premenopausal women reported a change in frequency and quality of their sexual relationships compared with 41% of postmenopausal patients.

Premature menopause with depleted supplies of estrogen and testosterone causes menopausal symptoms, sleep disturbances, and impairment in all three phases of the sexual response cycle: desire, excitement, and orgasm (Blume, 1993). These troubling effects are often neglected because patients are too embarrassed to approach the topic with the physician, fearing he/she may consider the patient's complaints as trivial. This can be a major source of stress to a woman who may already be emotionally vulnerable. A trusting, caring relationship encourages the open expression of their concerns. Estrogen deficiency causes vaginal dryness, burning, itching, dyspareunia, and eventual vaginal atrophy. Using a water-based vaginal lubricant such as Replens or Astroglide can decrease discomfort. Patients may initially require more frequent use until vaginal tissue becomes lubricated.

Fertility is a concern for younger women diagnosed with breast cancer. Patients who receive CMF are at risk for ovarian failure. Amenorrhea occurs in 53% of women less than 35 years old, 84% in women aged 35 to 44, and 94% of those 45 years or older. This ovarian failure will be permanent in 86% of women younger than 40 and 96% of women 40 years of age or older. Preliminary data comparing cyclophosphamide, methotrexate, and fluorouracil with doxorubicin and cyclophosphamide suggest that a greater percentage of patients receiving the latter will recover ovarian function once treatment has been completed (Cobleigh, Bines, Lincoln, & Wolter, 1994).

NEUROTOXICITY

Breast cancer drugs with dose-limiting neurotoxicity are vinblastine, paclitaxel, cisplatin, and navelbine. Most patients experience temporary neurotoxicity; however, these effects can be permanent. When patients are unable to perform fine coordinated movements such as buttoning clothing or writing, or are experiencing muscle pain, altering the dose is considered appropriate. Therapy can be reinstituted when symptoms abate at a 50% dose reduction (MacDonald, 1992).

The incidence of neurotoxicity is greatest in patients receiving paclitaxel in >200 mg/m^2 doses. These are usually cumulative and worsen with successive doses. Patients describe paresthesia and numbness in a "glove and stocking" distribution. Physical examination reveals distal sensory loss of both large- and small-diameter fibers (Meehan & Johnson, 1992). Amitriptyline has been used with moderate success for relief of neuropathic pain (Brown et al., 1991; Rowinsky, Eisenhauer, Chaudry, Arbuck, & Donehower, 1993).

Myalgias and arthralgias occur in 61% of patients receiving paclitaxel in doses of 175 mg/m^2 and are exaggerated during the time of granulocyte–colony stimulating factor administration (Reichman et al., 1993). Effects occur 48 to 72 hours after infusion and can persist for up to 7 days. Effects occur primarily in large joints, but can involve the whole body (Lubejko & Sartorius, 1993). Pharmacologic interventions such as nonsteroidal analgesics or narcotics are usually required. Seldane 60 mg twice daily has demonstrated efficacy in treating myalgias and arthralgias (Martoni, Zamagni, Gheka, & Pannuti, 1993).

FATIGUE

The problem of tiredness disrupts daily activities and patients' abilities to separate the chemotherapy experience from the rest of their life. Patients have described how the cumulative impact of multiple side effects outweighs any specific effect (Love, Leventhal, Easterling, & Nerenz, 1989). In two studies, tiredness was the most frequently reported side effect (Tierney et al., 1991; Knobf, 1986). Nurses play an important role in guiding and educating women with breast cancer in health-promoting behaviors to help minimize the problems associated with side effects. The development of more effective interventions could provide significant benefit to the patients, both psychologically and physically.

LATE EFFECTS OF ADJUVANT CHEMOTHERAPY

Acute myeloid leukemia (AML) after treatment with chemotherapeutic regimens containing alkylators is an uncommon but well-established risk (Levine & Bloomfield, 1992). It is thought that the risk of leukemia is overshadowed by the benefit of adjuvant therapy. The recent discovery of secondary AML in patients enrolled in NSABP trial B-25, where higher than standard doses of cyclophosphamide were used in combination with adriamycin and colony stimulating factors, is a reminder of this risk and that it may be amplified in intensified doses (Abrams, 1994). Bonadonna et al. reviewed 2,465 patients with operable breast cancer and noted that for those who received CMF there was no increased risk of second malignancies (Bonadonna, Valagussa, Moliterni, Zambetti, & Terenziani, 1993).

METASTATIC BREAST CANCER

In metastatic disease, treatment is considered palliative and therefore should have minimal side effects. However, many patients do well on higher dose therapy with multiple interruptive toxicities. Some require daily injections of growth factors to achieve the greatest results. Commonly prescribed combinations used to treat metastatic disease are CMF, CAF, and paclitaxel, which can result in overall response rates of 45% to 80% and median response duration of 5 to 13 months (Reichman et al., 1993).

SURVIVORSHIP

Completing treatment should be a day to celebrate life; however, many patients are apprehensive. They are fearful of a recurrence with less frequent visits. Many patients say that they will never be the same again; in fact, some say they are better. They have surprised themselves with their own strength, and now they look at life in a new way. Providing patients with information on wellness, survivorship, and follow-up gives them direction as they face the future.

SUMMARY

Educating breast cancer patients during treatment is a challenging and rewarding task. Providing patients with the information and the support they need to maintain maximum quality of life requires consistency and attention to details. Teaching patients about chemotherapy and the management of its side effects is a role for which the oncology nurse is eminently qualified.

References

Abrams, J. (1994) (Investigators letter). National Institute of Health. 1–4.

Beck, S. L. (1992). Prevention and management of oral complications in the cancer practice. *Current Issues in Cancer Nursing Practice Updates* (pp. 27–38). Philadelphia: Lippincott.

Blume, E. (1993). Sex after chemotherapy: A neglected issue (news). *Journal of the National Cancer Institute. 85* (10), 768–770.

Bonadonna, G., Valagussa, P., Moliterni, N., Zambetti, M., & Terenziani, M. (1993). Risk of acute leukemia and other malignancies following CMF-based adjuvant chemotherapy for breast cancer (Abstract). *Proceedings of the Annual Meeting of the American Society of Clinical Oncology, 12*, A45.

Bonneterre, J., Chevallier, B., Metz, R., Fargeot, P., Pujade–Lauraine, E., Spielmann, M., Tubiana-Hulin, M., Paes, D., & Bons, J. (1990). A randomized double–blind comparison of ondansetron and metoclopramide in the prophylaxis of emesis induced by cyclophosphamide, fluorouracil and doxorubicin or epirubicin chemotherapy. *Journal of Clinical Oncology, 8* (6), 1063–1069.

Brown, T., Havlin, K., Weiss, G., Cagnola, J., Koeller, J., Kuhn, J., Rizzo, J., Craig, J., Phillips, J., & Von Hoff, D. (1991). A phase I trial of taxol given by a 6-hour intravenous infusion. *Journal of Clinical Oncology, 9* (7), 1261–1267.

Camoriano, J. K., Loprinzi, C. L., Ingle, J. N., Therneau, T. M., Krook, J. E., & Veeder, M. H. (1990). Weight change in women treated with adjuvant therapy or observed following mastectomy for node positive breast cancer. *Journal of Clinical Oncology, 8*, 1327–1334.

Chlebowski, R. T., Rose, D., Buzzard, M., Blackburn, G. L., Insull, W., Grosvenor, M., Elashoff, R., & Wynder, E. L. (1991). Adjuvant dietary fat intake reduction in postmenopausal breast cancer patient management. *Breast Cancer Research and Treatment, 20*, 73–84.

Coates, A., Abraham, S., Kay, S. B., Sowerbutts, T., Frewin, C., Fox, R. M., & Tattersall M. H. (1983). On the receiving end—patient perception of the side effects of cancer chemotherapy. *European Journal of Cancer and Clinical Oncology, 19* (2), 203–208.

Cobleigh, M. A., Bines, J., Lincoln, S. T., & Wolter, J. M. (1994). Amenorrhea following adjuvant chemotherapy for breast cancer. *Proceedings from the American Association of Clinical Oncology, 13*, A55.

Demark-Wahnefried, W., Winer, E. P., & Rimer, B. K. (1993). Why women gain weight with adjuvant chemotherapy for breast cancer. *Journal of Clinical Oncology, 11* (7), 1418–1429.

Ferretti, G.A., Raybould, T. P., Brown, A. T., MacDonald, J. S., Greenwood, M., Maruyama, Y., Geil, J., Lillich, T. T., & Ash, R. C. (1990). Chlorhexidine prophylaxis for chemotherapy and radiotherapy induced stomatitis: A double blind trial. *Oral Surgery, Oral Medicine, Oral Pathology, 69*, 331–338.

Fischer, B., Redmond, C., Dimitrov N. V., Bowman, D., Legault-Poisson, S., Wickerham, K. L., Wolmark, N., Fischer, E. R., Margolese, R., & Sutherland, C. (1989). A randomized clinical trial evaluating sequential methotrexate and fluorouracil in the treatment of patients with node negative breast cancer who have estrogen receptor negative tumors. *New England Journal of Medicine, 320*, 473–478.

Foltz, A. T. (1985). Weight gain among stage II breast cancer patients: A study of five factors. *Oncology Nursing Forum, 12* (3), 21–26.

Gabrilove, J. L., Jakubowski, A., Scher, H., Sternberg, C., Wong, G., Grous, J., Yogoda, A., Fain, K., Moore, M. A. S., Clarkson, B., Oettgen, H. F., Alton, K., Welte, K., & Souza, L. (1988). Effect of granulocyte colony stimulating factor on neutropenia and associated morbidity due to chemotherapy for transitional-cell carcinoma of the urothelium. *The New England Journal of Medicine, 318,* 1414–1422.

Given, B. A., & Given, C. W. (1989). Compliance among patients with cancer. *Oncology Nursing Forum, 16* (1), 97–103.

Goodman, M. (1989). Managing the side effects of chemotherapy. *Seminars in Oncology Nursing, 5* (2), 29–52.

Goodwin, P. J., Panzarella, T., & Boyd, N. F. (1988). Weight gain in women with localized breast cancer: A descriptive study. *Breast Cancer Research and Treatment, 11,* 59–66.

Heasman, K. Z., Sutherland, H. J., Campbell, J. A., Elhakim, T., & Boyd, N. F. (1985). Weight gain during adjuvant chemotherapy for breast cancer. *Breast Cancer Research and Treatment, 5,* 195–200.

Holland, J. C., Morrow, G. R., Schmale, A., Derogatis, L., Stefanek, M., Berenson, S., Carpenter, P. J., Breitbart, W., & Feldstein, M. (1991). A randomized clinical trial of alprazolam versus progressive muscle relaxation in cancer patients with anxiety and depressive symptoms. *Journal of Clinical Oncology, 9* (6), 1004–1011.

Huntington, M.O. (1985). Weight gain in patients receiving adjuvant chemotherapy for carcinoma of the breast. *Cancer, 56,* 472–474.

Jacobsen, P. B., Andrykowski, M. A., Redd, W. H., Die-Trill, M., Hakes, T. B., Kaufman, R. J., Currie, V. E., & Holland, J. C. (1988). Nonpharmacologic factors in the development of posttreatment nausea with adjuvant chemotherapy for breast cancer. *Cancer, 61,* 379–385.

Jacobsen, P. B., Bovbjerg, D. H., & Redd, W. H. (1993). Anticipatory anxiety in women receiving chemotherapy for breast cancer. *Health Psychology, 12*(6), 469–475.

JNIH Consensus Development Conference Statement. (1989). Oral complications of cancer chemotherapies: Diagnosis, prevention, and treatment. *NCI Monographs, 9.*

Knobf, M.T. (1986). Physical and psychologic distress associated with adjuvant chemotherapy in women with breast cancer. *Journal of Clinical Oncology, 4,* 678–684.

Knobf, M., Mullen, J. C., Xistris, D., & Moritz, D. A. (1983). Weight gain in women with breast cancer receiving adjuvant chemotherapy. *Oncology Nursing Forum, 10* (2), 28–33.

Kris, M. G. (1994). Ondansetron: A specific serotonin antagonist for the prevention of chemotherapy induced vomiting. *Principles and Practice of Oncology: PPO updates, 8* (2), 1–11.

LeBonniec, M., Madelaine, I., Marty, M., Dieras, V., Extra, J. M., & Romain, D. (1990). Single–blinded randomized comparison study with cross over of granisetron versus standard antiemetics in the treatment of chemotherapy induced emesis (Abstract). *Proceedings of the Annual Meeting of the American Society of Clinical Oncology, 9,* A1277.

Levine, E., & Bloomfield, C. (1992). Leukemias and myelodysplastic syndrome secondary to drug, radiation, and environmental exposure. *Seminars in Oncology, 19,* 47–84.

Levine, E. G., Raczynski, J. M., & Carpenter, J. T. (1991). Weight gain with breast cancer adjuvant treatments. *Cancer, 67,* 1954–1959.

Levine, L. A., & Richie, J. P. (1989). Urological complications of cyclophosphamide. *Journal of Urology, 141* (5), 1063–1069.

Lindley, C. M, Bernard, S., & Fields, S. M. (1989). Incidence and duration of chemotherapy induced nausea and vomiting in the outpatient oncology population. *Journal of Clinical Oncology, 7,* 1142–1149.

Love, R. R., Leventhal, H., Easterling, D. V., & Nerenz, D. R. (1989). Side effects and emotional distress during cancer chemotherapy. *Cancer, 63,* 604–612.

Lubejko, B. G., & Sartorius, S. E. (1993). Nursing considerations on paclitaxel (Taxol) administration. *Seminars in Oncology, 20* (4), 26–30.

MacDonald, D. R. (1992). Neurotoxicity of chemotherapeutic agents. In M. C. Perry (Ed.), *The chemotherapy source book* (pp. 666–679). Baltimore: Williams & Wilkins.

MacVicar, M. G., Winningham, M. L., & Nickel, J. L. (1989). Effects of aerobic interval training on cancer patients' functional capacity. *Nursing Research, 38* (6), 348–351.

Mahood, D. J., Dose, A. M., Loprinzi, C. L., Veeder, M. H., Athmann, L. M., Therneau T. M., Sorenson, J. M., Gainey, D. K., Mailliard, J. A., Gusa, N. L. et al. (1991). Inhibition of fluorouracil-induced stomatitis by oral cryotherapy. *Journal of Clinical Oncology, 9* (3), 449–452.

Marschner, N. (1991). Antiemetic control with ondansetron in the chemotherapy of breast cancer: A review. *European Journal of Cancer, 27,* s15–17.

Martoni, A., Zamagni, C., Gheka, A., & Pannuti, F. (1993). Antihistamines in the treatment of taxol-induced paroxystic pain syndrome. *Journal of the National Cancer Institute, 85* (8), 676.

McCarthy, G. M., & Skillings, J. R. (1992). Orofacial complications of chemotherapy for breast cancer. *Oral Surgery, Oral Medicine, Oral Pathology, 74* (2), 172–178.

Meehan, J. L., & Johnson, B. L. (1992). The neurotoxicity of antineoplastic agents. *Current Issues in Cancer Nursing Practice Updates, 1* (8), 1–11.

Morrow, G. R. (1985). The effect of a susceptibility to motion sickness on the side-effects of cancer chemotherapy. *Cancer, 55,* 2766–2770.

Northouse, L. L., & Swain, M. A. (1987). Adjustment of patients and husbands to the initial impact of breast cancer. *Nursing Research, 36,* 221–225.

Perez, E.A. (1994). Prevention and control of chemotherapy induced emesis in the 1990's. *Mediguide to Oncology, 14* (2), 1–8.

Pisters, K. M. & Kris, M. G. (1992). Management of nausea and vomiting caused by anticancer drugs: State of the art. *Oncology 6* (Suppl. 2), 99–104.

Poland, J. (1991). Prevention and treatment of oral complications in the cancer patient. *Oncology, 5* (7), 45–50.

Razavi, D., Delvaux, N., Farvacques, C., De Brier, F., Van Heer, C., Kaufman, L., Derde, M. P., Beauduin, M., & Piccart, M. (1993). Prevention of adjustment disorders and anticipatory nausea secondary to adjuvant chemotherapy: A double-blind, placebo-controlled study assessing the usefulness of alprazolam. *Journal of Clinical Oncology, 11* (7), 1384–1390.

Reichman, B. S., Seidman, A. D., Crown, J. P. A., Heelan, R., Hakes, T. B., Lebwohl, D. E., & Gilewski, T. A. (1993). Paclitaxel and recombinant human granulocyte colony stimulating factor as initial chemotherapy for metastatic breast cancer. *Journal of Clinical Oncology, 11* (10), 1943–1951.

Roila, F., Tonato, M., Cognetti, F., Cortesi, E., Favalli, G., Marangolo, M., Amadori, D., Bella, M. A., Gramazio, V., Donati, D., et al. (1991). Prevention of cisplatin–induced emesis: A double–blind multicenter randomized crossover study comparing ondansetron and ondansetron plus dexamethasone. *Journal of Clinical Oncology, 9* (4), 675–678.

Rowinsky, E. K., Eisenhauer, E. A., Chaudry, V., Arbuck, S. G., & Donehower, R. C. (1993). Clinical toxicities encountered with paclitaxel (Taxol). *Seminars in Oncology, 20* (4, Suppl. 3), 1–15.

Seral, R. (1990). Management of acute viral infections. *National Cancer Institute Monograph, 9,* 107–110.

Soukop, M., McQuade, B., Hunter, E., Stewart A., Kay, S., & Cassidy, J. (1992). Ondansetron compared with metoclopramide in the control of emesis and quality of life during repeated chemotherapy for breast cancer. *Oncology, 49* (4), 295–304.

Tierney, A. J., Leonard, R. C., Taylor, J., Closs, S. J., Chetty, L. L., & Rodger, A. (1991). Side effects expected and experienced by women receiving chemotherapy for breast cancer. *British Medical Journal, 302* (6771), 272.

Tonato, M., Roila, F., & Del Favera, A. (1991). Methodology of antiemetic trials: A review. *Annals of Oncology, 2* (2), 107–114.

Toth, B. B., Martin, J. W., & Fleming T. J. (1990). Oral and dental care associated with cancer therapy. *The Cancer Bulletin, 43* (5), 397–402.

Twelves, C. J., & Seymour, A. M. (1991). Mouth cooling to prevent doxorubicin–induced stomatitis. *Annals of Oncology, 2,* 695.

Wadleigh, R. G., Redman, R. S., Graham, M. L., Krasnow, S. H., Anderson, A., & Cohen, M. H. (1992). Vitamin E in the treatment of chemotherapy induced mucositis. *The American Journal of Medicine, 92,* 481–483.

Warr, D., Willan, A., Fine, S., Wilson, K., Davis, A., Erlichman, C., Rusthoven, J., Lofters, W., Osoba, D., Laberge, F. et al. (1991). Superiority of granisetron to dexamethasone plus prochlorperazine in the prevention of chemotherapy induced emesis. *Journal of the National Cancer Institute, 83* (16), 1169–1173.

Wickham, R. (1989). Managing treatment related nausea and vomiting: State of the art. *Oncology Nursing Forum, 16,* 563–574.

Wilcox, P. M., Fetting J. H., Nettesheim, K. M., & Abeloff, M. (1982). Anticipatory vomiting in women receiving cyclophosphamide, methotrexate and fluorouracil (CMF) adjuvant chemotherapy for breast cancer. *Cancer Treatment Reports, 66,* 1601–1604.

Winningham, M. L., McVicar, M. G., Bondoc, M., Anderson, J. I., & Minton, J. P. (1989). Effect of aerobic exercise on body weight and composition in patients with breast cancer on adjuvant chemotherapy. *Oncology Nursing Forum, 16* (5), 683–689.

Young-McCaughan, S., & Sexton, D. L. (1991). A retrospective investigation of the relationship between aerobic exercise and quality of life in women with breast cancer. *Oncology Nursing Forum, 18* (4), 751–757.

CHAPTER 4 | Breast Cancer and the Role of Radiation Therapy

Nancy O'Rourke, RN, MSN
Lucette M.P. Robinson, RN, BSN

Breast cancer is a major and growing health concern for our society. The impact of breast cancer on women and their families is overwhelming. Physical and psychological adjustment to the diagnosis and treatment is an ongoing process. Most women actively participate in the decision-making process in selecting treatment and in the delivery of their care. Healthcare providers must meet the patient's need for information on the disease, as well as the options and implications of treatment.

Radiation therapy is a main treatment modality used in the management of breast cancer. It can play a role in primary, adjunctive, or palliative treatment. This chapter addresses:

1. the role of radiation therapy in breast cancer treatment,
2. the management of potential side effects of radiation therapy to the breast, and
3. the role of the oncology nurse as a member of the radiation oncology team.

HISTORICAL PERSPECTIVE

Use of radiation for cancer treatment began as early as 1896, 1 year after Willhelm Roentgen's discovery of radiation. Some of the early uses of radiation with x-ray machines began at Boston City Hospital, and by 1905, two thousand patients had been treated with radiation (Harris, 1991). The use of x-rays decreased the size of cancer growths or eliminated them entirely.

Earlier radiation treatments were limited due to equipment that delivered essentially 100% of the radiation dose to the skin. The radiation dose would then decrease, or fall off as it penetrated deeper tissues. Thus, doses were limited to skin tolerance, making it difficult to treat tumors located deep within tissue. Modern radiation equipment has a "skin sparing" effect that delivers maximum dose below the skin surface. In addition to improved equipment, dosing and treatment schedules were refined over the years as clinicians became more experienced with radiation. Dosing

43

schedules were modified to achieve tumor cell death while preserving skin tissue.

The most common treatment for breast cancer up until about 35 years ago was radical surgery. This surgical intervention involved removal of the entire breast, pectoral muscles, and axillary nodes, which left women disfigured and with other long-term complications. In the mid-1970s more surgeons began using a modified approach, and modified radical mastectomy became the standard operative procedure for breast cancer (Kinne, 1991).

There has been and continues to be a trend toward more breast-preserving options such as radiation therapy and conservative surgery for women with stages I and II breast cancers. The role of radiation therapy in breast cancer treatment has been fueled by an increased understanding of breast cancer, improved radiation equipment, and women's demand for a more acceptable alternative. Radiation therapy and conservative surgery is an alternative that improves cosmetic outcome and takes into consideration psychological and sexual concerns.

Radiation therapy following conservative surgery is a radical treatment used to improve local control. Research is ongoing to answer the questions regarding the exact amount of local radiation treatment required and sequencing of radiation therapy with chemotherapy. This chapter highlights the main aspects of radiation therapy as a radical treatment for breast cancer as well as its use for palliation in metastatic disease.

STAGE 0, NONINVASIVE CARCINOMA, DUCTAL CARCINOMA IN SITU

Historically, the standard treatment for ductal carcinoma in situ (DCIS) was mastectomy, which achieved excellent survival rates of 98% to 100% (Herbert, 1991). Based on research that demonstrated nearly equivalent survival rates when mastectomy for DCIS was compared with conservative surgery and radiation therapy, breast conservation is now a frequently recom-

mended treatment option for patients with DCIS. Conservative surgery with radiation therapy is a recommended treatment option for patients with a single, small, palpable mass of DCIS or a limited area of microcalcifications that has been excised with clear surgical margins. Due to the low incidence of axillary node involvement, axillary dissection or radiation therapy to the axilla is not included in the treatment plan (Herbert, 1991).

EARLY-STAGE BREAST CANCER

Breast conservation has become an acceptable alternative to mastectomy for patients with early-stage I and -stage II breast cancer. This technique includes the combination of conservative surgery to excise gross tumor and radiation therapy to eradicate microscopic residual disease. Surgery usually involves two procedures. *Lumpectomy* is the term most often used for the excisional biopsy. To ensure clear surgical margins, a re-excision of the biopsy area is often necessary. This may be accompanied by an axillary lymph node dissection, which provides prognostic and therapeutic information to establish which patients should receive adjuvant chemotherapy. The goals of breast conservation treatment are to achieve comparable long-term survival rates to mastectomy, maintain a high level of local control, and achieve an acceptable cosmetic outcome for the patient (Hassey, 1985; Harris & Recht, 1991; Herbert, 1991).

LOCALLY ADVANCED BREAST CANCER

Locally advanced breast carcinoma includes stage III disease and can be subgrouped into T3 tumors, T4 tumors with fixed nodes, supraclavicular nodes, and inflammatory breast carcinoma (Herbert, 1991; Morrow, Hoffman, & Weichselbaum, 1991). Due to poor local control of disease, surgery combined with radiation therapy is often the major local treatment. When radiation therapy is used as the primary treatment, typically doses as high as 65 to 80 Gy are required to improve local control. Doses in this range, unfortunately, increase the risk of fibrosis and soft tissue necrosis, leading to poor cosmetic outcomes. As a result, combinations of surgery with preoperative or postoperative radiation therapy are often used to improve local control and cosmetic outcome. For patients with stage III disease, systemic chemotherapy is also recommended due to the high incidence of distant metastases (Morrow et al., 1991).

POSTMASTECTOMY RADIATION THERAPY TO THE CHEST WALL

Radiation therapy to the chest wall following mastectomy improves local-regional control by eradicating residual microscopic disease that has spread beyond the margin of surgical resection. However, this technique has not improved overall survival due to the potential development of distant metastases. When radiation is used in conjunction with adjuvant chemotherapy, however, there is a greater likelihood of improving survival. To date, the role of radiation therapy and chemotherapy for the postmastectomy patient has not been firmly established (Harris, 1991).

RADIATION TREATMENT PROCESS

Consultation

A woman's first visit to the radiation therapy department is for consultation, physical assessment, and discussion of the specific role of radiation in the overall treatment plan. During this initial consultation, diagnostic studies and pathology may be further reviewed. This first visit can be a stressful appointment. It is often helpful to have family members and significant others present to clarify questions and reinforce information from the discussions. The woman is presented with information about radiation therapy as a treatment option. The treatment course and potential side effects of

treatment are explained. Patients are encouraged to ask questions, voice their concerns, and participate in the decision making. Ideally, the presence of a radiation oncology nurse is critical for the patient to use as an identifiable resource for questions, emotional support, and assistance in managing the side effects of radiation therapy and the sequelae of the cancer diagnosis.

Treatment Planning

Before treatments begin, a radiation treatment planning or "simulation" appointment is scheduled. The goals of treatment planning are to maximize the radiation dose to the specific treatment area and to minimize the dose to other normal tissues, such as lung and heart. Treatment planning can take approximately 1 hour. Radiation therapists and radiation oncologists measure the breast and axilla and take x-rays on the simulator machine to carefully delineate the breast and draining lymph node areas. To serve as daily landmarks for the treatment positions, markings are placed directly on the patient's skin. Physicists use this information to calculate and map out the specific treatment field. To ensure consistent patient positioning for treatments, immobilization devices using styrofoam casts for the patient's head and arm are also fashioned (Hassey, 1985).

Patients may find this experience frightening and impersonal. Thus, patient education about the planning appointment should focus on an explanation of the procedure. Reassurance should be given that the planning is not painful. However, it may be uncomfortable to lie on a hard table in the same position for an hour.

Treatment

The radiation treatment plan includes external beam therapy to the entire breast and often an additional boost to the primary tumor site. External beam is delivered by using high-energy photons from a linear accelerator.

Some institutions may still use cobalt treatment units. The entire breast, the underlying chest wall, and the lower axilla are typically treated with opposing tangential fields. Tangential fields minimize lung and heart exposure (Harris & Recht, 1991). If the upper axillary and supraclavicular areas are to be treated, a third anterior field is added. According to Harris & Recht (1991), it is generally agreed that the whole breast dose should be 45 to 50 Gy. Typically, patients receive a daily dose of 180 to 200 cGy over 4-1/2 to 5 weeks.

Radiation boosts to the breast can be delivered by electron beam or temporary iridium-192 implants. Boosts are delivered to the primary tumor site to increase local control without decreasing cosmetic outcome.

Electron boosts are performed on an outpatient basis. The electron beam penetrates tissue to a specific depth, which allows treatment of the tumor bed while sparing underlying lungs and ribs from radiation. A boost generally consists of an additional five to eight daily fractions of 200 cGy to bring the total dose to the primary tumor site to 60 cGy or higher (Harris & Recht, 1991).

An alternative but less frequently used method for delivering the boost is the interstitial implantation of iridium-192. This is an invasive procedure and requires a 2- to 3-day hospital stay. During the implantation, nursing care focuses on managing the mild discomfort associated with the procedure; maintaining radiation safety precautions for hospital staff, family members, and visitors; and providing emotional support to the patient.

Patient and Family Education

The education of patients receiving radiation therapy is directed toward anticipating the potential side effects of treatment, dealing with the treatment experience, and providing patient and family education on the early assessment of side effects and side effect management. Recognizing the patient and family as active participants in the care process is crucial, as radiation therapy is an outpatient treatment and patients perform self-care interventions in the home setting. Department and emergency telephone numbers should be provided. Patients and family members are encouraged to approach the radiation oncology team members as questions and concerns arise.

In preparing the patient for daily radiation treatments, description of the treatment course should be provided. The nurse can "walk the patients through a treatment" by explaining the number of treatments they will receive and what can be expected in the treatment room. Patients are reassured that they will not feel discomfort during the treatments and that the radiation therapists will work closely with them during the course of their therapy. Most of the approximately 15 minutes spent in the treatment room is used to set up accurate positioning. Actual treatment time is approximately 3 minutes.

Radiation therapy is a local treatment and side effects are limited to the treatment field. Thus, only the breast area is affected. Emphasis should be placed on the local effects of treatment, as patients and families frequently expect the side effects of radiation to be similar to the systemic side effects of chemotherapy. In addition, patients often harbor fears of radiation stemming from their knowledge of radiation in the setting of nuclear radioactivity. This may be influenced by media reports of nuclear accidents and an association with the potential systemic side effects of chemotherapy. Many patients receiving breast radiation often need reassurance they will not be radioactive and will not experience systemic side effects such as hair loss.

They may also express fear that they will experience nausea or "severe burns," which are very uncommon. Helpful strategies to reinforce site-specific effects are to show the patient the prescription, which clearly outlines the treatment field, or to have the patient use the permanent markings on their skin as a visual way to identify the treatment field. Clarifying information, dispelling misconceptions, and helping patients and families understand what to expect or not to expect is extremely important throughout the treatment course. Providing written instructions is essential and helps reinforce points of emphasis.

Some radiation oncology departments have used clinical pathways to prospectively map out the major aspects of a radiation treatment course. Increasing attention is being focused on using these pathways as a patient educational tool. In addition, critical pathways may promote consistency of information provided to patients regarding the management of side effects and what can be expected during treatment. Quality improvement activities to evaluate the outcome in clinical practice as a result of using this tool are ongoing.

Radiation therapy is unique in the need for daily treatment over several weeks. This provides the team with an opportunity to assess the patient's psychosocial status over time. For example, when beginning treatment, many patients may not want to participate in support groups or see a social worker. Ongoing assessment allows the nurse to provide emotional support and to connect the patient with additional supports at critical points when concerns regarding treatment, uncertainty about the future, fertility, and financial issues, and overall adjustment to the disease arise. In addition, patients are often resourceful themselves. Often, they bring in various creams for skin care to be reviewed by the nurse and share feedback on what community resources have been most helpful for them. Some patient recommendations include mind-body programs, exercise, visualization and guided imagery classes, and relaxation techniques. Including patients as active participants in the care process provides a sense of control over their care. In addition, openness to their suggestions has the potential of enhancing care for other patients. It is hoped that more nursing research will incorporate patient-generated care measures that can be scientifically evaluated for effectiveness.

SIDE EFFECTS OF BREAST IRRADIATION

Side effects that occur in the treatment field are caused by radiation cellular damage. This damage is the result of radiation's effect on DNA synthesis and cell division. Normal tissues can recover more easily from the effects of radiation, while cancer cells die. Radiation side effects may be categorized as acute or late. Acute side effects develop during treatment and up to 6 months after. Late side effects occur after 6 months. Cell lines that have higher mitotic activity, such as the skin and the hair follicles, demonstrate changes more rapidly. Early effects are thought to be related to parenchymal cell loss. These effects generally resolve within approximately 2 weeks after completion of treatment. Cellular destruction ends and cellular renewal properties begin to return to normal. Late effects are felt to be caused by injury to stromal vasculature and endothelial cells. Unlike acute side effects, late effects are often permanent (Strohl, 1988).

Acute Side Effects

The most common acute side effects of radiation therapy to the breast are skin reactions; intermittent aches and pains in the treated breast, chest wall, or axilla; breast edema; and fatigue. These reactions are normal and begin to resolve when treatment is completed. Table 4-1 summarizes the acute side effects of radiation therapy to the breast.

Skin Reactions.   As a result of megavoltage equipment with skin-sparing effects, the degree of skin reactions today are less severe than the reactions seen in the past. Skin reactions to radiation therapy include erythema, increased pigmentation, folliculitis with pruritus, hair loss in the treated area, dry desquamation (dry peeling), and moist desquamation (moist peeling). The degree of skin reaction is variable from patient to patient. There are several factors that may influence the de-

Table 4-1 Potential Acute Side Effects of Radiation Therapy to Breast/Chest Wall

Side Effect	Average Onset	Usual Duration	Appearance/Presentation	Intervention
Skin erythema	Approximately 2 weeks after start of treatment.	Resolution usually within 10 days to 2 weeks after end of treatment.	Variable. Mild redness to brisk or bright redness. Mild-moderate discomfort.	Unscented hydrophilic creams such as Aquaphor, Eucerin, Lubriderm Unscented, 99-100% pure aloe vera gel (no added perfumes, colors). Avoid tight bras; underwire bras.
Hyperpigmentation	Approximately 2 weeks after start of treatment. May be more pronounced in darker pigmented women.	Resolves slowly after end of treatments. Mild hyperpigmentation may last for months.	Presents as mild to deep tanning of the skin. May be associated with mild discomfort.	As above
Itching/folliculitis (Irritation of hair follicles)	Approximately 10 days to 2 weeks after start of treatment.	Variable—may start to resolve at end of treatment course to entire breast (before start of boost treatment) usually much improved by end of treatment course.	Itchy skin appears slightly red and dry. Folliculitis appears as small red dots often in sternal, infraclavicular, and supra clavicular area. Occasionally found on back below clavical 20 exit dose. May cause mild discomfort and itching.	Oatmeal colloidal based soaps (such as Aveeno). Make paste and apply to affected area, let dry for 3-5 minutes and rinse off with cool water. Oatmeal Colloidal based bath products may be added to tub bath. 99-100% pure aloe vera gel (no added dyes or perfumes). Unscented hydrophilic creams such as those listed above for erythema. Diphenhydramine—25 mg may be taken at night for severe itching.
Fatigue	Highly variable approximately 2-3 weeks after start of treatment. May be an increased effect with previous or concurrent chemotherapy.	Fatigue may last up to 2-3 weeks after finishing radiation treatments. Average is 10 days to 2 weeks. May be more prolonged if patient is receiving chemotherapy.	Increased tiredness late afternoon or early evening. Most women are able to continue their usual routines.	Earlier bedtime, late afternoon or early evening rest period. Good nutrition—avoid dieting during course of treatment. Conserve energy by having family and friends help as needed. Moderate exercise such as walking has been found to help energy levels.

Dry desquamation	Approximately 3 weeks after starting radiation.	Usually resolves within 2 weeks of finishing radiation treatments.	Dry flaking or peeling of skin frequently associated with erythema or hyper-pigmentation of skin.	Use of highly moisturizing hydrophilic creams such as Aquaphor and Eucerin.
Moist desquamation	4-5 weeks after start of radiation therapy.	Usually completely healed within 2-3 weeks after end of radiation treatments.	Moist peeling of the skin with associated erythema. Area may ooze or weep. May be associated with mild-moderate discomfort depending on severity of reaction. Increased reaction is possible if patients is receiving concurrent chemotherapy. Often occurs in areas with increased shearing friction such as intramammary fold and axilla.	Gentle rinsing with drying antibacterial solutions such as Hibiclens/chlorhexidine gluconate or 1/4-1/2 strength H202. Pat dry with soft clean towel 2-3 times a day. Above can be followed by application of unscented hydrophilic cream such as Aquaphor, followed by nonadherent dressing such as Aquaphor gauze, covered with a soft ABD pad and held in place by a bra or large size body netting. Moist soaks can be used such as aluminum acetate solutions: Bluboro and Domeboro for 20 minutes 3 times a day. Moisture vapor permeable dressing may be used such as Op-site, although they can be difficult to adhere in skin folds. Avoid use of tape on irritated skin. Patient can use gentle lukewarm shower spray to help debride the skin. Allow area to be open to air whenever possible. If pain is moderate or severe use of NSAID, or mild narcotic may be indicated.

Table 4-1 Continued

Side Effect	Average Onset	Usual Duration	Appearance/Presentation	Intervention
Intermittent aches and pains in breast	May occur approximately 1 week after start of radiation.	Can persist for months after radiation finishes although usually with decreased frequency.	Patients often describe pain as intermittent sharp twinge in the breast.	Reassurance that this is a normal occurrence and may be alleviated with use of NSAID.
Breast Edema	As above.	Can persist for months after radiation.	Slight-moderate swelling of treated breast. Breast may feel full or heavy.	As above. Wearing a supportive bra may improve comfort.
Hair loss in treatment portal (fine hair of breast, nipple, and possibly small amount of axillary hair)	Usually starts 3-4 weeks at doses of 30–35 Gy.	Variable. May take 1-6 months for hair to grow back.	Typically not very noticeable or bothersome to patients except when associated with folliculitis or itching.	Follow interventions for itching/folliculitis.

gree of skin reaction for the patient receiving radiation treatments to the breast or chest wall. Patients receiving concurrent chemotherapy may experience an enhanced skin reaction, including moist desquamation (O'Rourke, 1987). Skin folds in the treatment field, such as the axilla and inframammary fold, warrant careful assessment. These skin shearing areas, due to warmth, moisture, and decreased aeration, may exhibit an increased skin reaction (Hilderley, 1983). The radiation type and energy may intensify the reaction. The electron beam, "boost," delivers higher doses to the skin. For patients receiving chest wall radiation, an enhanced skin reaction is intended. This effect is achieved using boluses, which are materials placed on the skin during treatment. The bolus promotes an increased absorption of the radiation dose by the skin, thereby increasing the reaction (Sitton, 1992a). If the supraclavicular region and axillary nodes are in the treatment field, skin reactions may occur at the beam exit site, which is the upper back.

To date, many of the skin care regimens for patients receiving breast irradiation are nonresearch based. In general, recommendations are dependent on what has worked most effectively in clinical practice, and on institutional policies (See Table 4-2). Some studies have evaluated aloe vera gel and the use of various dressings to manage skin reactions to radiation.

Witt, McDonald-Lynch, and Lydon (1990) evaluated a product containing aloe vera and D-panthenol. Thirty-two women receiving radiation to the breast or chest wall participated in this study. Serving as their own controls, women were instructed to follow routine skin care on one half of their breast and the study product on the other half. The researchers noted that the product did not change erythema or desquamation. However, using the product resulted in less pruritus, improved skin texture, and increased skin and nipple comfort.

Margolin et al. (1990) conducted a noncomparative study of 20 patients using hydrocolloid occlusive dressing in the treatment of moist desquamation. Results showed no wound infections and indicated that the dressing can be effective in healing. The major disadvantage reported was the containment of melted gel. This resulted in the need for frequent dressing changes and was a source of concern for half of the patients in the study.

Shell, Stanutz, and Grimm (1986) conducted a pilot study comparing conventional dressings to moisture vapor permeable (MVP) dressings for skin reactions. Researchers reported comparable results in healing time. An advantage of MVP dressings is that, unlike conventional dressings, MVP dressings did not act as a bolus and could remain on during treatment. The disadvantages included difficulty in securing dressings in areas with skin folds and the dressing's occlusive properties, which may lead to skin maceration.

Currently, a multi-site, double-blind comparison study is being conducted to determine whether there is a noticeable difference among three skin creams in preventing or minimizing skin reactions in patients receiving radiation therapy for breast cancer (McDonald et al., unpublished research). Developing skin care regimens from scientific investigations will enhance patient care outcomes, justify nursing recommendations, and contribute to nursing knowledge.

Intermittent Twinges and Shooting Pains. Intermittent twinges and shooting pains in the treated breast, chest wall, or axilla are common after surgery and radiation therapy. The shooting pains are transient in nature and do not usually require intervention. Providing reassurance that these discomforts are normal and expected can help allay a patient's anxiety over their occurrence. They may last for months to years and may be alleviated with analgesics.

Breast Edema. Edema of the breast is a response to radiation treatments and can affect a patient's perception of the cosmetic outcome. In retrospective studies of cosmetic outcomes

Table 4-2   General Skin Care Guidelines for Radiation Treatment to the Breast/Chest Wall

General skin care guidelines are provided to patients at the beginning of the course of radiation and are as follows:

1. Keep breast or chest wall clean and dry.
2. Cleanse the treated area with gentle soap such as Ivory, Basis, Pears, Neutrogena, or unscented Dove.
3. Avoid the use of creams, lotions, perfumes, or deodorant in the treatment area unless directed by a radiation oncologist, nurse, or radiation therapist.
4. Avoid extremes of temperature such as heating pads, hot water bottles, and ice packs in the treatment area. Jacuzzis and saunas should be avoided during treatment.
5. Avoid excess friction or rubbing that may be caused by tight clothing or underwire bras.
6. Use an electric razor to shave under the arm on the side receiving treatment.
7. Protect the skin in the treatment field from exposure to direct sunlight by either covering the skin or using a sunblock with SPF of 15 or greater.

Aftercare
Once the radiation therapy course is completed, patient education should focus on aftercare instructions. General aftercare instructions include the following:

1. Occasional aches and pains in the treated breast/chest wall may continue for weeks or months after finishing radiation therapy. If this occurs, use of an NSAID such as Tylenol or Ibuprofen may be helpful.
2. Skin changes will gradually improve over the 1 to 2 weeks following completion of treatment. The skin may look tanned in the area of treatment.
3. The breast tissue may feel thicker and more firm after radiation therapy. The patient should continue self breast exams monthly in order to remain familiar with the feel of the breast tissue. The patient should call her health care provider with any concerns or questions.
4. The skin may feel dry after radiation therapy. Use of a moisturizer on the skin for at least 2 weeks after completion of radiation is beneficial, and continued moisturization can help prevent dryness.
5. If previously irradiated skin is exposed to direct sunlight, it should be either covered or protected with SPF 15 or higher.
6. Should the patient develop any areas of redness, heat, or swelling in the breast, hand, or arm on the affected side, the health care providers must be notified.

The following information should be included if patients have had an axillary dissection and/or radiation therapy to the axilla.

7. The patient must wear gloves when gardening or using harsh chemicals.
8. The patient must avoid carrying heavy packages for a long period of time with the arm/hand on the affected side.
9. If the patient gets a cut or burn on the arm/hand on the affected side, she must wash it well and apply antibacterial cream.
10. The arm on the untreated side should be used for blood drawing, blood pressures, and vaccinations or injections.

---

following conservative surgery and radiation therapy, breast edema was included as a measured parameter (Harris & Recht, 1991). Breast edema was most prominent in the first year following treatment completion. Axillary node dissection was a significant factor in the occurrence of breast edema. This reaction may take up to 3 years or longer to resolve (Harris & Recht, 1991). Patients often report mild breast discomfort and feelings of fullness in the treated breast. Nonsteroidal anti-inflammatory drugs can be recommended to promote comfort. Cotton sport bras also provide additional support for the breast.

Fatigue.   Fatigue is a major symptom of cancer and is a high priority for research. Winningham et al. (1994) provide a comprehensive literature review on fatigue and the cancer experience. Etiologic factors and correlates of fatigue associated with radiation therapy have not been identified. Although it is not well understood, fatigue is a common reaction reported by patients receiving radiation therapy (King, Nail, Kreamer, Strohl, & Johnson, 1985). Fatigue appears to be multifactorial. Hilderley (1992) describes several factors that may contribute to fatigue for the patient receiving radiation therapy: recovering from recent surgery, receiving previous or concurrent chemotherapy, tumor burden, medications that may increase drowsiness such as antiemetics or analgesics, and malnourishment. These factors all compound the inherent treatment-related fatigue.

For women receiving radiation therapy to the breast or the chest wall, the demands of the treatment experience may influence fatigue. Daily trips to the radiation oncology department for a period of 5 to 6 weeks may become taxing on energy levels and time commitments. Women attempt to incorporate the treatment schedule into their busy lifestyles with family and work responsibilities. For women receiving concurrent chemotherapy, blood counts should be monitored for anemia during radiation therapy, which may intensify the degree of fatigue experienced. However, some women who are otherwise healthy may not feel tired during treatment.

Hilderley (1992) also notes a relationship of fatigue to radiation dose and field location. For example, women receiving palliative radiation therapy for metastatic breast cancer to the brain exhibit a greater degree of fatigue than women receiving radiation therapy to the breast.

Helping women manage and cope with fatigue is a major goal of the radiation oncology team. Setting expectations that fatigue may occur as a result of treatment is important. Many patients may interpret fatigue as a symptom of disease progression. It should be emphasized that each patient reacts differently to the treatment and may experience fatigue in varying degrees of intensity. Generally, with radiation therapy to the breast, fatigue can range from none at all to moderate fatigue. Often, it is described as a need to take a nap in the afternoon or to go to bed earlier than usual. Patients should be reassured that fatigue will begin to resolve once treatment ends, usually, within weeks. However, it may take longer for energy levels to return to the pretreatment baseline.

Bone Marrow Suppression.   When patients are receiving breast radiation, blood counts are not significantly affected due to the limited amounts of bone marrow in the radiation field. Blood counts may be taken only once or twice while the patient is undergoing therapy to the breast or chest wall. However, if a patient has an underlying medical condition or has received previous chemotherapy, lab values should be monitored more closely. It is important to establish baseline lab values and monitor counts at least twice weekly (more frequently if results indicate) if someone is receiving concurrent chemotherapy or has had a recent bone marrow transplant. Radiation may be stopped temporarily if blood counts fall significantly to allow for rebound of the values in question.

Emotional Response to Radiation Treatment

It is important to highlight that there are often emotional reactions when patients complete treatment. Many women find reassurance in being closely followed during the treatment course and are anxious in anticipation of less frequent visits. Sometimes they report uncertainty over the treatment's effectiveness and their ability to return to their lifestyles. During the treatment course, they may have established supportive relationships with other patients on treatment. Often, informal support groups are formed in the treatment waiting area. It is important to acknowledge the issues and losses and provide increased emotional support. If the patient is not involved with a support group or does not have an individual counselor/social worker, referrals to these resources can be offered again and should be encouraged.

A thorough follow-up plan is individually determined for each patient and often includes appointments with surgeons and medical oncologists, as well as the radiation oncologist. Patients should be encouraged to call the department with any questions. The primary nurse often plays a pivotal role in triaging patient concerns and coordinating care after treatment. Although the treatment course has been completed, the relationship with the radiation oncology team continues.

Late Effects of Treatment

With careful surgical and radiotherapeutic techniques, late reactions to radiation therapy are minimized. Late reactions to radiation therapy may include rib fractures, arm edema, pneumonitis, soft tissue fibrosis, and brachial plexopathy.

Rib Fractures.   Rib fractures occur in the radiated field in approximately 1% of patients due to a slight weakening of the ribs underlying the treated breast. This most often occurs if a patient sustains trauma to this area. Patients are usually asymptomatic or experience only mild discomfort. Nonnarcotic analgesics and anti-inflammatory agents may alleviate discomfort. It is important to inform patients that a rib fracture does not represent bony metastases (Herbert, 1991).

Arm Edema.   Arm edema is noted in less than 10% of patients treated and is related to the extent of axillary dissection, use of chemotherapy, and radiation to the axillary region (Herbert, 1991). This is a distressing reaction both psychologically and physically for the patient. Interventions to decrease swelling are aimed at preventing venous stasis. Physical therapy, nonrestrictive clothing, elevation, and the use of a compression sleeve can promote comfort and decrease swelling. To prevent infection in

patients with arm edema, careful instructions should be given to the patient to avoid any cuts or burns in the treated arm.

Pneumonitis.   Radiation pneumonitis occurs in 1% of patients treated. Usually, patients present with a cough, low-grade fever, and shortness of breath 6 to 18 months after treatment. Symptoms may be transient in nature or if more severe, may require treatment with steroids. The risk of pneumonitis is increased with treatment to the supraclavicular region and axillary nodes, especially with concurrent chemotherapy (Harris & Recht, 1991).

Soft Tissue Fibrosis.   The degree of soft tissue fibrosis is related to the total radiation dose and fractionation schedule. The skin may feel hard, with telangiectasia present. Telangiectasiae appear as spidery purple-red vessels in the treated area, due to dilatation of the capillaries and increased pressure of blood flowing through superficial vessels. In addition, fibrotic changes in the skin decrease the skin's ability to respond to trauma, such as excessive exposure to direct sunlight. With skin-sparing effects and moderate-dose radiotherapy, these effects are rarely seen (Sitton, 1992a). Patient education should focus on protecting the irradiated skin from sun exposure with sunscreen products and minimizing trauma (Sitton, 1992b).

Brachial Plexopathy.   Brachial plexopathy, while rare, can occur as a result of radiation treatment to the axillary and supraclavicular regions. Influencing radiation factors for brachial plexopathy are total dose and fractionation schedule. Brachial plexus syndromes are either transient or more progressive and irreversible. Signs and symptoms of this syndrome are mild discomfort in the shoulder and arm, and paresthesias and weakness in the arm and hand. It is often difficult to differentiate this syndrome from tumor involvement. Treatment is directed toward relieving arm and hand pain (McGrath, 1992).

Health care providers routinely assess physical complications to treatment. Long-term follow-up should also focus on a patient's on-going psychosocial adjustment to having had breast cancer and treatment. Uncertainty over treatment effectiveness and fear of recurrence are major concerns for patients (Loveys & Klaich, 1991). Greater attention needs to be paid to the patients' perceived rehabilitative needs and their ability to integrate this experience into their lives (Kostka, 1990). Emotional support and factual information should be consistently provided. Research studies designed to address the concerns of patients will enhance a health care provider's ability to implement strategies that will improve quality of life.

ROLE OF RADIATION THERAPY IN PALLIATION OF METASTATIC DISEASE

Some of the common sites of breast cancer metastases are the bone, spinal cord, brain, chest wall, and axilla. Radiation therapy can be used in the treatment of metastases to these areas. Palliative radiation is usually effective in reducing the distressing symptoms of metastases, and may be given in an emergency for these purposes.

Bone Metastasis

Patients with metastases to bone usually present with pain and possible loss of mobility in the involved extremity. This diagnosis can often be confirmed by a physical exam and bone scan or plain film. If the involved area cannot be seen by either of these tests, the patient may need a CT scan or MRI to locate the lesion. Goals of radiation treatment to bone are to improve mobility, decrease pain, prevent fracture, and return the patient to an acceptable quality of life. Side effects in patients treated to an extremity may include skin erythema in the area of treatment, and mild to moderate fatigue.

Spinal Cord Metastases and Spinal Cord Compression

More than two thirds of patients with breast cancer will eventually develop bone metastases with the most common site of these metastases being the spinal cord (Henderson, Harris, Kinne, & Hellman, 1989). A patient may experience mild to severe pain in the area of metastasis. In certain circumstances, spinal cord metastasis can cause spinal cord compression. Compression can be caused by tumor growth putting pressure on the cord, or fracture of the vertebrae weakened by tumor cells. Spinal cord compression is one of the most serious complications of breast cancer metastases. Spinal cord compression can present with numbness, weakness, or paralysis of an extremity and possible loss of bladder or bowel sphincter control. The patient may experience moderate to severe pain.

Spinal cord compression requires emergency treatment. The goal of immediate treatment is to prevent further damage or to restore function to the spinal cord, and to decrease pain. Skin care instructions should follow the general skin care guidelines as outlined previously. Patients treated to the spinal cord may have mild to moderate side effects, depending on the bodily structures in the path of the radiation beam. For example, a patient receiving radiation to the cervical spine may get slight dysphagia associated with radiation treatments because the esophagus may be in the path of the radiation beam.

Patients with painful bone metastases require an effective pain control regimen. Nonopioid analgesics such as nonsteroidal anti-inflammatory medication are often highly effective for the management of bone pain. If this does not provide sufficient pain relief, patients should be medicated appropriately with an opioid analgesic (narcotic). Frequently a combination of opioid and nonopioid (NSAID) medication provides the greatest pain control. Assistive devices, such as canes and walkers, can be very helpful for problems with mobility due to bone metastases.

Patients with diffuse painful metastases to bone may benefit from a new form of radiation therapy called strontium 89. Strontium 89 is a radioactive isotope given by intravenous injection. This radioactive isotope deposits in bony areas where there is osteoblastic activity. This new form of therapy may help provide relief for patients with diffuse metastases.

Brain Metastasis

Breast cancer can also metastasize to the brain, causing sensory-perceptual changes. The patient and family may report changes in orientation or personality. Symptoms of brain metastases often include headache, dizziness, visual changes, gait changes, mental status changes, and weakness. In extreme cases, a patient can present with convulsions or seizures. As soon as brain metastases are confirmed by CT scan or MRI, steroids should be given to reduce intracranial pressure. In some cases, a patient may need antiseizure medications.

Side effects in patients receiving radiation to the brain include hair loss, skin erythema (especially in forehead and periauricular areas), increased fatigue, and potential transient increase of neurological symptoms with the initiation of radiation. Skin care guidelines should be followed as well as the following: use a mild shampoo such as baby shampoo with gentle rinsing and towel drying; avoid hair dryers, curling irons, and harsh chemicals (such as those used for dyeing and perming). Patient teaching should include information regarding wigs, scarves, and protection of the scalp from summer sun or winter cold. It is important to assess the patient's safety and present living situation if there is significant cognitive impairment. Steroids are often tapered at the end of the treatment course. Support to patient and family is critical during this difficult time.

Chest Wall Recurrence

Recurrent breast cancer of the chest wall is most often treated with surgical excision if possible and radiation therapy, chemotherapy, or both if indicated (Chaglassian & McCormack, 1991). If radiation therapy is given to this area, potential side effects are primarily to the skin.

ROLE OF RADIATION ONCOLOGY NURSES

The role of the radiation oncology nurse has been evolving since the early 1970s. The role has grown from task oriented to one that encompasses many dimensions of patient care in an interdisciplinary setting (Hilderley, 1980). Oncology nurses in radiation departments are increasing in numbers, strength, and professionalism, creating a unique subspecialty practice.

The Oncology Nursing Society established special interest groups (SIGs) in 1990 and the Radiation Oncology SIG became one of the largest and first to be formally recognized (Hilderley & Dow, 1991). In addition, the American Society of Therapeutic Radiology and Oncology (ASTRO) recently began recognizing radiation oncology nurses as associate members. Nurses participate in ASTRO conferences on a national level.

Radiation oncology nurses frequently work with many varied health care providers, including radiation oncologists, radiation therapists, administrative support staff, social workers, nutritionists, physicists, and medical and surgical oncologists. As nursing presence increases in this integrated setting, nurses play a critical role in improving patient care through management of side effects, support, teaching, and coordination. These interventions strongly impact the patient treatment experience and contribute to positive patient outcomes.

SUMMARY

Breast cancer often requires the use of radiation therapy. There is a trend toward more breast-preserving options, such as radiation therapy, for women with stages I and II breast cancer. Radiation therapy is also an option in treating patients after mastectomy or in cases of locally advanced breast cancer. Health care providers who care for breast cancer patients have a responsibility to understand what is involved in the course of radiation treatment and the common side effects of this therapy. Providers are encouraged to work with the radiation oncology staff to educate patients and families regarding self-care measures. As radiation oncology develops as a specialty, nurses are able to care for patients at a critical point in the cancer experience. Increased development of research-based interventions and support will benefit our patients and contribute to the advancement of the oncology nursing profession.

ACKNOWLEDGMENT

To Judy Kostka, our manager, mentor, and friend.

References

Chaglassian, T., & McCormack, P. (1991). Reconstruction following necrosis or local recurrence. In J. R. Harris, S. Hellman, I. C. Henderson, & D. W. Kinne (Eds.), *Breast diseases* (2nd ed., pp. 840–848). Philadelphia: J.B. Lippincott.

Hassey, K. M. (1985). Radiation therapy for breast cancer: A historic review. *Seminars in Oncology Nursing, 1* (3), 181–188.

Harris, J. R. (1991). Postmastectomy radiotherapy. In J. R. Harris, S. Hellman, I. C. Henderson, & D. W. Kinne (Eds.), *Breast diseases* (2nd ed., pp. 373–387). Philadelphia: J. B. Lippincott.

Harris, J. R., & Recht, A. (1991). Conservative surgery and radiotherapy. In J.R. Harris, S. Hellman, J.C. Henderson, & D.W. Kinne (Eds.), *Breast Disease* (2nd ed., pp. 388–419). Philadelphia: J. B. Lippincott.

Henderson, I. C., Harris, J. R., Kinne D. W., and Hellman, S. (1989). Cancer of the breast. In V. T. DeVita, Jr., S. Hellman, & S. A. Rosenberg (Eds.), *Cancer principles and practice of oncology* (3rd ed., pp. 1197–1261). Philadelphia: J. B. Lippincott.

Herbert, S. H. (1991). Breast cancer. In L. R. Coio & D. J. Moylan (Eds.), *Introduction to clinical radiation oncology* (pp. 161–185). Madison, WI: Medical Physics Publishing.

Hilderley, L. (1980). The role of the nurse in radiation oncology. *Seminars in Oncology, 7,* 39–47.

Hilderley, L. (1983). Skin care in radiation therapy. *Oncology Nursing Forum, 10* (1), 51–56.

Hilderley, L. (1992). Pain and fatigue. In K. Hassey-Dow & L. J. Hilderley (Eds.), *Nursing care in radiation oncology.* (pp. 57–68). Philadelphia: W. B. Saunders.

Hilderley, L. J., & Dow, K. H. (1991). Radiation oncology. In S. Baird, R. McCorkle, & M. Grant (Eds.), *Cancer nursing: A comprehensive textbook* (pp. 246–265). Philadelphia: W. B. Saunders.

King, K. B., Nail, L. M., Kreamer, K., Strohl, R. A., & Johnson, J. E. (1985). Patient's descriptions of the experience of receiving radiation therapy. *Oncology Nursing Forum, 12* (4), 55–61.

Kinne, D. W. (1991). Primary treatment of breast cancer. In J. R. Harris, S. Hellman, I. C. Henderson, & D. W. Kinne (Eds.), *Breast diseases* (2nd ed., pp. 347–373). Philadelphia: J. B. Lippincott.

Kostka, J. A. (1990). *Rehabilitation needs of early stage breast cancer patients.* Unpublished master's thesis, University of Massachusetts, Worcester.

Loveys, B. J., & Klaich, K. (1991). Breast cancer: Demands of illness. *Oncology Nursing Forum, 18* (1), 75–80.

Margolin, S. G., Breneman, J. C., Denman, D. L., La Chapelle, P., Weckbach, L., & Aron, B. S. (1990). Management of radiation induced moist skin desquamation using hydrocolloid dressing. *Cancer Nursing, 13* (2), 71–80.

McDonald, A., Cotanch, P., Kostka, J., Giselle, J., Sitton, E., & Jeffrey-Irwin, D. *Preventing radiology skin reactions in patients with breast cancer: Double blind comparison of three products.* Unpublished research, in progress.

McGrath, E. B. (1992). Myelopathy, brachial plexopathy, and osteoradionecrosis. In K. Hassey-Dow & L. J. Hilderley (Eds.), *Nursing care in radiation oncology* (pp. 334–341). Philadelphia: W. B. Saunders.

Morrow, M., Hoffman, P., & Weichselbaum, R. (1991). Locally advanced breast cancer. In J. R. Harris, S. Hellman, I. C. Henderson, & D. W. Kinne (Eds.), *Breast disease* (2nd ed., pp. 767–774). Philadelphia: J.B. Lippincott.

Nielson, B. B, & East, D. (1990). Advances in breast cancer: Implications for nursing care. *Nursing Clinic of North America, 25* (2), 365–375.

O'Rourke, M. E. (1987). Enhanced cutaneous effects in combined modality therapy. *Oncology Nursing Forum, 15* (4), 429–434.

Shell, J. A., Stanutz, F., & Grimm, J. (1986). Comparison of moisture vapor permeable (MVP) dressings to conventional dressings for management of radiation skin reactions. *Oncology Nursing Forum, 13* (1), 11–16.

Sitton, E. (1992a). Early and late radiation-induced skin alterations Part I: Mechanisms of skin changes. *Oncology Nursing Forum, 19* (5), 801–807.

Sitton, E. (1992b). Early and late radiation induced skin alterations Part II: Nursing care of irradiated skin. *Oncology Nursing Forum, 19* (6), 907–912.

Strohl, R. A., (1988). The nursing role in radiation oncology: Symptom management of acute and chronic reactions. *Oncology Nursing Forum, 15* (4), 429–434.

Winningham, M. L., Nail, L. M., Burke, M. B., Brophy, L.,

Cimprich, B., Jones, L. S., Pickard-Holley, S., Thodes, V., St. Pierre, B., Beck, S., Glass, E. C., Mooney, K. H., & Piper, B. (1994). Fatigue and the cancer experience: The state of the knowledge. *Oncology Nursing Forum, 21* (1), 23–36.

Witt, M. E., McDonald-Lynch, A., and Lydon, J. (1990). Enhancing skin comfort during radiation therapy. *Oncology Nursing Forum, 17* (2), 266–267.

CHAPTER 5 | Tamoxifen in Perspective
Benefits, Side Effects, and Toxicities

Jennifer L. Aikin, RN, MSN, OCN

Tamoxifen citrate (Nolvadex, Zeneca Pharmaceuticals, Wilmington, DE) is the most widely prescribed drug for the treatment of breast cancer (Fisher et al., 1994; Jordan, 1992). Synthesized in 1966 and introduced into the clinical setting in the early 1970s, tamoxifen has a significant role in treating women with advanced, node-positive and node-negative breast cancer. Years of clinical experience have shown that tamoxifen is well tolerated, as demonstrated by compliance rates as high as 95% (Love, 1989). This fact, combined with the effectiveness of tamoxifen in reducing the incidence of contralateral breast cancers, has become the rationale for its use in cancer prevention.

While the benefits of tamoxifen are considerable, recent data regarding the associated incidence of endometrial cancers have caused concern for health care providers and the public. Furthermore, other toxicities such as thromboembolic events, ophthalmic abnormalities, and questionable liver toxicities have been described. These reports have resulted in a re-examination of the risk/benefit ratio in the use of tamoxifen for breast cancer prevention. Health care providers have also begun to recognize the importance of educating patients about potential side effects and toxicities. There is consensus, however, that when tamoxifen is prescribed appropriately and careful follow-up is conducted to assure early attention to side effects and toxicities, this agent will remain an important cornerstone for the treatment of breast cancer in the 1990s.

PHARMACOLOGY/MECHANISM OF ACTION

Tamoxifen is classified as a synthetic, nonsteroidal, antiestrogen (Zeneca Pharmaceuticals, 1994). Mechanisms of action are complex since the drug possesses both antiestrogenic and estrogenic features, depending on the target tissue (Jordan, 1991). Tamoxifen works primarily as an estrogen antagonist by blocking estradiol from binding to estrogen receptors located on breast cancer cell membranes, thus inhibiting the growth of malignant cells (Rich, 1993). The estrogen agonist activities are demonstrated by effects on bone and endometrial cells and appear to be the source of some of the toxicities associated with tamoxifen (Gould, Gates, & Miaskowski, 1994; Jordan, 1992).

In addition to estrogen blockade, it is believed that tamoxifen has other significant mechanisms of action that may account for its activity in women regardless of estrogen receptor status. Cell proliferation may be inhibited by modulating the production of transforming growth factors and by increasing the levels of natural killer (NK) cells (National Surgical Adjuvant Breast and Bowel Project [NSABP], 1994). These mechanisms may explain tamoxifen's effect in preventing contralateral breast cancers for women with node-negative breast cancer.

Tamoxifen is rapidly absorbed, but slowly excreted. Maximum blood levels are achieved 4 to 7 hours after the medication is taken, and its half-life is about 7 days (Zeneca, 1994). Tamoxifen is metabolized in the liver and is eliminated primarily in the feces. A steady blood concentration is achieved after 4 weeks of therapy (NSABP, 1994). When tamoxifen is discontinued, 4 to 6 weeks may elapse before the drug has cleared completely from the body. The most effective dose has not been determined; however, most adjuvant trials use tamoxifen 10 mg twice daily (bid) (Love, 1992). Studies are currently underway to determine the optimum duration of therapy.

RESEARCH EVALUATING TAMOXIFEN

Animal Studies

Tamoxifen inhibits both the initiation and promotion of mammary tumors in rats. When tamoxifen was withdrawn in animal studies, regrowth of tumors occurred in the presence of estrogen. Scientists concluded that tamoxifen's action was cytostatic rather than tumoricidal (Love, 1989). The dose of tamoxifen in early animal experiments greatly exceeded standard doses given to humans, and a worrisome toxicity was the development of secondary hepatic cancers (Love, 1989; Zeneca, 1994).

Human Studies

In the 1970s and 1980s, 30,000 women received tamoxifen in clinical trials conducted in the United States and Europe. In 1992 the Early Breast Cancer Trialists' Collaborative Group (EBCTCG) published a meta-analysis describing the effects of tamoxifen and other therapies in the treatment of early breast cancer, which was defined as node-positive or node-negative breast cancer. In these trials, adjuvant tamoxifen was compared with no tamoxifen, as a single agent or in conjunction with chemotherapy. The results were highly favorable for the use of tamoxifen for women with both node-negative and node-positive breast cancer. At 10 years, the overall recurrence-free survival was 51.2% for women treated with tamoxifen compared with 44.7% for women who did not receive tamoxifen. Overall survival benefits were also significant: 58.8% for the tamoxifen group and 52.6% for the control group (EBCTCG, 1992). Some of the key studies that contributed to the results of this meta-analysis include the following.

Node-Positive Breast Cancer.   A number of trials evaluated the use of tamoxifen versus no tamoxifen in the treatment of node-positive breast cancer. The Stockholm, Danish, Scottish, and Nolvadex Adjuvant Trial Organisation [NATO] trials showed a significant benefit in disease-free survival for women receiving tamoxifen, while only the NATO trial demonstrated a significant benefit for survival (Breast Cancer Trials Committee, 1987; NATO, 1985; Wallgren et al., 1985). Furthermore, the NATO trial was the only study that included premenopausal women. The duration of tamoxifen administration varied from 1 to 5 years.

Node-Negative Breast Cancer. The largest trial evaluating tamoxifen in the treatment of node-negative breast cancer was conducted by the NSABP. In NSABP Protocol B-14, 2,892 women with positive estrogen receptors were randomized to receive either 20 mg of tamoxifen or a placebo for 5 years (Fisher et al., 1989). While there was no survival benefit observed during the first 4 years of follow-up, there was a significant increase in disease-free survival for women who received tamoxifen (83%) compared with the placebo group (77%), regardless of age. Another important finding of this study was the decreased incidence of contralateral breast cancers for women who received tamoxifen as compared with those who received placebo (Fisher et al., 1989; NSABP, 1994).

Other important studies that evaluated the use of tamoxifen in the treatment of node-negative breast cancer were the Stockholm, NATO, and Cancer Research Campaign and Scottish trials (Love, 1989). Like NSABP B-14, each of these reported benefits in disease-free survival for women who received tamoxifen. Only the NATO trial demonstrated a significant benefit in survival.

Tamoxifen in Combination with Chemotherapy. The use of tamoxifen with chemotherapy has yielded mixed results. Two studies have demonstrated benefit when tamoxifen was added to adjuvant chemotherapy for postmenopausal women, or women older than 60 years. In NSABP B-09, tamoxifen did not provide any additional benefit for women less than 50 years old and appeared to be dependent on estrogen and progesterone status for women 50 to 59 years of age (Fisher et al., 1986).

Other Tamoxifen Benefits

Initially, there was concern that tamoxifen would have an adverse effect on bone density and cardiovascular health due to antiestrogenic mechanisms of action. Recent studies suggest that tamoxifen exerts estrogen agonist effects resulting in important benefits related to cardiovascular disease and osteoporosis.

Cardiovascular Disease. In 1991, Love et al. published the results of a 2-year placebo controlled trial to determine the effects of tamoxifen on risk factors for cardiovascular disease. Postmenopausal women receiving tamoxifen had a decrease of 12% in total cholesterol and a 20% decline in low-density lipoprotein (LDL) levels. An increase in high-density lipoproteins (HDL) has been observed in other studies (NSABP, 1994).

Rutqvist and Mattsson (1993) reported that women receiving tamoxifen as adjuvant therapy for early-stage breast cancer had a reduced incidence of hospital admissions due to cardiac disease. Furthermore, there was a statistically significant cardiovascular benefit among women taking tamoxifen for 5 years compared with 2 years. The authors advocated further trials of tamoxifen in women with early-stage breast cancer as well as chemoprevention trials.

Osteoporosis. A number of studies have demonstrated favorable results in the use of tamoxifen for the prevention of bone loss. In 1990, Fornander et al. published a report in which bone mineral density (BMD) was measured in 75 postmenopausal women who had participated in a trial in which they received either tamoxifen 40 mg daily for 2 to 5 years or no adjuvant endocrine therapy. No difference in BMD between the two groups was noted, leading the investigators to conclude that bone loss was not accelerated by tamoxifen use in these women. Other trials have yielded similar results, suggesting that tamoxifen may actually protect the bone (NSABP, 1994).

Some experts have suggested that women with breast cancer for whom estrogen replacement therapy is contraindicated may benefit from tamoxifen as an alternative hormone replacement therapy (Love, 1992). The benefits of tamoxifen in relation to cardiovascular disease and osteoporosis have paved the way for more widespread applications for the drug.

ONGOING RESEARCH INVOLVING TAMOXIFEN

Future Uses for Tamoxifen

Questions remain as to other uses for tamoxifen. For example, how long should tamoxifen be administered? NSABP B-14 registered an additional 1,220 women to receive tamoxifen so that after 5 years of therapy, women who had received tamoxifen could be rerandomized to receive an additional 5 years of therapy or placebo. When complete, this trial will provide insight into the benefits of extended treatment with tamoxifen in relation to toxicities that may occur over 10 years.

Other questions that remain include whether tamoxifen is of value in treating small occult tumors (<1 cm in size) and ductal carcinoma in situ (DCIS). Perhaps the most intriguing question is whether tamoxifen will prove to be of benefit in the prevention of breast cancer.

Breast Cancer Prevention

In 1992 the NSABP launched the first large-scale cancer prevention trial in the United States and Canada, the Breast Cancer Prevention Trial (BCPT). The primary objective of this ongoing study is to evaluate the effectiveness of tamoxifen in preventing the occurrence of invasive breast cancer and reducing mortality from breast cancer. Secondary aims are to evaluate the effectiveness of tamoxifen in reducing mortality due to cardiovascular disease, and reducing the incidence of bone fractures. In this trial, 16,000 healthy women, at significant risk for breast cancer, will be randomized to receive tamoxifen 10 mg or placebo twice daily for 5 years (NSABP, 1994). Risk is estimated using the Gail model, which considers risk factors such as age, family history of breast cancer, number of breast biopsies, number of pregnancies, and age at first menstrual period.

The BCPT, however, has been the source of significant controversy. The project is supported and sponsored by the National Cancer Institute but has received criticism from some

Table 5-1   NSABP B-14: Adverse Effects

Adverse Effect	Percent of Women	
	Nolvadex^R (n = 1424)	Placebo (n = 1440)
Hot flashes	63.9	47.6
Weight gain (>5%)	38.1	40.1
Fluid retention	32.4	29.7
Vaginal discharge	29.6	15.2
Nausea	25.7	23.9
Irregular menses	24.6	18.8

Reprinted with permission: Zeneca Pharmaceuticals, 1994. *Professional Information Brochure.*

scientists and some women's activist groups. The major debate lies in the potential risks that women may incur from tamoxifen compared with the potential benefits that may be experienced in terms of breast cancer, cardiovascular events, and bone fractures.

SIDE EFFECTS

While tamoxifen has been well tolerated by the majority of women receiving it, side effects may be disturbing for others. Table 5-1 outlines the adverse effects experienced by the group of women who received tamoxifen compared with those who received placebo in the NSABP B-14 trial.

Three statistically significant side effects were attributed to tamoxifen: hot flashes, vaginal discharge, and irregular menses (NSABP, 1994). The incidence of nausea, fluid retention, and skin changes was not statistically significant for women receiving tamoxifen in this study (Zeneca, 1994). Other studies have revealed similar findings, but have reported the discontinuation of therapy due to symptoms such as nausea, vaginitis, depression, edema, rash, and migraine headaches (Love, 1989; NATO, 1985). The incidence of depression associated with tamoxifen is rare. However, it can be severe and should be treated promptly (Love, 1989). Recently, hair loss and hair thinning have also been associated with tamoxifen use (Zeneca, 1994).

Laboratory values may be influenced by tamoxifen. Elevations in liver enzymes, T_4, and triglyceride levels, and a decrease in platelet counts (same as thrombocytopenia) have been reported, (Zeneca, 1994). In response to these alterations in laboratory tests, the BCPT has instituted specific guidelines for the temporary discontinuation of tamoxifen/placebo therapy in the presence of elevated liver functions (transaminases greater than 2.5 times normal values) and thrombocytopenia (platelets less than 75,000) (NSABP, 1994). As another precaution, women who participate in the BCPT who are on thyroid replacement therapy are mandated to have their thyroid functions evaluated at regular intervals so that adjustment in the medication may be made accordingly.

TOXICITIES

For the purpose of this chapter, toxicities are distinguished from side effects due to their potential for producing more serious and potentially life-threatening consequences. The following toxicities have been associated with tamoxifen: endometrial cancers, other secondary cancers, thromboembolic events, and ocular toxicities.

Endometrial Cancers

In the spring of 1994, controversy surrounded the release of data concerning an increased incidence of endometrial cancers in women receiving tamoxifen in NSABP B-14 (Fisher et al., 1994). While other studies had reported a greater incidence of endometrial cancers associated with tamoxifen therapy, the NSABP data sparked concern about potential risks for participants in the BCPT (Friedman, Trimble, & Abrams, 1994).

The number of endometrial cancers in participants in NSABP B-14, and the number of deaths associated with these cancers are outlined in Table 5-2. Of note, two cases of endometrial cancer reported for the placebo group occurred in women who received

Table 5-2 Endometrial Cancers in NSABP B-14

	Placebo Patients (n = 1424)	Randomly Assigned to Tamoxifen (n = 1419)	Registered to Tamoxifen (n = 1220)
No. of endometrial cancers: 2		15	8
No. of deaths attributed to endometrial cancers: 0		4*	1

* One patient never received tamoxifen.

Note. Adapted from "Endometrial Cancer in Tamoxifen-treated Breast Cancer Patients: Findings from the National Surgical Adjuvant Breast and Bowel Project (NSABP) B-14" by B. Fisher, et al., *Journal of the National Cancer Institute, 86,* (7), pp. 527–537.

tamoxifen subsequent to enrolling in the study: one for recurrent breast cancer and the other after diagnosis with secondary colon cancer. In addition, one of the women in the randomly assigned tamoxifen group never received tamoxifen, but later developed endometrial cancer and died.

Overall, the average annual hazard rate of endometrial cancer in NSABP B-14 was .2/1,000 for women in the placebo group and 1.6/1,000 for women randomized to receive tamoxifen (Fisher et al., 1994). According to Friedman, Trimble, and Abrams, the relative risk is therefore two- to three-fold greater for women with breast cancer who receive tamoxifen than for those who never receive tamoxifen (1994).

While an earlier report by Magriples, Naftolin, Schwartz, and Carcangiu (1993) posed some concern that the endometrial cancers associated with tamoxifen were more aggressive and yielded a poorer prognosis, the B-14, Stockholm, and Netherlands studies did not support this conclusion (Fornander, Hellstrom, & Moberger, 1993; Magriples, Naftolin, Schwartz, & Carcangiu, 1993; van Leeuwen et al., 1994).

Recommendations have been made regarding the most appropriate detection methods for following women receiving tamoxifen. The NSABP advocates, at minimum, yearly gynecologic exams (Fisher et al., 1994). Others have suggested vaginal ultrasonography as a means of detecting endometrial thickening, or yearly endometrial sampling (Cohen et al., 1994; Friedman, Trimble, & Abrams, 1994). There is agreement, however, that women must be educated to report abnormal vaginal bleeding and obtain yearly gynecologic exams.

Other Secondary Cancers

In light of the hepatic cancers observed in the laboratory, scientists have anticipated the occurrence of liver cancer in women receiving tamoxifen therapy for breast cancer. To date, however, only three cases of liver cancer have been linked to tamoxifen use. These cases were observed in the Swedish trial using tamoxifen at doses of 40 mg/d for 2 to 5 years (Wallgren et al., 1985). No cases of liver cancer were observed in NSABP B-14. Fisher et al. also concluded that there was no increased incidence of gastrointestinal, urinary tract, or other genital cancers associated with tamoxifen in this trial (Fisher et al., 1994).

Thromboembolic Events

The prevalence of thromboembolic toxicity associated with tamoxifen is controversial (Rutqvist & Mattsson, 1993). NSABP B-14 reported an increased incidence of deep vein thrombosis (DVT), pulmonary embolism, and superficial phlebitis associated with tamoxifen (Zeneca, 1994). (See Table 5-3.) Other researchers have failed to demonstrate a significant correlation between tamoxifen and thromboembolic activity (Auger & Mackie, 1988; Rutqvist & Mattsson, 1993).

Ocular Toxicities

The structure of tamoxifen is similar to other drugs that are known to cause ocular side effects (NSABP, 1993). A number of studies since 1978 have implicated tamoxifen as the cause of retinopathy, characterized by decreased visual acuity and macular edema. In 1992 Pavlidis et al. published a prospective study of

Table 5-3   Thrombotic Events in NSABP B-14

	Nolvadex[R] (n = 1424)	Placebo (n = 1440)
Deep vein thrombosis	.8	.3
Pulmonary embolism	.4	.1
Superficial phlebitis	.3	0.0

Reprinted with permission: Zeneca Pharmaceuticals, 1994. *Professional Information Brochure.*

63 women who had received tamoxifen 20 mg daily for a mean duration of 25 months. Four patients (6.3%) were found to have retinopathy with macular edema and yellow-white dots in the paramacular and fovea areas. After discontinuation of tamoxifen, the ocular changes appeared to resolve.

In 1993, the NSABP launched protocol P-1E to evaluate the prevalence of ophthalmic abnormalities associated with long-term, low-dose tamoxifen (NSABP, 1993). This ongoing study is unique in that it is a placebo-controlled trial involving 500 women originally enrolled in NSABP B-14. These women receive a complete clinical examination and an extensive evaluation of visual function. In addition, a complete ophthalmic history is obtained. When complete, this study will provide the most definitive data to date regarding the incidence and character of ocular toxicities associated with tamoxifen.

IMPLICATIONS FOR HEALTH CARE PROVIDERS

Given the extensive experience with tamoxifen over the past two decades, much is known about benefits as well as risks associated with its use in the treatment of breast cancer. Since women, as consumers of health care, expect a full and accurate explanation of any proposed treatment, it is essential that health care providers be thoroughly acquainted with these risks and benefits. In addition, nurses and physicians have an opportunity to impact positive quality of life and compliance when they possess knowledge of strategies available to help women cope with side effects attributed to tamoxifen therapy.

Risk/Benefit Ratio in Women with Breast Cancer

When re-examining the risk/benefit ratio for tamoxifen therapy, there is agreement among experts that the benefits of tamoxifen continue to outweigh potential toxicities for women with breast cancer (Fisher et al., 1994; Friedman et al., 1994; Love, 1992). The amount of benefit may be more or less dependent on the stage of disease and estrogen receptor status. Love describes an approach weighing the benefits of tamoxifen against the risk of second breast cancers, cardiovascular disease, and osteoporosis, against the risk of uterine cancer for women with node-negative breast cancer (1992). The benefits for postmenopausal women outweigh the risks. However, the benefits for premenopausal women may not be as significant. Furthermore, tamoxifen might not be the treatment of choice in situations when personal risks for complications are significant, or when severe side effects are experienced on beginning treatment (Love, 1992).

The risk/benefit ratio is more difficult to define when tamoxifen is considered for breast cancer prevention. Until the BCPT is complete, only estimates of the benefits of tamoxifen for prevention can be determined statistically. In 1993, Bush and Helzlsouer criticized the BCPT and the assumptions made regarding risks and benefits. Their recalculations determined the net benefit to be significantly smaller than originally calculated by NSABP investigators. Fisher et al. maintain their thesis that the benefits of tamoxifen significantly outweigh the risks for women participating in the trial.

The NSABP and the National Cancer Institute continue to support the BCPT with built-in safeguards to protect women from potential toxicity. These include monitoring with annual gynecologic examinations, educating women about the urgency of reporting any abnormal bleeding, excluding women with a

Table 5-4   Interventions for Hot Flashes

1. Wear absorbent cotton clothing.
2. Dress in layers, so that clothing may be removed during a hot flash.
3. Lower thermostat in home.
4. Learn relaxation techniques to alleviate anxiety in stressful situations.
5. Limit intake of caffeine and spicy foods.
6. Exercise regularly.

history of previous thromboembolic events or macular degeneration, and using regular laboratory testing to monitor liver functions and hematological parameters.

Many women have fears, often generated by alarming media reports, of secondary cancers and other toxicities associated with tamoxifen. When benefits and risks are explained in numerical terms when possible, much of this anxiety can be alleviated and women are able to participate in decisions regarding treatment options.

Helping Women Cope with Side Effects

Side effects attributed to tamoxifen must be recognized promptly so that interventions can be initiated early. The following discussion provides some practical interventions for the most commonly experienced side effects.

Hot Flashes. Sixty-four percent of the women who received tamoxifen in NSABP B-14 experienced hot flashes. While most women continue with therapy, this symptom has the potential to affect quality of life adversely. Since treatment with estrogen replacement therapy is contraindicated in most cases, health care providers must work closely with women to address this side effect in other ways. Nurses may suggest some practical, nonpharmacologic interventions that enhance comfort. These are listed in Table 5-4.

A number of nonhormonal pharmacologic agents have also been found to provide some relief for women who experience hot flashes

Table 5-5 Nonhormonal Pharmacologic Agents for Hot Flashes

Drug	Dose/Schedule
Vitamin E	400 IUs bid
Vitamin B-6	200 mg daily
Peridin C	2 tablets tid
Clonidine	.1-mg patch weekly,
(Catapres Transderm)	apply at hs
Bellergal-S	1 po every hs
Aldomet	250 mg bid

(Bergmans, Merkus, Corbey, Schellekens, & Ubachs, 1987; Nagamani, Kelver, & Smith, 1987; Smith, 1964; Young, Kumar, & Goldzieher, 1990). Table 5-5 outlines the doses and schedules for the agents.

Vaginitis/Vaginal Discharge. As a result of estrogen blockade, women who receive tamoxifen experience vaginal symptoms that mimic menopause. Vaginal dryness is associated with lack of lubrication as well as thinning of the vaginal mucosa, while vaginal discharge is often caused by infection. These symptoms may interfere with sexual intimacy due to irritation and pain with intercourse. Hormonal interventions are usually discouraged, so other strategies need to be instituted to provide comfort.

Women who experience vaginal dryness may benefit from using a water-soluble lubricant with intercourse such as K-Y Jelly (Johnson & Johnson, Skillman, NJ), and Astroglide (BioFilm, Inc., Vista, CA). Other products designed to provide more prolonged action include Replens (Park-Davis, Morris Plains, NJ), Gyne-Moistrin (Schering-Plough, Memphis, TN), and Lubrin (Kenwood Laboratories, Fairfield, NJ), vaginal suppositories. These products are available without a prescription.

Over-the-counter antifungal vaginal creams may provide some relief for women who experience vaginal discharge associated with infection. It is important, however, to rec-

ommend that a patient see her gynecologist if symptoms do not resolve.

Irregular Menses. Premenopausal women may experience irregular menses associated with tamoxifen use. Accompanying symptoms such as bloating, abdominal discomfort, or back pain may also occur. Pregnancy must be ruled out, as tamoxifen may cause fetal harm (Zeneca, 1994). When a woman is not pregnant and symptoms are disturbing, tamoxifen may be temporarily discontinued for 4 to 6 weeks and an attempt made to rechallenge with the medication after a break.

Abnormal bleeding in postmenopausal women must be reported immediately. An endometrial biopsy is generally required and decisions are made whether to continue therapy when the results of the biopsy are available.

CONCLUSION

This chapter has outlined important issues related to the use of tamoxifen in the treatment of breast cancer. While extensive research has demonstrated tamoxifen's effectiveness for both node-positive and node-negative disease, experience has also shown side effects and toxicities associated with tamoxifen use. The toxicity of greatest concern is endometrial cancer, which has been the source of recent controversy among health care professionals. While most experts agree that the benefits of tamoxifen outweigh risks for women who have breast cancer, there is debate regarding its use for breast cancer prevention.

Health care providers who work with women receiving tamoxifen experience both a challenge and an opportunity. The challenge lies in explaining risks and benefits in a manner that women can understand, thus allowing them to participate actively in decisions regarding their care. An opportunity exists to enhance quality of life by recommending specific strategies to assist women in coping with side effects. When these two issues are addressed, patients will be in the best position to receive maximum benefit from treatment with tamoxifen.

References

Auger, M. J., & Mackie, M. J. (1988). Effects of tamoxifen on blood coagulation. *Cancer, 61,* 1316–1319.

Bergmans, M. G. M., Merkus, J. M. W. M., Corbey, R. S., Schellekens, L. A., & Ubachs, J. M. H. (1987). Effect of bellergal retard on climacteric complaints: A double-blind, placebo-controlled study. *Maturitas, 9,* 227–234.

Breast Cancer Trials Committee. (1987). Adjuvant tamoxifen in the management of operable breast cancer: The Scottish trial. *The Lancet,* July 25, 171–175.

Bush, T. L., & Helzlsouer, K. J. (1993). Tamoxifen for the primary prevention of breast cancer: A review and critique of the concept and trial. *Epidemiologic Reviews, 15*(1), 233–243.

Cohen, I., Rosen, D. J. D., Shapira, J., Cordoba, M., Gilboa, S., Altaras, M. M., Yigael, D., & Beyth, Y. (1994). Endometrial changes with tamoxifen: Comparison between tamoxifen-treated and nontreated asymptomatic, postmenopausal breast cancer patients. *Gynecologic Oncology, 52,* 185–190.

Early Breast Cancer Trialists' Collaborative Group [EBCTCG]. (1992). Systemic treatment of early breast cancer by hormonal, cytotoxic, or immune therapy. *The Lancet, 339*(8784), 1–15, 71–85

Fisher, B., Constantino, J., Redmond, C., Poisson, R., Bowman, D., Couture, J., Dimitrov, N. V., Wolmark, N., Wickerham, D. L., Fisher, E. R., Margolese, R., Robidoux, A., Shibata, H., Terz, J., Paterson, A. H. G., Feldman, M. I., Farrar, W., Evans, J., Lickley, H. L., & Ketner, M. (1989). A randomized clinical trial evaluating tamoxifen in the treatment of patients with node-negative breast cancer who have estrogen-receptor-positive tumors. *The New England Journal of Medicine, 320*(8), 479–484.

Fisher, B., Redmond, C., Brown, A., Fisher, E. R., Wolmark, N., Bowman, D., Plotkin, D., Wolter, J., Bornstein, R., Legault-Poisson, S., & Saffer E. A. (1986). Adjuvant chemotherapy with and without tamoxifen in the treatment of primary breast cancer: 5-year results from the National Surgical Adjuvant Breast and Bowel Project. *Journal of Clinical Oncology, 4*(4), 459–471.

Fisher, B., Constantino, J. P., Redmond, C. K., Fisher, E. R., Wickerham, D. L., & Cronin, W. M. (1994). Endometrial cancer in tamoxifen-treated breast cancer patients: Findings from the National Surgical Adjuvant Breast and Bowel Project (NSABP) B-14. *Journal of the National Cancer Institute, 86*(7), 527–537.

Fornander, T., Hellstrom, A., & Moberger, B. (1993). Descriptive clinicopathologic study of 17 patients with endometrial cancer during or after adjuvant tamoxifen in early breast cancer. *Journal of the National Cancer Institute, 85*(22), 1850–1855.

Fornander, T., Rutqvist, L. E., Sjöberg, H. E., Blomqvist,

L., Mattsson, A., & Glas, U. (1990). Long-term adjuvant tamoxifen in early breast cancer: Effect on bone mineral density in postmenopausal women. *Journal of Clinical Oncology, 8*(6), 1019–1024.

Friedman, M. A., Trimble, E. L., & Abrams, J. S. (1994). Tamoxifen: Trials, tribulations, and trade-offs. *Journal of the National Cancer Institute, 86*(7), 478–479.

Gould, K., Gates, M. L., & Miaskowski, C. (1994). Breast cancer prevention: A summary of the chemoprevention trial with tamoxifen. *Oncology Nursing Forum, 21*(5), 835–840.

Jordan, V. C. (1991). Chemosuppression of breast cancer with long-term tamoxifen therapy. *Preventive Medicine, 20,* 3–14.

Jordan, V. C. (1992). The strategic use of antiestrogens to control the development and growth of breast cancer. *Cancer 70*(4) (Suppl 1), 977–982.

Love, R. R. (1989). Tamoxifen therapy in primary breast cancer: Biology, efficacy, and side effects. *Journal of Clinical Oncology, 7*(6), 803–815.

Love, R. R. (1992). Tamoxifen in axillary node-negative breast cancer: Multisystem benefits and risks. *Cancer Investigation, 10*(6), 587–593.

Love, R. R., Wiebe, D. A., Newcomb, P. A., Cameron, L., Leventhal, H., Jordan, V. C., Feyzi, J., & DeMets, D. L. (1991). Effects of tamoxifen on cardiovascular risk factors in postmenopausal women. *Annals of Internal Medicine, 115*(11), 860–864.

Magriples, U., Naftolin, F., Schwartz, P. E., & Carcangiu, M. L. (1993). High-grade endometrial carcinoma in tamoxifen-treated breast cancer patients. *Journal of Clinical Oncology, 11*(3), 485–490.

Nagamani, M., Kelver, M. E., & Smith, E. R. (1987). Treatment of menopausal hot flashes with transdermal administration of clonidine. *American Journal of Obstetrics and Gynecology, 156,* 561–565.

National Surgical Adjuvant Breast and Bowel Project [NSABP]. (1993). *A protocol to evaluate the prevalence and detection of ophthalmic abnormalities associated with long-term, low-dose tamoxifen administration.* NSABP Protocol P-1E. Pittsburgh: NSABP.

National Surgical Adjuvant Breast and Bowel Project [NSABP]. (1994 rev.). *A clinical trial to determine the worth of tamoxifen for preventing breast cancer.* NSABP Breast Cancer Prevention Trial. Pittsburgh: NSABP.

Nolvadex Adjuvant Trial Organisation [NATO]. (1985). Controlled trial of tamoxifen as single adjuvant agent in management of early breast cancer. *Lancet,* April 13, 836–840.

Pavlidis, N. A., Petris, C., Briassoulis, E., Klouvas, G., Psilas, C., Rempapis, J., & Petroutsos, G. (1992). Clear evidence that long-term, low-dose tamoxifen treatment can induce ocular toxicity. *Cancer, 69*(12), 2961–2964.

Rich, S. E. (1993). Tamoxifen and breast cancer—from palliation to prevention. *Cancer Nursing, 16*(5), 341–346.

Rutqvist, L. E., & Mattsson, A. (1993). Cardiac and thromboembolic morbidity among postmenopausal women with early stage breast cancer in a randomized trial of adjuvant tamoxifen. *Journal of the National Cancer Institute, 85*(17), 1398–1405.

Smith, C. J. (1964). Non-hormonal control of vaso-motor flushing in menopausal patients. *Chicago Medicine, 67*(5), 193–195.

van Leeuwen, F. E., Benraadt, J., Coebergh, J. W. W., Kiemeney, L. A. L. M., Gimbrère, C. H. F., Otter, R., Schouten, L. J., Damhuis, R. A. M., Bontenbal, M., Diepenhorst, F. W., van den Belt-Dusebout, A. W., & van Tinteren, H. (1994). Risk of endometrial cancer after tamoxifen treatment of breast cancer. *The Lancet, 343,* 448–452.

Young, R. L., Kumar, N. S., & Goldzieher, J. W. (1990). Management of menopause when estrogen cannot be used. *Drugs, 40*(2), 220–230.

Wallgren, A., Baral, E., Carstensen, J., Friberg, S., Glas, U., Hjalmar, M. L., Kaigas, M., Norkenskjöld, B., Skcog, L., Theve, N. O., & Wilking, N. (1985). Adjuvant 'Nolvadex' treatment in postmenopausal breast cancer: The Stockholm experience. *Reviews on Endocrine-Related Cancer, 17* (Suppl.), 35–37.

Zeneca Pharmaceuticals. (1994). *Professional Information Brochure 3/94.* Wilmington, DE: Zeneca.

CHAPTER 6 | Issues in New Treatment Modalities

Patricia M. Clark, RN, MSN, CS, AOCN

Women with breast cancer face an exceedingly complicated spectrum of treatment options. Medical literature is easily accessible and interpreted widely in various media venues, creating confusion for those who could most benefit. It falls to oncology nurses and other providers to clarify the latest treatment options, providing a perspective for the woman facing choices about her breast cancer treatment. This chapter presents new options for systemic treatment of breast cancer and revisits familiar therapies from a new viewpoint. Issues of high-dose therapy and associated supportive care will be addressed as will the role of the oncology nurse in medical clinical trials.

Changes in breast cancer therapy over the last 15 to 20 years have focused on minimizing local damage to the breast, and determining dose and schedule for systemic therapies. Although advances have been made in these areas, current treatment options carry significant limitations. Clearly, surgery and radiation

therapy are beneficial in control of local disease. Less clear is the definitive combination of these therapies that will most benefit women. The trend is toward breast-conserving surgery combined with radiation therapy. Surgical techniques have become more precise and spare the brachial plexus nerve with the use of selective axillary node dissection. When breast-conserving surgery is not possible, the option of immediate reconstruction is available. Although options for reconstruction are limited by available autologous tissue and the safety of artificial implants, most women undergoing reconstruction are pleased with the cosmetic results. Local treatment was refined further by advances in radiation therapy field techniques. Organs and tissue that once were routinely part of the radiation field with resultant long-term sequelae are now receiving only a fraction of prior radiation exposure.

Systemic therapy in the form of chemotherapy or hormonal therapy has demonstrated benefit for women with disease involving axillary lymph nodes. Systemic therapy in node-negative women is controversial. Several promising tumor markers are available that may aid in decision making in this often confusing clinical situation. The choice of systemic therapy is still made primarily by considering menopausal, hormonal receptor, and lymph node status. Although choices in hormonal manipulation are relatively standard, the choices in primary chemotherapy cover a broad spectrum in type and toxicity. Recurrence rates increase in a linear fashion with the number of involved lymph nodes. Recurrence is high among women with ten or more positive lymph nodes, so they may be offered adjuvant marrow ablative therapy in the attempt to achieve a longer disease-free survival. Effective, less toxic systemic therapies are needed as well as more accurate predictors for recurrence.

The suggestion that a woman's breast cancer can be characterized from the outset as likely or not likely to recur is especially attractive in the node-negative setting in which the use of systemic therapy is debatable. In addition to a suspicious histological picture, overexpression of oncogenes, the presence of specific surface proteins on breast cancer cells, or the number of blood vessels associated with a tumor may help in determining criteria for such difficult treatment decisions. The use of tumor markers is being studied carefully. In the case of the proto-oncogene *HER-2/neu*, targeted therapy is also becoming a reality.

Another avenue of exploration is the upfront treatment of micrometastases. The knowledge that recurrence is more likely with positive lymph nodes makes high-dose, upfront chemotherapy an acceptable risk to some women. Hematopoietic growth factors and peripheral blood stem cells for marrow support make the use of marrow ablative therapy in the early stages of breast cancer possible.

Finally, the control of macrometastases is of great concern. The creative use of old drugs in new combinations or with adjunctive therapies has provided new choices for medical providers and patients. New chemotherapeutic agents have shown promising responses. The use of supportive therapies such as granulocyte colony stimulating factor has helped ensure that clinicians can deliver full chemotherapy doses.

With innovation in medical treatment comes the translation of these new treatments to the clinical setting and to the understanding of the client. The role of the oncology nurse in the doctor's office, the infusion room, the exam room, and the O.R. suite, has become critical in helping women with breast cancer and their families understand the available choices. Advocacy in this decision making often falls to the oncology nurse. It is critical that the oncology nurse possess an understanding of treatment choices, the goal of treatment, and the availability of clinical trials.

NODE-NEGATIVE BREAST CANCER

The previously held opinion that breast cancer proceeded from the breast to the local-regional lymph nodes and to the rest of the body in an orderly fashion led to the recommendation of radical breast surgery. The current knowledge that breast cancers have been present for many years at the time of their discovery and that there is a high likelihood that invasive cancers have spread systematically at the time of diagnosis puts a new perspective on local therapy (Goodman, 1991). For women with stage I or II breast cancer, breast conservation therapy is an appropriate primary treatment. It provides equivalent survival to total mastectomy and axillary dissection while preserving the breast (National Institutes of Health, 1990). While wide excision and subsequent radiation therapy may provide local control, the histological characteristics of even small tumors may suggest the high likelihood of local recurrence if not systemic involvement with disease. Prognostic indicators of various types are currently being studied to help clarify the need for systemic therapy. With the broad use of screening mammography, this population tends to be younger and healthier. The use of certainly toxic and possibly sterilizing systemic therapy in such a population without objective evidence of metastatic disease makes the use of prognostic indicators an important adjunct in decision making.

Prognostic Indicators and Treatment Decisions

The most commonly used prognostic markers in breast cancer are size of tumor, lymph node involvement, and hormone receptor status. Larger tumors and small tumors with nodal involvement are predictors of poor outcome. However, even small tumors may have invasive histological features that raise the possibility of systemic involvement. Extensive in situ carcinoma (EIC) and lymphatic vascular invasion (LVI) are two such characteristics. Unfortunately, these markers are very subjective in interpretation, with poor agreement even among pathologists. More objective markers are currently under study.

Estrogen and progesterone receptor assays are thought to be predictors of early systemic relapse (Ravdin, 1994). They are also thought to be indicative of growth rate (Hayes, 1993). One of their most valuable uses is in deciding when hormonal therapy is a viable option in adjuvant therapy or as therapy for metastatic disease.

Other prognostic indicators that have come into common use are the S-phase fraction (SPF) and ploidy analysis. As an indicator of cellular proliferation, SPF has been associated with longer disease-free survival in some studies (Clark et al., 1992). Ploidy, the characterization of DNA content of breast cancer cells may represent aggressive disease (Madeya & Pfab-Tokarsky, 1992). Aneuploid cells have been associated with HER-2/Neu over-expression (Bacus, Bacus, Slamon, & Press, 1990). This proto-oncogene, which is overexpressed in 25% to 30% of breast and ovarian cancers in women, has been positively associated with a poor prognosis in node-positive women (Slamon et al., 1987). Its use in node-negative women as a prognostic factor is less certain but, in some se-

ries, HER-2/Neu has been more predictive of overall survival than lymph node status, ER/PR receptor status, and size of tumor or age at diagnosis (Slamon et al., 1987).

Not only does this oncogene predict for survival, it also may indicate poor response to cyclophosphamide, methotrexate, 5-fluorouracil (CMF) chemotherapy. Women with an excess of HER-2/Neu seem to have a pattern of drug resistance similar to women who have failed combination chemotherapy (Porter-Jordan & Lippman, 1994). The choice between CMF and a doxorubicin-containing regimen might be clearer in this population. This oncogene has also been associated with poorer response to hormonal therapy in some studies (Wright et al., 1992). Another prognostic factor, Cathepsin D, has been linked with a poorer prognosis. This enzyme may help cancer invade surrounding tissue. The data are mixed, with some studies showing that women with lower levels are more susceptible to relapse. In other studies, using different techniques, Cathepsin-D demonstrated the opposite effect (Porter-Jordan & Lippman, 1994). Conflicting data illustrate that many prognostic factors have yet to consistently show significance in predicting a systemic outcome and therefore are probably best put to use in conjunction with more standard prognostic factors.

Some prognostic markers may identify micrometastases or minimal residual disease. Lymph nodes treated with monoclonal antibodies to cytokeratins may show micrometastases, as have other organs treated in this manner. The use of polymerase chain reaction (PCR), which is currently used in lymphomas and leukemias to spot genetic mutations and translocations, is now being used in research to determine genetic abnormalities in breast cancer cells (Hayes, 1993). When such unique cellular anomalies can be identified in breast cancer, this technology may also be applicable in detecting minimal metastatic breast disease and provide a more definitive argument for treating node-negative disease.

Menopausal Status and Treatment Decisions

Although breast cancer is still primarily a disease of women over 50, premenopausal women are increasingly being diagnosed with breast cancer. Exposing women to cytotoxic systemic therapy at any point in life carries some disadvantages. Exposure in premenopausal women carries the extra risk of amenorrhea. In women who receive cyclophosphamide, methotrexate, and 5FU, the incidence of permanent loss of menstrual periods ranges from 40% to 77%. In women over 40 years old, this incidence reaches 90% (Shapiro & Henderson, 1994). There may be some advantage to ovarian ablation in premenopausal women with hormonally sensitive tumors, but whether this is effective has yet to be defined. In one trial conducted by the Scottish Cancer Trials Breast Group, 332 women with node-positive breast cancer were randomized to receive either ovarian oblation or chemotherapy (Scottish Cancer Trials Breast Group, 1993). After a 12-year follow-up, this trial showed that the two treatments were similar in relapse rates. Patients with ER-positive tumors benefited from ovarian oblation and those with ER-negative tumors benefited from CMF when survival was used as the endpoint.

Although women may benefit from these therapies by gaining years of disease-free survival, both chemotherapy and ovarian ablation exact the price of permanent sterility. For the premenopausal woman who has not yet started her family, this can be too high a price to pay in the absence of positive nodes and distant metastases. One option may be the use of gonadotropin-releasing hormone (GnRH) agonists. The mechanism of action of GnRH agonists is to suppress ovarian function. Their appeal is that the suppression is reversible and they have shown some favorable responses in hormonally sensitive advanced breast cancers (Dixon et al., 1990). Several clinical trials are underway to compare adjuvant chemotherapy with or without a GnRH agonist with the use of the GnRH agonist alone. These drugs may

be especially appealing among the node-negative premenopausal women who may be able to delay but not abandon child-bearing.

Postmenopausal women have a wider range of treatment options. In the case of the pathologically suspicious but node-negative breast cancer, hormonal manipulation may provide a tolerable treatment in this age group. In a trial conducted by the National Surgical Adjuvant Breast and Bowel Project (NSABP) published in 1989, a significant overall disease-free survival was noted in women over 50 years of age who received tamoxifen compared with those who did not. These women had both fewer local-regional and distant relapses (Fisher, Costantino, & Redmond, 1989). Studies are ongoing to examine the use of adjuvant therapy in very small node-negative tumors in this age group. This issue remains a controversial one, as many women may not realize a survival benefit with systemic therapy. Most postmenopausal women with ER-positive tumors, regardless of the size, can expect to receive tamoxifen. Careful explanation regarding the role of hormonal manipulation is important for all women receiving this therapy, but especially for those whose physician does not recommend any systemic cytotoxic therapy. The recent controversy regarding the increased incidence of uterine cancer in women on tamoxifen requires that providers educate women carefully on the need for routine gynecologic follow-up and that they provide perspective to the risks and benefits of taking this drug.

NODE-POSITIVE DISEASE: HIGH-RISK TREATMENT AND TOXICITIES

Node-positive breast cancer warrants systemic therapy because the disease is capable of spreading outside the breast. The use of chemotherapy in premenopausal women and hormonal therapy (usually tamoxifen) in ER-positive, postmenopausal women has demonstrated disease-free and overall survival advantages (Early Breast Cancer Trialists' Collaborative Group, 1992). In patients with a high number of positive lymph nodes, the question is not *if* they should receive adjuvant systemic therapy but *what* type and *how* much.

Adjuvant High-Dose Chemotherapy

Although there has been some evidence for a steep dose-response curve in animal models, the evidence for this phenomenon within the usual range of adjuvant chemotherapy doses has been generally lacking or inferred from retrospective studies. The Cancer and Leukemia Group B (CALGB) published a trial in 1992 that compared three dose levels of cyclophosphamide, doxorubicin, and 5-fluorouracil (CAF). The highest level was two times larger than the low-dose arm; the middle level provided the same total dose of chemotherapy as the high-dose arm over a prolonged time period. After a 3-year follow-up, the high-dose regimen showed a statistical advantage in disease-free and overall survival. The differences between the high and moderate doses were not statistically significant. Importantly, the patients in the high-dose CAF arm had a higher rate of myelosuppression and more often required hospitalization for fevers in the setting of neutropenia (Budman et al., 1992).

Marrow Ablative Therapy

Although the CALGB study looked at higher dose level, these levels are still well within the range considered standard chemotherapy. Higher doses of chemotherapy, requiring autologous marrow or peripheral stem cell support, are also under study. One such study involves young women with ten or more involved positive lymph nodes. Subjects receive four cycles of standard-dose CAF followed by high-dose cyclophosphamide, cisplatin, and carmustine followed by autologous marrow support. At 30 months, the event-free survival was 72% and overall survival was 79% in this young, rigorously screened cohort of women. Toxicity included a 22% hospitalization rate

for febrile neutropenia and ten deaths due to treatment-related toxicities (Peter et al., 1993). Adjuvant therapy that carries with it a 12% mortality requires careful consideration and longer follow-up to determine the survival advantage against long-term toxicities.

Supportive Therapies

The advent of marrow ablative therapies has necessitated creative ways to provide cellular support during marrow repopulation and recovery. Two ways of accomplishing this support are pan-marrow stimulation and lineage-specific cellular repopulation.

The incidence of documented infection in the face of neutropenia is well established. Longer neutropenic episodes are associated with culture-negative infections and with a high rate of fungal infection. The ability to supplement the leukocyte defenses with hematopoietic growth factors such as granulocyte colony stimulating factor (G-CSF) and granulocyte-macrophage colony stimulating factor (GM-CSF) has allowed clinicians to deliver full doses of standard chemotherapy regimens. These agents not only allow a more tolerable course during high-dose chemotherapy, they also stimulate marrow release of progenitor cells into the peripheral blood supply, offering a possible alternative to bone marrow harvesting.

Cytokine research is a promising area in supportive therapy. The use of a well-known red cell stimulant, erythropoietin (EPO), to ameliorate chemotherapy-induced anemia has not completely obviated the need for blood transfusions; but in some studies, the number of transfusions has decreased (Abels, Larholt, Krantz, & Bryant, 1991). The major benefit is decreased financial cost as well as personal cost to the patient in terms of time and risk of exposure to pathogens. The use of EPO in combination with other cytokines is currently under study (Demetri, 1994). Platelets also require support during both standard and high-dose chemotherapy. Potentially life-threatening events such as cerebrovascular accident may be decreased by maintaining a platelet count above 10,000/mm³. Currently, the treatment most often used for thrombocytopenia is transfusion of platelets. This intervention carries inherent risks of reaction and the possibility of antibody development that make future transfusions difficult if not impossible. The availability of platelets in the local care setting and their short shelf life after collection often require linkages with larger acute care hospitals for needed transfusions. The logistics of arranging transfusions places considerable stress on the patient and clinician alike.

The ability to give a growth factor that might decrease the need for platelet transfusions is an attractive one. Both interleukin-3 (IL-3) and IL-6 have been evaluated in phase I studies and have been shown to increase circulating platelet counts after high-dose chemotherapy (Demetri, Samuels, & Gordon, 1992; Ganser et al., 1990). PIXY 321 is a newer agent that combines IL-3 with GM-CSF. In trials involving the use of this fusion protein in breast cancer and sarcoma, reductions in neutropenia and cumulative thrombocytopenia were noted (Vadhan-Raj et al., 1993; Jakubowski et al., 1992).

Other promising cytokines being studied for their effectiveness in decreasing the need for platelet transfusions include: IL-1, leukemia inhibitory factor (LIF), IL-11, and the c-kit ligand, also known as stem cell factor. Reported side effects of cytokines have included constitutional symptoms of myalgias, arthralgias, and fever along with local skin reactions. Recovery of all marrow cell lines in several studies has not demonstrated the phenomenon of a growth factor "stealing" uncommitted cells from one lineage to support another (Demetri, 1994). Overall, these hematopoietic growth factors seem to be well tolerated and show promise in ongoing studies.

Another "rescue" after marrow ablative therapy is the infusion of cytokine-mobilized circulating progenitor cells, better known as peripheral blood stem cells. After marrow stimulation with cytotoxic agents, cytokines,

or both, progenitor cells are released into peripheral circulation in what has been termed a "rebound" effect (Schwartzberg et al., 1992). Leukopheresis captures these cells, which are then frozen and reinfused after high-dose chemotherapy. Although the exact number of cells needed to accomplish repopulation of the marrow is unknown, studies have shown this to be a feasible procedure. Peripheral progenitor cell reinfusion after a single high-dose regimen of chemotherapy (Elias et al., 1992) and a regimen that provides the same total dose of drug over a longer period of time with multiple reinfusions of peripheral progenitor cells (Shapiro et al., 1994) have been studied, and both regimens are feasible. While follow-ups to evaluate efficacy have not determined any advantage over conventional treatment, several studies have shown promising measurable benefits in rapid recovery from severe thrombocytopenia, shorter duration of severe anemia, and some improvement in leukocyte recovery times (Demetri & Elias, 1994).

An even more select cellular population, the CD34+ peripheral blood progenitor cell, is now within reach of the investigator through leukopheresis followed by identification and separation of these cells in the laboratory. CD34+ cells include the multilineage hematopoietic progenitor cells. Of particular interest is that breast cancer cells are not CD34+. The risk of reinfusion of breast cancer cells released by a contaminated bone marrow in standard peripheral blood stem cell collection has not yet been quantified. Whether the elimination of circulating tumor cells by the infusion of a more pure progenitor cell population affects relapse remains to be seen (Demetri & Elias, 1994).

In harvesting peripherally circulating stem cells or forcing them from the marrow with hematopoietic growth factors, there is a concern of depleting the stem cell pool. One possible solution to this problem could be the stem cell factor (c-kit ligand) mentioned earlier in the treatment of thrombocytopenia. Studies have shown that unlike G-CSF or GM-CSF, stem cell factor expands all three lineages of primitive cells. Side effects of this growth factor included localized skin reactions and moderate to severe upper respiratory symptoms most likely related to mast cell effect (Demetri et al., 1993).

The question regarding high-dose chemotherapy remains the same: Is *more* treatment better than standard treatment? Certainly, in women with metastatic breast cancer who have failed standard chemotherapy, the possibility exists that a threshold of drug and dose resistance needs to be crossed to provide tumor control. In women without distant metastases, the need to overcome this resistance is less clear. As noted earlier, these treatments and their support can be inconvenient at least and toxic at worst, with long-term implications that have yet to be fully appreciated. In many cases women may face a range of choices from tamoxifen to transplant without clear indication of which would be the most beneficial. Exploring each of the possibilities in relationship to the individual, her life goals, her family, and her coping abilities takes time, but is absolutely necessary when considering a marrow ablative therapy with uncertain outcome and certain toxicity. The trade-off involved is a relatively short period of intense therapy with significant side effects for the possibility of extended life, which presents no dilemma to some. Others prefer to stick to the standard therapy and save the high-dose therapy or clinical trial for another, more compelling time. One way of helping women through this decision-making process is to enlist the assistance of a marrow transplant or high-dose chemotherapy veteran who is willing to be candid about her experience. This provides a unique source of information from one who "has been there." Finally, it is important that high-dose therapies be conducted in the setting of a very carefully monitored clinical trial. The answers to the efficacy and advantages of high-dose therapy can only be answered in this critical setting.

MANAGEMENT OF MACROMETASTASES

New Versions of Old Therapies

There are several options for women with metastatic breast cancer that exploit both new and old therapies. One strategy that combines old therapies is modulation or potentiation of a chemotherapeutic agent. First noted in colon cancer, the combination and sequencing of 5-fluorouracil (5FU) and leucovorin has shown some success in breast cancer. There are several regimens using this combination, but the basic premise in all of them is that leucovorin potentiates the cytotoxic activity of 5FU (Loprinzi, 1989). Although the dose of 5FU remains relatively constant, the leucovorin dose in these regimens varies, as does the method of administration, usually either IV bolus or continuous infusion. This combination has shown a 20% to 25% response rate even in those women already treated with 5FU (Hainsworth, Andrews, Johnson, & Greco, 1991). The most common dose-limiting side effect is stomatitis; diarrhea is also a side effect, but is controlled easily. This regimen has also been combined with other therapies, such as mitoxantrone. This increases the side effect profile, adding myelosuppression as a dose-limiting side effect, but may also increase effectiveness. In one study, the response rate was 65%, with a median duration of response of 6 months (Hainsworth et al., 1991).

Other drugs have been used as potentiators including verapamil, phenothiazines, and tamoxifen. These potentiators take advantage of the multiple drug resistance gene (MDR1). One of the ways that this gene works is to signal a rapid release of drug from tumor cells, leaving little time for cellular damage to take place. Verapamil, phenothiazines, and tamoxifen may prevent this efflux of drugs such as doxorubicin and therefore may increase the potency of chemotherapeutics (Vogel, 1991).

New Drugs

Although it was first isolated in 1967, paclitaxel (Taxol, Bristol-Myers, Princeton, NJ) is a new and now widely used drug in the treatment of metastatic breast cancer. Although related to the vinca alkaloids, it has a different mechanism of action. Paclitaxel interferes with cellular division by disrupting the equilibrium of microtubule assembly (Arbuck, Dorr, & Friedman, 1994). Administration of this drug has generally been either over 24 hours in continuous infusion, or infusion over a 3-hour period. Preliminary data show a response rate in pretreated patients of 33% in one study in which the drug was administered over 24 hours. Preliminary data in a study randomizing women between 135 mg/m^2 and 175 mg/m^2 over 3 hours reveal a pooled response rate of 27% (Arbuck et al., 1994). It is clear that this drug has some response rate in pretreated women. Side effects include hypersensitivity reactions, which are controlled by premedication with dexamethasone and histamine-2 blockers. A variety of cardiac arrhythmias have also been noted, most commonly bradycardia, which is reversible by decreasing the rate of infusion. Nausea and vomiting are usually controlled with oral antiemetics; other gastrointestinal (GI) symptoms such as mild diarrhea have been reported. Typhilitis has been reported when paclitaxel is used in combination with doxorubicin. This necrotizing inflammation of the lower GI tract is manifested by fever, possible neutropenia, right lower quadrant abdominal pain with accompanying nausea, vomiting, rebound tenderness, diarrhea, and guiac-positive stools. Both myelosuppression and neurological toxicity can be dose limiting and are reversible with discontinuation of the drug. Myalgias and arthralgias are also common and usually begin 2 to 4 days after treatment and may last 1 to 3 days (Rogers, 1993). Resistance to other drugs, especially doxorubicin, does not seem to predict resistance to paclitaxel. However, paclitaxel does have some characteristics of drugs that induce multidrug resistance (MDR) in cancer cells.

One way of overcoming MDR is to add another agent to the chemotherapeutic regimen to overcome resistance. A study is underway that looks at the addition of R-verapamil to paclitaxel in patients with tumors that have progressed while on treatment. This has increased hematologic and neurologic toxicity of paclitaxel, but the combination can be given. Response data are not yet available for this combination (Tolcher et al., 1994).

The use of paclitaxel in combination with other drugs is also currently under study. Drug combinations being studied include paclitaxel and carboplatin, cyclophosphamide, edatrexate, etoposide, 5FU (with and without leucovorin), ifosfamide, methotrexate, estramustine, and topotecan. Phase II studies with paclitaxel and cisplatin are underway, taking advantage of documented synergy between these two drugs (Arbuck et al., 1994).

A semisynthetic version of paclitaxel has been developed. Known as docetaxel (Taxotere), it is derived from the needles of the European yew tree. Again, responses have been documented in heavily pretreated patients with similar toxicities, as were noted with paclitaxel. One difference has been the occurrence of pleural effusions and peripheral edema, which have not readily been explained and are still being studied (Arbuck et al., 1994).

Navelbine is a semisynthetic vinca alkaloid that has been tested both orally and intravenously in breast cancer. Unlike vinblastine, its dose-limiting toxicity is neutropenia rather than thrombocytopenia. While neuropathy was observed in phase I trials, it has not necessitated dose reductions. Phase II studies have suggested that navelbine is at least equivalent to other vinca alkaloids in antitumor activity. It has shown promise in non-small cell lung cancer and is currently being studied both alone and in combination with cisplatin in advanced breast cancer (Jones & Smith, 1994). The ability to give navelbine orally makes it especially appealing as a new agent for advanced disease.

Another new class of drugs is being studied in breast cancer. Anthrapyrazoles are related to the anthracycline antibiotics such as doxorubicin and its analog, mitoxantrone. Their pattern of activity is related to doxorubicin but appears to be less cardiotoxic. The drug currently under consideration is biantrazole. It has shown no clinically significant cardiovascular events so far and its dose-limiting toxicity is leukopenia. Interestingly, only 32% of patients treated with this drug had alopecia requiring the purchase of a wig. Nausea and vomiting were mild and easily controlled (Jones & Smith, 1994). Although still in very preliminary use, this drug presents another promising avenue of breast cancer treatment.

NURSE AS GUIDE IN DECISION MAKING

The role of the oncology nurse in assisting the woman with breast cancer to make thoughtful, informed decisions regarding her treatment is an important one. It is essential that the nurse involved understand the full scope of options being offered to patients and therefore be involved in initial discussions among the physician, the patient, and family members. The range of options may be a wide one, depending on the clinical circumstances. In the case of the node-positive, perimenopausal woman who is physiologically young, the options may range from tamoxifen to marrow transplant. Nurses need to understand and be able to articulate the risks and benefits of each choice. This is not to say that the nurse or other provider should not offer an opinion regarding the appropriate treatment in any one circumstance. It is a disservice to patients to present them with a "menu" without any guidance in decision making. Few patients will have the medical background to make such decisions. It is the responsibility of the health care professional to assess the patient's physical and emotional condition, present the available options, and from those options, provide a recommendation. If the patient does not agree with the provider's recommendation, assistance in finding another provider or initiating a negotiation

until a satisfactory and appropriate treatment plan is in place is appropriate.

One intervention that has been suggested by Neufeld, Degner, and Dick (1993) is a preliminary assessment by the nurse of how a particular patient has made decisions in the past by using "preference cards" that enumerate specific roles that the treatment team and the patient could possibly play in decision making. The nurse, after meeting with the physician to discuss the preferred method of decision making, remains with the patient throughout the exam and discussion of treatment options, acting as a "coach" to facilitate questions. The nurse also sees the patient alone after the physician has completed his or her discussion to give the patient additional time to ask questions. This particular strategy has been used with women making initial treatment decisions.

Another instrument has been used with women considering adjuvant chemotherapy for node-negative breast cancer (Levine, Gafni, Markham, & MacFarlane, 1992). Scenarios were written for the available treatment options that described the option and the possible outcome in terms of toxicity and response. The use of a decision board allowed the treatment choice and probable outcomes to be visually considered by the patient and provider alike. The potential toxicity and benefits of treatment were also included and a take-home decision board was given to the patient to facilitate additional thought and question formation. This technique facilitates clear communication between health care provider and patient as well as shared decision making. It is inexpensive and can be modified as new treatments are available.

Hughes (1993) reported that women making decisions about primary treatment of breast cancer received much of their information prior to their initial consultation, especially in the case of women who chose mastectomy as their primary treatment. Women obtained most information from friends, family, and popular media sources. It may be that this type of information is valued more highly by women than health care providers are aware. Asking what information the patient has obtained and from what sources gives the opportunity to clarify any misconceptions. This study found that style of presentation and amount of information were less important. The finding of poor patient recall of information is not suprising, considering the anxiety that these decisions provoke. The opportunity to ask questions and to repeat information to the patient is essential for informed consent.

When a woman is given the option of participating in a clinical trial, not only is understanding of the specific procedures, medications, and schedule important, but the goals of the trial should be explained in detail. The goal of a phase I trial, safety, is very different than the goal of a randomized phase III trial, which compares interventions for efficacy. A woman's understanding of where she is on the continuum of breast cancer is essential to her understanding of the reasons for and possible benefits of participating in a clinical trial. Advantages to participation include access to new treatments or treatments that are otherwise not used in a clinical setting, careful monitoring during and after the trial, and the opportunity to realize the altruistic contribution of helping women in the future who have breast cancer. Possible disadvantages include frequent visits to the clinic, multiple blood testing and other testing, and the uncertainty of outcome. In some trials, the uncertainty of treatment may pose a disadvantage to some women. Careful explanation of randomization is an important part of informed consent that the nurse can reinforce. Feelings of regret or anger at the randomization may contribute to depression and anxiety.

THE FUTURE IN BREAST CANCER

The future of treatment in breast cancer promises to be an interesting one. The issue of high-dose therapy in both the adjuvant and metastatic settings continues to be studied with great interest. The further refinement of hematopoietic growth factors as supportive treatment for both high-dose and standard-dose therapies will make this research much more palatable for both provider and patient.

New treatments will certainly be of interest, but it is the genetic characterization of breast cancer that may represent the most exciting progress in the years to come. The identification of the proto-oncogene HER-2/Neu has provided us with one target for treatment. The identification of a gene on chromosome 17 could potentially provide another more specific target for therapy.

Unlike other cancers that have been genetically characterized, breast cancer seems to result from multiple mutations possibly on multiple chromosomes (King, 1991). If several "hits" are necessary to cause breast cancer, they may represent targets for disabling the genetic machinery that causes this disease. This futuristic therapy may eventually become reality with the help of continued basic research in genetics. Some of this research is in the area of antisense RNA that interferes with protein transcription (Morrison, 1994). This type of targeted treatment could be used to disable oncogenes.

As discussed earlier, the over-expression of the HER-2/Neu oncogene has been linked with a poor prognosis in breast cancer. Antibodies have been produced against the HER-2 receptor and are being tested in clinical trials in combination with cisplatin. If these clinical trials mirror preclinical data, this combination may help overcome resistance to cisplatin therapy in pretreated patients (Tripathy & Benz, 1994).

Angiogenesis relates to the development of blood vessels that nourish a tumor and provide a pathway for metastasis. Another appealing therapeutic option is the possibility of using an antiangiogenesis factor in treatment of breast cancer. Some antiangiogenesis agents include: corticosteriods, antiestrogens, and medroxyprogesterone acetate. However, experience with these agents clinically limits their successful use in patients with ER- and PR-positive tumors, suggesting that they are working against breast cancer in some other way than to prevent angiogenesis. Other agents with antiangiogenesis properties that have been evaluated in the laboratory caused unacceptable toxicity in animal models and suggest that a combination of agents will be more effective than a single agent alone (Hayes, 1994). Studies are being carried out to establish clinical usefulness of angiogenesis as a prognostic factor (Hayes, 1994). In concert with other prognostic factors, it might assist women with node-negative disease in making treatment decisions.

Another possible genetic target could be the p53 gene, which is deranged in approximately 30% of human breast tumors. As an anti-oncogene, p53 is active in tumorigenesis when its function is lost. Gene therapy to replace p53 in deficient cells or attempting to find a surrogate activator for those genes that p53 turns on will be occupying basic science in this arena.

The p53 anti-oncogene is also used as a prognostic indicator. Its detection in primary breast tumors has been associated with a poor prognosis (Allred et al., 1993).

Nursing in Medical Clinical Trials

Translation of basic science to the clinical setting requires the coordinating efforts of a variety of both basic scientists and clinical providers. Nursing has a critical role in clinical applications of new therapies. As the team members who spend the most time with the patient, oncology nurses have a unique opportunity to see first hand the effects of new therapies and to report them accurately. A grounding in the scientific process enables the nurses not only to contribute effectively to medical clinical trials, but also to develop associated nursing trials that can answer important questions about new therapies. Quality of life and symptom management are only two of many areas in which nursing has made great contributions. How women decide to enter clinical trials and how they make decisions among complicated treatment choices deserve

more study; this would assist all caregivers in providing timely and useful guidance for women with breast cancer. The role of the advanced practice nurse in delivering care to women with breast cancer is another important area of investigation. The trend toward nurse practitioners in oncology is novel. Defining this role requires careful thought not only to assure quality nursing practice in a collegial setting with physicians and other nurses, but also to ensure patient satisfaction in a changing health care environment.

References

Abels, R. I., Larholt, K. M., Krantz, K. D., Bryant, E. C. (1991). Recombinant human erythropoietin (r-HuEPO) for the treatment of the anemia of cancer. In *Blood cell growth factors: Their present and future use in hematology and oncology.* Dayton, OH. Alpha Med Press.

Allred, D. C., Clark, G. M., Eddedge, R., Fuqua, S. A. W., Brown, R.W., Chamness, G. C., Osborne, C. K., & McGuire, W. L. (1993). Association of p53 protein expression with tumor cell proliferation rate and clinical outcome in node-negative breast cancer. *Journal of the National Cancer Institute, 85,* 200–206.

Arbuck, S. G., Dorr, A., & Friedman, M. A. (1994). Paclitaxel (Taxol) in breast cancer. *Hematology /Oncology Clinics of North America, 8* (1), 121–140.

Bacus, S. S., Bacus, J. W., Slamon, D. J., & Press, M. F. (1990). HER-2/Neu oncogene expression and DNA ploidy analysis in breast cancer. *Archives of Pathological Laboratory Medicine, 114,* 164–169.

Budman, D. R, Wood, W., Henderson, I. C., Korzun, A. H., Cooper, R., Younger, J., Hart, P. D., Moore, A., Ellerton, J., Norton, L., Ferree, C., & McIntyre, O.R. (1992). Initial findings of CALGB 8541: A dose and dose intensity trial of cyclophosphamide, doxorubicin and 5-fluorouracil as adjuvant treatment of Stage II, node +, female breast cancer. *Proceedings of the American Society of Clinical Oncology, 11,* 51.

Clark, G. M., Mathieu, M. C., Owens, M. A., Dressler, L. G., Eudey, L., Tormey, D. C., Osborne, C. K., Gilchrist, K. W., Mansour, E. G., Abeloff, M. D., & McGuire, W. L.(1992). Prognostic significance of S-phase fraction in good-risk, node-negative breast cancer patients. *Journal of Clinical Oncology, 10* (3), 428–432.

Demetri, G. D. (1994). The use of hematopoietic growth factors to support cytotoxic chemotherapy for patients with breast cancer. *Hematology/Oncology Clinics of North America, 8 (1),* 223–249.

Demetri, G. D., Costa, J., Hayes, D., Sledge, G., Galli, S., Hoffman, R., Merica, E., Rich, W., Harkins, B., Mcguire, B., & Gordon, M. (1993). A phase I trial of recombinant methionylhuman stem cell factor (SCF) in patients with advanced breast carcinoma pre- and post-chemotherapy (chemo) with cyclophosphamide (C) and doxorubicin (A). *Proceedings of the American Society of Clinical Oncology, 12,* 142.

Demetri, G. D., & Elias, A. D. (1994). Current understanding of PBPCs and hematopoietic growth factors. *Advances in Oncology, 10,* 11–19.

Demetri, G. D, Samuels, B., & Gordon, M. (1992). Recombinant human interleukin-6 (IL-6) increases circulating platelet counts and C-reactive protein levels in vivo: Initial results of a phase I trial in sarcoma patients with normal hemopoiesis. *Blood, 80* (Suppl 1).

Dixon, A. R., Robertson, J. F. R., Jackson, L., Nicholson, R. I., Walker, K. J., & Blamey, R. W. (1990). Goserelin (Zoladex) in premenopausal advanced breast cancer: Duration of response and survival. *British Journal of Cancer, 62,* 868.

Early Breast Cancer Trialists' Collaborative Group. (1992). Systemic treatment of early breast cancer by hormonal, cytotoxic, or immune therapy: 133 randomised trials involving 31,000 recurrences and 24,000 deaths among 75,000 women. *Lancet, 339,* 1–15, 71–85.

Elias, A. D., Ayash, L., Anderson, K. C., Hunt, M., Wheeler, C., Schwartz, G., Tepler, I., Mazanet, R., Lynch, C., Pelaer, I., Reich, E., Critchlow, J., Demetri, G., Bibbo, J., Schnipper, L., Griffin, J. D., Frei, E., & Antman, K. (1992). Mobilization of peripheral blood progenitor cells by chemotherapy and granulocyte-macrophage colony-stimulating factor for hematologic support after high-dose intensification for breast cancer. *Blood, 79,* 3036–3044.

Fisher, B., Costantino, J., & Redmond, C., (1989). A randomized clinical trial evaluating tamoxifen in the treatment of patients with node-negative breast cancer who have estrogen-receptor-positive tumors. *New England Journal of Medicine, 320,* 473–478.

Fisher, B., Wickerham, D. L., & Redmond, C. (1992). Recent developments in the use of systemic adjuvant therapy for the treatment of breast cancer. *Seminars in Oncology, 19* (3), 263–277.

Ganser, A., et al. (1990). Effects of recombinant human interleukin-3 in patients with normal hematopoiesis and in patients with bone marrow failure. *Blood, 76,* 666–676.

Goodman, M. (1991). Adjuvant systemic therapy of stage I and II breast cancer. *Seminars in Oncology Nursing, 7* (3), 175–186.

Hainsworth, J. D., Andrews, M. B., Johnson, D. H., & Greco, F. A. (1991). Mitoxantrone, fluorouracil, and high-dose leucovorin: An effective, well-tolerated regimen for metastatic breast cancer. *Journal of Clinical Oncology, 9* (10), 1731–1735.

Hayes, D. F. (1993). Tumor markers for breast cancer. *Annals of Oncology, 4,* 807–819.

Hayes, D. F. (1994). Angiogenesis and breast cancer. *Hematology/Oncology Clinics of North America, 8* (1), 51–71.

Hughes, K. K. (1993). Decision making by patients with breast cancer: The role of information in treatment selection. *Oncology Nursing Forum, 20* (4), 623–628.

Jakubowski, A., et al. (1992). A phase I/II trial of PIXY 321 (PIXY) in patients (pts) with metastatic breast cancer receiving doxorubicin and thiotepa. *Blood, 80* (Suppl 1), 88a.

Jones, A. L., & Smith, I. E. (1994). Navelbine and the anthrapyrazones. *Hematology/Oncology Clinics of North America, 8* (1), 141–152.

King, M. L. (1991). Localization of the early-onset breast cancer gene. *Hospital Practice, 10,* 89–94.

Levine, M. N., Gafni, A., Markham, B., & MacFarlane, D. (1992). A bedside decision instrument to elicit a patient's preference concerning adjuvant chemotherapy for breast cancer. *Annals of Internal Medicine, 117,* 53–58.

Loprinzi, C. L. (1989) 5-Fluorouracil with leucovorin in breast cancer. *Cancer, 63,* 1045–1047.

Madeya, M. L., & Pfab-Tokarsky, J. M. (1992). Flow cytometry: An overview. *Oncology Nursing Forum, 19* (3), 459–463.

Morrison, B. (1994). The genetics of breast cancer. *Hematology/Oncology Clinics of North America, 8,* (10), 15–27.

National Institutes of Health. (1990). *Treatment of early-stage breast cancer.* NIH Consensus Development Conference Consensus Statement, 8, 1–19.

Neufeld, K. R., Degner, L. F., & Dick, J. A. M. (1993). A nursing intervention strategy to foster patient involvement in treatment decisions. *Oncology Nursing Forum, 20* (4), 631–635.

Peters, W. P., Ross, M., Vredenburgh, J. J., Meisenberg, B., Marks, L. B., Winer, E., Kurtzberg, J., Bast, R. C., Jones, R., Shpall, E., Wu, K., Rosner, G., Gilbert, C., Mathias, B., Coniglio, D., Petros,W., Henderson, I. C., Norton, L., Weiss, R. B., Budman, D., & Hurd, D. High-dose chemotherapy an autologous bone marrow support as consolidation after standard-dose adjuvant therapy for high-risk primary breast cancer. *Journal of Clinical Oncology, 11,* 1132–1143.

Porter-Jordan, K., & Lippman, M. E. (1994). Overview of the biologic markers of breast cancer. *Hematology/Oncology Clinics of North America, 8* (1), 73–100.

Ravdin, P. M. (1994). A practical view of prognostic factors for staging, adjuvant treatment planning, and as baseline studies for possible future therapy. *Hematology/Oncology Clinics of North America, 8* (1), 197–211.

Rogers, B. (1993). Taxol: A promising new drug of the '90s. *Oncology Nursing Forum, 20* (10), 1483–1489.

Schwartzberg, L., West, W., Tauer, W., Altemose, R., George, C., & Birch, R., (1992). Cyclophosphamide, etoposide, cisplatin plus G-CSF (CEP+G) for peripheral blood stem cell (PBSC) mobilization. *Proceedings of the American Society of Clinical Oncology, 11,* 402.

Scottish Cancer Trials Breast Group (1993). Adjuvant ovarian ablation versus CMF chemotherapy in premenopausal women with pathological stage II breast carcinoma: The Scottish trial. *The Lancet, 341* (8856), 1293–1298.

Shapiro, C. L., & Henderson, I. C. (1994). Adjuvant therapy of breast cancer. *Hematology/Oncology Clinics of North America, 8* (1), 213–231.

Shapiro, C. L., Hurd, D., Clark, P., Demetri, G. D., Ayash, L., Blumsack, R., Gelman, R., Cruz, J., Antman, K., Elias, A., Hayes, D., Duggan, D., & Henderson, I. C. (1994). Repetitive cycles of cyclophosphamide, thiotepa and carboplatin (CTCb) intensification with peripheral blood progenitor cells (PBPC) and Filgrastim (G-CSF) in advanced breast cancer patients (Pts.). *Proceedings of the American Society of Clinical Oncology, 13,* 66.

Slamon, D. J., Clark, G. M., Wong, S. G., Levin, W. J., Ulrich, A., & McGuire, W. L. (1987). Human breast cancer: Correlation of relapse and survival with amplification of the HER-2/*neu* oncogene. *Science, 235,* 177–182.

Tolcher, A. W., Cowan, K. H., Solomon, D., Berg, S., Venzon, D., Goldspiel, B., & O'Shaughnessy, J. A. (1994). A phase I study of paclitaxel (T) with r-verapamil (RV), in metastatic breast cancer (MBC). *Proceedings of the American Society of Clinical Oncology, 13,* 139.

Tripathy, D., & Benz, C. (1994). Growth factors and their receptors. *Hematology/Oncology Clinics of North America, 8* (1), 29–50.

Vadhan-Raj, S., Papadoupoulos, N., Burgess, M., Patel, S., Linke, K., Plager, C., Hayes, C., Arcenas, A., Kudelka, A., Williams, D., Garrison, L., & Benjamin, R. (1993). Optimization of dose and schedule of PIXY321 (GM-CSF/IL-3 fusion protein) to attenuate chemotherapy (CT)-induced multilineage myelosuppression in patients with sarcoma. *Proceedings of the American Society of Clinical Oncology, 12,* 470.

Vogel, C. L. (1991). Treatment of metastatic breast cancer. *Seminars in Oncology Nursing, 7* (3), 194–198.

Wright, C., Nicholson, S., Angus, B., Sainsbury, J. R. C., Farndon, J., Cairns, J., Harris, A. L., & Horne, C. H. W. (1992). Relationship between c-*erb* B-2 protein product expression and response to endocrine therapy in advanced breast cancer. *British Journal of Cancer, 65,* 118–121.

PART 3 | **Survivorship Issues**

CHAPTER 7 | Menopausal Symptoms Associated with Breast Cancer Treatment

M. Tish Knobf, RN, MSN, FAAN

The estimated 182,000 new breast cancer cases diagnosed in the United States in 1995 account for 32% of all new cases of cancer (Wingo, Tong & Bolden, 1995). The majority of these new breast cancer cases will be diagnosed as "early-stage" (stage I or stage II) disease, with approximately 20% of women being diagnosed under the age of 50 years. Prognosis is related to several factors, the most significant of which are tumor size and axillary node involvement. In the past, systemic therapy (following primary local-regional treatment) was used only in patients with a high risk for recurrence, large tumors, and/or positive axillary lymph nodes. However, mounting evidence has shown that adjuvant systemic therapy (either chemotherapy, hormone therapy, or a combination) results in prolonged disease-free periods and overall survival rates (Early Breast Cancer Trialist's Collaborative Group, 1992a, 1992b). This treatment now is considered increasingly for women at lower risk for recurrence.

Approximately 25% to 30% of stage I (node-negative) patients will experience a recurrence of, and ultimately die of, their breast cancer. Because it is difficult to identify patients who are at the greatest risk for relapse, almost all women with negative node disease are considered candidates for adjuvant systemic therapy (Davidson & Abeloff, 1992). Thus the overwhelming majority of women diagnosed with breast cancer today are candidates for systemic therapy following their primary local regional treatment, either mastectomy (with or without reconstruction) or breast conservation surgery with radiation.

Physical and psychological sequelae associated with adjuvant therapy represent a wide variety of symptoms. Patients rate the severity along a continuum from mild to severe (Ehlke, 1988; Greene et al., 1994; Knobf, 1986; Knobf, 1990; Maguire et al., 1980; Nerenz, Leventhal, & Love, 1982). Common symptoms include fatigue, nausea, insomnia, weight gain, hair loss, anorexia, taste change, and menopausal symptoms. The type of adjuvant treatment (hormonal or chemotherapy), the specific drug regimen, drug dose, the duration of therapy, and patient factors such as menopausal status and psychological profile appear to influence the incidence, severity of symptoms, and perceived symptom distress (Greene, Nail, Fieler, Dudgen & Jones, 1994; Hull, 1993; Knobf, 1990; Sinsheimer & Holland, 1987).

Menopausal symptoms associated with drug-induced ovarian failure have been more commonly reported in the last decade by premenopausal women treated for breast cancer. Symptoms including hot flashes, sweats, headaches, vaginal dryness, dyspareunia, menstrual irregularities, and amenorrhea have been reported as toxicity data from clinical trials and cited in the clinical literature, although these data are limited in scope and specificity (Aikin, 1994; Chamorro, 1991; Feldman, 1989; Fisher et al., 1989; Hull, 1993; Legha, 1988; Love, Leventhal, & Easterling, 1989; Tarpy & Rothwell, 1983). Preliminary published data on women with breast cancer who experience menopausal symptoms suggest that these symptoms disrupt routine activities, interfere with sleep and rest, and may affect the quality and frequency of their sexual relationship (Chapman, 1982; Derogotis, 1980; Knobf, 1986; Ringer,1983; Schover, 1991; Young-McCaughan, 1995). These data primarily reflect clinical observations or incidental findings from larger studies on adjuvant therapy, quality of life, or sexuality. Only recently have prospective studies of premenopausal women on adjuvant therapy been initiated, to assess menopausal symptoms (Headley, 1994; Roy, Pritchard, Sawka, & Franssen, 1994).

PERIMENOPAUSE

Perimenopause covers the phase in a woman's life from a beginning decline in ovarian function through several years after cessation of menses (Fogel & Woods, 1995; Lorrain, Ravnikar, & Charest, 1994; McKinlay, Brambilla, & Posner, 1992; Utian, 1980c). Menopause occurs during the perimenopausal transition and is defined clinically as the occurrence of amenorrhea for 12 months or longer. Perimenopause may begin up to 10 years before menopause and continues for a period of years after menopause.

Physiologic Changes

The ovarian reproductive cycle will be briefly described here, because it provides the foundation for understanding the transition to menopause. The function of the ovary is to produce eggs and sex steroids (estrone, estradiol, and progesterone). The ovarian reproductive cycle, or menstrual cycle, is not solely dependent on ovarian function but involves a complex interaction between the ovary, pituitary, hypothalamus, and gonadal hormones (Hatcher et al., 1994; Speroff, Glass, & Kase, 1994). The hypothalmus integrates information from the environment through the central nervous system and stimulates the pituitary through the gonadotropin-releasing hormone (GnRH). The pituitary is also influenced by a complex inhibitory-stimulating input from the ovarian steroids (Goodman, 1994). The two pituitary gonadotropins, follicle stimulating hormone (FSH) and luteinizing hormone (LH), stimulate ovarian steroid production. They are also regulated largely by the ovarian steroid hormones.

The blood levels of hormones during the menstrual cycle depend on the phase of the cycle (follicular, mid-cycle, peak, or luteal). Estradiol, the dominant estrogen, is lowest during the follicular phase (25-75 pg/ml) and highest at the mid-cycle peak (200–600 pg/ml). Levels of FSH and LH are generally less than 10 IU/L, except at the mid-cycle peak (often called the "surge") where values increase significantly, to 20 to 60 IU/L for FSH and 30 to 70 IU/L for LH (Chang, Plouffe, & Schaeffer, 1994).

At birth, the female is endowed with 2 to 4 million primordial ovarian follicles. The majority of these follicles undergo a degenerative change called atresia, leaving approximately 200,000 to 400,000 follicles at puberty (Goodman, 1994). At the beginning of the menstrual cycle, a group of follicles are recruited for development into mature oocyte. One follicle becomes dominant, and the others undergo atresia. During a woman's reproductive life span, only about 500 follicles will result in mature oocytes. The process of atresia is continuous, reflected by a progressive decrease in the number of oocytes as a woman ages. (Utian, 1980a). The ovarian reproductive cycle will continue as long as there are primordial ovarian follicles. As the ovarian follicles are depleted, the cycle will fail and changes in hormonal production and secretion will be evident (Utian, 1980b).

The transition from the ovulatory reproductive cycle to menopause reflects declining ovarian function, and may precede the actual cessation of menses by 4 to 8 years (Utian, 1980b; Goodman, 1994). This period of transition, prior to actual cessation of menses is often characterized by changes in menstrual bleeding patterns and alterations in cycle length.

Menopause, the actual cessation of menses, can be described simply by four sequential steps (Utian, 1990):

1. **Morphologic change in the ovary.** Once menses cease, the ovaries become smaller, fibrotic, and devoid of any functional follicles.
2. **Change in the hormonal profile.** Estradiol, the dominant source of estrogen for the premenopausal woman, dramatically declines. Estrone becomes the principal source of estrogen for the postmenopausal woman, which is primarily derived from peripheral conversion of androstenedione. The production of androstenedione lessens in postmenopausal women, but the conversion rate to estrone is significantly higher (Chang et al., 1994). The levels of gonadotrophins (FSH, LH) rise significantly after menopause due to estrogen loss and, thus, alteration in the feedback mechanisms regulating these gonadotropins. The increase in FSH levels is much greater than LH levels, and conse-

quently, FSH is accepted as the most common measure to establish menopause in clinical practice.
3. **Target tissues response to altered hormone levels.** The decline in circulating estrogen affects the tissues of the urogential tract, skin, mucous membranes, the skeleton, and cardiovascular system, and may affect the central nervous system, resulting in mood or behavioral changes.
4. **Clinical signs and symptoms.** Patients may present with subjective complaints related to altered estrogen levels, or may demonstrate objective findings in target organs.

Menopause either occurs naturally, as part of the physiologic aging process described above, or is artifically induced. Radiation therapy to the pelvic area, surgical removal of the ovaries, or the use of drugs that produce gonadal toxicity all can induce premature menopause. In industrialized countries, the onset of natural menopause occurs at 50 to 51 years of age, on average. Artifically induced menopause may occur at any age, but the age of the patient will influence fertility, incidence and severity of menopausal symptoms, and the long-term effects of low estrogen levels.

Menopausal Symptoms

The perimenopause may or may not be associated with bothersome symptoms. However, symptoms are experienced by 50% to 90% of women in the years preceding, during, and after cessation of menstrual periods, and approximately 30% will seek medical care for symptomatology (Treolar, 1982; Belchetz, 1994). The characteristic menopausal symptoms were historically referred to as the "menopause syndrome." These symptoms are the result of decreasing estrogen levels and changes in the endocrine balance of a woman's system, but are also influenced by psychological and sociocultural factors. Vasomotor symptoms (hot flashes, sweats) and changes in the vaginal epithelium

Table 7-1   Target Organ Responses and Symptoms Associated with Menopause

Organ/System	Response/Symptoms
Vagina	Shorter, more narrow, increased pH, decreased elasticity and rugae. Discomfort, dyspareunia, and proneness to to infection may result.
Ovary	Becomes smaller and fibrotic.
Vulva	Gradual atrophy with a decrease in subcutaneous tissue, progressive hair loss, and thinning of the skin. Pruritus and dyspareunia common.
Uterus	Decrease in size and weight; thinning of the walls, yet endometrium maintains ability to respond to estrogen; decrease in size and atrophy of the cervix; cervical mucous decreases with eventual disappearance. Irregular menses with subsequent amenorrhea are characteristic, and dysfunctional uterine bleeding may occur.
Breasts	Decrease in size and shape due to atrophy of glandular tissue; nipples become smaller and more flat.
Bladder/Urethra	Atrophic changes which may be associated with aging or hormonal changes on the epithelium, but not definitely related to menopause.
Skin	Thinning of the epidermis and dermis, and decline in the function of sweat and sebaceous glands.
Cardiovascular	Changes in the lipid profile.
Skeleton	Decreased bone mineral density resulting in osteoporosis with an increased risk of fractures.
Nervous/Endocrine	Instability which may result in symptoms such as hot flashes, palpitations, anxiety, mood alterations, changes in cognitive function, headaches, nervous tension, and changes in libido.,

Note. Data from "Target Tissue Response to Ovarian Failure" by W. H. Utian, 1990. In *Menopause in Modern Perspective: A Guide to Clinical Practice* (pp. 47–61). New York: Appleton Century Crofts; and "Women at Midlife: Hormone Replacement Therapy" by M. A. Maddox, 1992, *Nursing Clinics of North America, 27,* pp. 959–969.

are the most common and immediate responses to reduced estrogen levels. Subjective symptoms associated with the menopause transition (Table 7-1) have been categorized as somatic, psychological, psychosomatic, or neurological (Greene, 1976; Kaufert & Syrotuik, 1981; Neugarten & Kraines, 1965). The etiology of psychological and somatic complaints (irritability, fatigue, nervousness, insomnia, and/or mood changes) is controversial. These symptoms may be related to vasomotor symptoms (insomnia and irritability related to sleep interruptions from night sweats), or sociocultural, environmental, or occupational aspects of a woman's life. The symptoms may also be a response to the body's struggle to adapt to the endocrine imbalance. Utian (1980c; 1980d) conceptualizes the body's response to decreased estrogen into early and late symptoms. Early symptoms include menstrual irregularities, the hot flash vasomotor symptom, vaginal dryness, and other subjective symptoms. The late symptoms are not actual symptoms, but the effects of decreased estrogen on target tissues. Late symptoms may or may not be associated with subjective symptoms (Table 7-1).

The hot flash is the most frequent symptom of menopause and appears to be unique to the individual. It varies from transient episodes of feelings of warmth to episodes of intense overheating, which may be accompanied by sweats, palpitations, anxiety, and chills (Kronenberg, 1990). Most women report experiencing a premonition or aura right before the hot flash. Heart rate and skin blood flow increase, and distribution of the heat sensation is primarily to the upper body. The hot flash occurs at various times in a 24-hour period, with no particular established pattern (Kronenberg, 1990; Voda, 1981). Self-report is a valid index of the presence of the symptom. Approximately 60% of women report experiencing hot flashes for 1 to 5 years, and 10% to 15% report experiencing hot flashes for more than 10 years (Feldman, Voda, & Gronseth, 1985; Kronenberg, 1990). They are more frequent and intense during the first 1 to 2 years, with 10% to 26% of women rating them as severe in intensity (Feldman et al., 1985; Kronenberg, 1990; Voda, 1981). Surgical oophorectomy can result in vasomotor symptoms within days of the procedure. A higher percentage of women on whom a surgical castration was performed report symptoms, and the symptoms are reported as more severe. For those women who experience moderate to severe hot flashes during the night, the major consequence is sleep deprivation, which can lead to fatigue and irritability and may affect occupational and social activities (Kronenberg, 1990; Sarrell, Rouseau, Mazur, & Glazer, 1990).

Vasomotor Symptoms. The phenomenon of vasomotor symptoms is not fully understood. Alteration of estrogen levels is a critical factor, but the lack of estrogen alone does not fully explain the phenomena of the hot flash (Feldman et al., 1985; Huddleston & McElmurray, 1990; Kronenberg, 1990; Sarrel, Rouseau, Mazur, & Glazer, 1990; Sherman, Wallace, Bean, Chang, & Schalabaugh, 1981; Utian, 1980c). The key factor is the withdrawal of estrogen, not low estrogen level. The observations that vasomotor symptoms can be alleviated by estrogen replacement,

hot flashes decrease in frequency and intensity over time, and women with low estrogen levels due to endocrine disorders do not experience hot flashes support the hypothesis that withdrawal of estrogen is a precipitating factor.

Other precipitating factors are not clearly established, but ambient temperature, hot drinks, hot foods, alcohol, emotional upset, weather, and caffeine appear to influence the frequency and severity of hot flashes (Greenwood, 1984). In attempts to achieve thermal comfort, women turn down thermostats, wear lighter clothing and cotton materials, fan themselves, and avoid outside hot temperatures. Many of these self-care measures are challenged by the work and home environments. This natural menopausal symptom was covered in more detail because it also appears to be the predominant menopausal symptom complaint of women who experience artificial (drug-induced) menopause.

Menopause Research

To understand the experience of premature menopause and menopausal symptoms in women treated for breast cancer, it is helpful to reflect on the research that has been conducted on natural menopause and womens' health. Historically, menopause has been viewed from a medical model perspective as a disease deficiency state, specifically an estrogen deficiency state. The dominant medical perspective of menopause as a deficiency disease requiring treatment provided the direction for research. Many of the early studies focused on assessment of symptom response to hormone replacement therapy in women who sought consultation for menopausal symptoms. Much, if not most, of that early menopause research suffers from significant flaws in design and methodology, including lack of definitions of menopause, heterogeneous samples of women in studies (before/after menopause, surgically induced, wide age ranges), self-report symptoms based on instruments developed on patients who sought treatment, and few biological parameters (i.e., serum hormone levels) to correlate symptoms (Archer, 1982; Glazer & Rozman, 1991; Goodman, 1982; Huddleston & McElmurray, 1990; Rausch, 1994; Voda & George, 1986; Woods, 1982). Attempts have been made to approach menopause more holistically, but unfortunately many of these studies are also plagued by design and methodologic problems characteristic of earlier research. Variables which have been studied include mood, psychological response, knowledge, attitudes, perceptions, life situation/change, stage of child rearing, age, marital adjustment, self-esteem, ability to cope, sexuality, sexual interest/activity, culture, ethnicity, and socioeconomic status (Bernhard & Sheppard, 1992; Dosey & Dosey, 1981; Frey, 1981; Glazer & Rozman, 1991; Holte & Mikklesen, 1991; Hunter, Battersby, & Whitehead, 1986; Huddleston & McElmurray, 1990; La Rocca & Polit, 1980; Polit & La Rocca, 1980; Uphold & Susman, 1981; Voda & George, 1986).

More recent investigations conducted by nurse researchers have captured a broader perspective of menopause by women who experience this mid-life transition (Dickson, 1994; McElmurray & Huddleston, 1991; Quinn, 1991). Hormone replacement therapy and symptoms represent concerns of women interviewed, but aging, adjustment to bodily changes, lack of information about menopause, self-care issues, and limited communication and support were equally important issues for women who experience menopause.

In summary, the research on natural menopause provides some data on the incidence of and experience of menopause for women, such as mechanism of endocrine alterations, age of onset, variability of symptoms among women, variability of the experience of women of different cultural or ethnic backgrounds, and issues for women during this mid-life transition. These data are relevant to the woman with artificially induced menopause. It is critical, however, to remember that a woman newly diagnosed and treated for breast cancer is challenged to cope with the diagnosis and treatment, as well as a variety of side effects, one of which may be premature menopause with associated symptomatology. The nursing profession must integrate the perimenopausal experience of healthy women into the assessment of the woman with breast cancer, for premenopausal as well as postmenopausal patients, recognizing the uniqueness of and the challenge posed by the breast cancer experience.

CHEMOTHERAPY-INDUCED OVARIAN FAILURE

The etiology of early menopausal symptoms related to chemotherapy is gonadal damage, specifically ovarian fibrosis and follicular destruction. Alkylating agents are the chemotherapy drugs associated with gonadal toxicity, specifically ovarian failure in the female (Chapman, Sutcliffe, & Malpas, 1979; Fisher et al., 1979; Horning et al., 1981; Koyama et al., 1977; Rivkees & Crawford, 1988; Rose & Davis, 1977; Rose & Davis, 1980; Samaan et al., 1987). Age and corresponding ovarian function are important factors in predicting ovarian dysfunction, and whether or not the toxicity will be reversible. There is an inverse relationship between age and the incidence of drug-induced menopause. In contrast, the closer a woman is to natural menopause (average age 51 years), which reflects a continuing reduction in the number of ovarian follicles, the more likely she is to experience ovarian dysfunction, demonstrated by menstrual irregularities or amenorrhea (Brinker, Rose, & Rank, 1987; Gershenson, 1988; Schilsky et al., 1980; Rose & Davis, 1977). The number of cycles of chemotherapy a woman undergoes also influences the incidence and degree of toxicity to the gonads. Amenorrhea is reported in 65% to 75% of premenopausal women treated with chemotherapy for six cycles (Bianco et al., 1991; Goldhirsh, Gelber, & Castiglione, 1990; Mehta, Beattie, & DasGupta, 1991; Reyno, Levine, Skingley, Arnold, & Abuzara, 1992; Rose & Davis, 1977; Rose & Davis, 1980; Samaan, DeAsis, Buzdar, & Blumenshein, 1987). The longer the treatment, the more likely amenorrhea will occur.

Symptoms associated with drug-induced ovarian failure in women with breast cancer are similiar to those described for natural menopause. The severity may be greater—analogous to surgically induced menopause. There is a more rapid decline in estrogen, versus the gradual decline in women who experience natural menopause. Hot flashes, sweats, headaches, decreased vaginal lubrication, painful intercourse, generalized aches and pains, and menstrual irregularities are reported in women who receive adjuvant chemotherapy for breast cancer (Bonadonna et al., 1985; Fisher et al., 1979; Knobf, 1986; Love, Leventhal, Easterling, & Nerenz, 1989; Rose & Davis, 1980; Samaan et al., 1987; Tarpy & Rothwell, 1983; Tormey et al., 1984). Drug-induced sterility and premature menopause are common concerns for women treated for breast cancer (Hull, 1993). The incidence of associated menopausal symptoms varies but have been reported to disrupt normal activities and sleep patterns (Knobf, 1986; Ringer, 1983). In clinical practice, hot flashes and night sweats are commonly reported as distressful symptoms, for which many patients seek interventions and treatment.

Oncology nurses view treatment-induced menopause as a significant clinical practice issue, and have recognized the need for research to define the problem and develop a database for nurses to assess and manage symptoms. (Aikin, 1994; Feldman, 1989; Headley, 1994; Hull, 1993; Knobf, 1990). Long-term side effects of decreased estrogen levels, such as changes in lipid profile and decreased bone mineral density, are also emerging concerns for long-term survivors.

ADJUVANT ENDOCRINE THERAPY

Hormonal therapy for breast cancer in the adjuvant setting consists primarily of the use of tamoxifen. It is a synthetic antiestrogen, but not a pure antagonist because it has known weak estrogenic properties (Jordan, 1990). The antitumor effect is achieved through competing for and binding to the estrogen receptors of the tumor and, most likely, through the in-

hibition of growth factors. The antiestrogen effect appears target site-specific, with the estrogenic effects seen in the bones, lipids, liver, and endometrium. In postmenopausal women, decreased circulating gonadotropins, increase in sex-hormone-binding globulin, a change in circulating proteins and a positive (estrogen-like) effect on the vaginal epithelium have been observed (Jordan, 1990).

The effect on the premenopausal woman is less well understood. Amenorrhea occurs in about 20% to 30% of women, with menstrual irregularities seen in the majority of women (Legha, 1988). Tamoxifen appears to stimulate ovarian steroidogenesis, which results in high estrogen levels. It is believed to occur due to interference with the normal negative feedback mechanism within the pituitary (Ravdin, Fritz, Tormey, & Jordan, 1988; Santen, Manni, Harvey, & Redmond, 1990). Symptoms associated with tamoxifen include hot flashes, fluid retention, nausea, skin rashes, mood alterations, headache, fatigue, vaginal discharge, and decrease in libido (Mortimer, Knapp, Fracasso, Rowland, & Kornblith, 1994; Varricchio & Johnson, 1993). Tamoxifen alone is indicated as adjuvant therapy for some patients, and is also being studied in clinical trials in combination with chemotherapy or following chemotherapy.

Tamoxifen does not provide complete estrogen suppression. Analogs of gonadotropin releasing hormone (GnRH), however, provide a more complete suppression of ovarian function, thus producing an effective medical oophorectomy or medical castration (Santen, Manni, & Harvey, 1986; Santen et al., 1990). The most popular GnRH analog in clinical practice and in clinical trials is goserelin (Zoladex). Hot flashes are reported, but data are sparse on symptoms and symptom distress. Part of the limited data may relate to use of GnRH analogs in combination with or following chemotherapy, or with or following tamoxifen. The approach of combining GnRH analogs with an antiestrogen to produce a maximum supression or blockade of estrogen is under investigation in clinical trials, but the symptom profile and impact on the woman's quality of life have yet to be determined (Buzzoni et al., 1994).

MANAGEMENT OF EARLY MENOPAUSAL SYMPTOMS WITHOUT ESTROGEN

Symptom management has focused primarily on relief of vasomotor symptoms and vaginal dryness. Hot flashes and night sweats are the most frequent and distressing symptoms. They may interfere with sleep patterns, routine activities, and functional ability at work, often resulting in irritability, fatigue, and mood changes. A considerable number of nonestrogenic drugs have been considered for vasomotor symptom relief, including sedatives, nonestrogen steroid hormones, nonsteroidal anti-inflammatory agents, α-adrenergics, antidopaminergics, beta-blockers, opiate receptor agonists, and aromatic amino acid decarboxylase inhibitors (Young, Kumar, & Goldzieher, 1990). The efficacy of many of these drugs, as indicated by relief of symptoms, was questionable when compared with a placebo. In practice, most prescriptives include progestins and clonidine (α-adrenergic). Bellergal, which is a preparation of ergotamine tartrate, belladonna alkaloids, and phenobarbitol, has also been used. Due to potential addictive risk and the availability of safer alternatives, however, its use is not recommended (Walsh & Schiff, 1990).

Progestins, specifically medroxyprogesterone acetate (Provera) and megesterol acetate (Megace) have been successful in relief of hot flashes. Low-dose Megace (20 mg) has been reported to significantly reduce hot flashes (Loprinzi et al., 1994). Progestins are associated with menstrual bleeding, and patients may also complain of breast tenderness, mood changes, and abdominal bloating, all of which may affect acceptability and compliance. (Walsh & Schiff, 1990).

Clonidine is the most common α-adrenergic agonist used for the relief of hot flashes. Low-dose clonidine (0.1 mg/day), adminis-

tered either in pill form or by transdermal patch, reduces the frequency and severity of vasomotor symptoms (Clayden, Bell, & Pollard, 1974; Goldberg et al., 1992; Erlik, Meldrum, & Judd, 1982; Nagamani, Kelver, & Smith, 1987; Plowman, 1988; Yanes, Ross, & Yanes, 1987). Escalation of the dosage is associated with improved response, although side effects of dizziness, nausea, dry mouth, and headache make higher doses unacceptable for some women. Clonidine in much higher doses is used to treat hypertension, but little or no changes in blood pressure have been noted in patients treated for vasomotor symptoms with the low-dose regimen.

Benadryl, with its antihistamine and sedative properties, is a reasonable alternative to the aforementioned drugs. It may be useful at bedtime in attempting to minimize sleep deprivation due to hot flashes. While there is no research available to support the use of Benadryl, clinical experience suggests benefit in some patients.

Vitamin E is frequently used by women for menopausal symptoms. Its efficacy in relieving a wide variety of menopausal symptoms is controversial, but it appears to decrease hot flashes in selected women (Blatt, Weisbader, & Kupperman, 1953). Recommended doses vary but are in the range of 200–800 mg/day (Costlow, Lopex, & Taub, 1989; Landau, Cyr, & Moulton, 1994; Barbach, 1993; Kronenberg, Hudson, & Lark, 1995). Vitamin E has also been used as a lubricant or suppository to relieve vaginal dryness symptoms. For women with heart disease, diabetes, or hypertension, vitamin E should *not* be taken without physician knowledge and supervision (Landau et al., 1994). Clinical experience with women treated for breast cancer who experience hot flashes demonstrates relief of symptoms with Vitamin E, although response and quality of the symptom relief varies considerably. But, Vitamin E is relatively inexpensive, with no significant side effects at doses in the range of 200 to 600 mg per day (Bieri, Corash, & Hubbard, 1983).

Vaginal dryness can result in general discomfort and painful intercourse. Water-soluble lubricants have been the historical intervention when estrogen (systemic or cream) is contraindicted. Newer topical lubricants, such as Replens and Astroglide, are reported by patients as superior to more standard KY Jelly. Replens has been reported to increase vaginal moisture and elasticity and return vaginal pH to premenopausal state (Nachtigall, 1994). Vaginal dryness is a very important issue, because dyspareunia is associated with changes in sexual function and satisfaction (Young-McCaughan, 1995).

Management of menopausal symptoms with hormone replacement therapy for women with breast cancer is generally contraindicated, although the absolute nature of that contraindication has been challenged. Hormone replacement therapy for women with a history of breast cancer has become a prominent clinical practice issue and clinical trials are strongly recommended (Gambrell, 1995; Cobleigh, et al. 1994; Sands, Boshoff, Jones, & Stadd, 1995). As in women who experience natural menopause, a major indication for HRT is prevention or risk reduction of osteoporosis and cardiovascular disease in the future. Management of early symptoms and prevention of late symptoms also includes "alternative therapies." These approaches include homeopathy, herbs, diet, exercise, and Chinese medicine such as acupuncture (Kronenberg, 1995; Barbach, 1994; Costow, Lopez, & Taub, 1989). A full discussion of these approaches is beyond the scope of this chapter but is important for nurses in both clinical practice and research settings because they help promote a healthy lifestyle and self-care behaviors in women.

RECOMMENDATIONS FOR PRACTICE AND RESEARCH

The initial nursing intervention for women is informing the patient of the potential for drug-induced ovarian failure and menopausal symptoms (Aikin, 1994; Feldman, 1989). Information can reduce anxiety and will help empower the patient to ask questions and, with the nurse, be proactive with interventions. Breast cancer treatment affects a woman's body image and overall sexuality, and menopausal symptoms may exacerbate these effects and challenge the woman's coping ability, and/or influence her adherence to treatment (Finney, 1992; Schover, 1991).

Routine follow-up assessment of women is the second important activity for nurses, because the ovarian failure and associated symptoms may occur over several months, depending on the age of the woman. These effects may not be evident in some women until their adjuvant therapy is completed. Menopausal symptoms may then become their priority problem. Nursing assessment is critical in follow-up as well as during active treatment. As in natural menopause, symptoms may persist for years, with individual variation in intensity.

Natural menopause is recognized as a complex biosocial, biophysical, and biopsychological phenomenon in healthy women (Goodman, 1982). Some research has identifed the problem of artificially induced menopause and menopausal symptoms in women with breast cancer, but it is limited in scope (Knobf, 1986; Tarpy & Rothwell, 1983). Research efforts directed at symptom identification, from within a physiologic and psychological context of the endocrine system, are needed for this complex population of women. The occurrence of premature menopause with or without menopausal symptoms for the woman newly diagnosed and treated for breast cancer may compound her stress and adaptive challenges. The impact of the experience of menopausal symptoms and premature menopause warrants investigation to identify the scope of the problem, symptom distress, the outcome of interventions, and the effect on quality of life. Variables identified from the natural menopause research, such as psychological adjustment, marital satisfaction, functional ability, sleep deprivation, and sexuality, may be considered for clinical practice assessment and in the design of research. Longitudinal designs are recommended to capture the process of recovery and symptom patterns, and quality of life instruments can help us identify adaptation and adjustment (Knobf, Sexton, Fox, Lenox, Miano, & Donlick, 1994; Woods, 1988).

Other important areas of research for these women will be the long-term side effects of treatment, such as osteoporosis, and increase in cardiovascular risk due to decreased bone mineral density and changes in lipids as a consequence of menopause.

References

Aikin, J. L. (1994). Menopausal symptoms resulting from cancer therapies: Helping women cope. *Oncology Nursing Forum, 21*(2), 381.

Archer, D. F. (1982). Biochemical findings and medical management of the menopause. In A. M. Voda, M. Dinnerstein, & S. R. O'Donnell (Eds.), *Changing perspectives on menopause* (pp. 39–50). Austin: University of Texas Press.

Barbach, L. (1993). *The pause.* New York: Penguin Books.

Belchetz, P. E. (1994) Hormonal treatment of postmenopausal women. *New England Journal of Medicine, 330,* 1062–1072.

Bernhard, L. A., & Sheppard, L. (1992). Health, symptoms, self-care and dyadic adjustment in menopausal women. *Journal Obstetrics, Gynecology Neonatal Nursing, 22,* 456–461.

Bianco, A. R., DelMastro, L., Gallo, C., Perrone, F., Matano, E., Pagliarulo, C., & De Placido, S. (1991). Prognostic role of amenorrhea induced by adjuvant chemotherapy in premenopausal patients with early breast cancer. *British Journal of Cancer, 63,* 799–803.

Bieri, J. G., Corash, L., & Hubbard, V. S. (1983). Medical uses of Vitamin E. *New England Journal of Medicine , 308,* 1063–1071.

Blatt, M. H., Weisbader, H., & Kupperman, H. S. (1953). Vitamin E and the climacteric syndrome. *AMA-Archives Internal Medicine, 91,* 792–799.

Bonadonna, G., Valagussa, P., Rossi, A., Tancini, G., Brambilla, C., Zambetti, M., & Veronessi, U. (1985). Ten-year experience with CMF-based adjuvant chemotherapy in resectable breast cancer. *Breast Cancer Research & Treatment, 5,* 95–115.

Boring, C. C., Squires, T. S., Tong, T. & Montgomery, S. (1994). Cancer statistics 1994. *Ca—A Journal for Clinicians, 44,* 7–26.

Brinker, H., Rose, C., & Rank, F. (1987). Evidence of castration-mediated effect of adjuvant cytotoxic chemotherapy in premenopausal breast cancer. *Journal of Clinical Oncology 5,*1771–1778.

Buzzoni, R., Bajetta, E., Biganzoli, L., Zampino, M. G., Formasiero, A., Arcangell, G., Farina, G., Barni, S., Schieppaati, G., Celo, L., & Martinetti, A. (1994). Combined Goserelin plus Tamoxifen treatment in premenopausal advanced breast cancer. *Proceedings American Society Clinical Oncology, 13, 56.*

Chamorro, T. (1991). Gonadal and reproductive sequelae of cancer therapy. In S. M. Hubbard, P. M. Green, & M. T. Knobf (Eds.), *Current issues in cancer nursing practice* (pp. 1–15). Philadelphia: J. B. Lippincott.

Chang, R. J., Plouffe, L., & Schaeffer, K. (1994). Physiology of menopause. In J. Lorrain, L. Plouffe, V. Ravnikar, L. Speroff, & N. Watts, (Eds.), *Comprehensive management of menopause* (pp. 3–13). New York: Springer-Verlag.

Chapman, R. M., Sutcliffe, M. B., & Malpas, J. S. (1979). Cytotoxic-induced ovarian failure in women with Hodgkin's disease. *Journal American Medical Association, 242,* 1877–1881.

Chapman, R. M. (1982). Effect of cytotoxic therapy on sexuality and gonadal function. *Seminars in Oncology, 9,* 84–94.

Clayden, J. R., Bell, J. W., & Pollard, P. (1974), Menopausal flushing: Double blind trial of a non-hormonal medication. *British Medical Journal, 1,* 409–412.

Cobleigh, M. A., Bems, R. F., Bush, T., Davidson, N., Robert, N. J., Sparano, J. A., Tormey, D. C., & Wood, W. C. (1994). Estrogen replacement therapy in breast cancer survivors. *Journal of the American Medical Association 272* (7), 540–545.

Costlow, J., Lopez, M. C. & Taub, M. (1989). *Menopause: A selfcare manual.* Santa Fe, NM: Santa Fe Health Education Project.

Davidson, N. E., & Abeloff, M. A. (1992). Adjuvant systemic therapy for node negative breast cancer. In V. T. DeVita, S. Hellman, S. A. Rosenberg (Eds.), *PPO updates.* Philadelphia: J. B. Lippincott.

Derogotis, L. R. (1980). Breast and gyn cancers. *Frontiers Radiation Therapy & Oncology, 14,* 1–11.

Dickson, G. L. (1994). Fifty-something: A phenomenological study of the experience of menopause. In P. L. Murhall (Ed.), *Women's Experience* (pp. 117–157). New York: National League for Nursing Press.

Dosey, M. A., & Dosey, M. F. (1980). The climacteric woman. *Patient Counseling, 2,* 14–21.

Early Breast Cancer Trialists Collaborative Group. (1992a). Systemic treatment of early breast cancer by hormonal, cytotoxic or immune therapy, Part I. *Lancet, 339,* 2–15.

Early Breast Cancer Trailists Collaborative Group. (1992b). Systemic treatment of early breast cancer by hormonal, cytotoxic or immune therapy, Part II. *Lancet, 339,* 71–85.

Ehlke, G. A. (1988). Symptom distress in breast cancer patients receiving chemotherapy in the outpatient setting. *Oncology Nursing Forum, 15,* 343–346.

Erlik, Y., Meldrum, D. R., & Judd, H. L. (1982). Estrogen levels in postmenopausal women with hot flashes. *Obstetrics & Gynecology, 59,* 403–407.

Feldman, J. E. (1989). Ovarian failure and cancer treatment: Incidence and interventions for the premenopausal woman. *Oncology Nursing Forum, 16,* 651–657.

Feldman, B. M., Voda, A., & Gronseth, E. (1985). The prevalence of hot flash and associated variables among perimenopausal women. *Research Nursing & Health, 8,* 261–268.

Finney, K. P. (1992). Self-care in women with breast cancer: Adherence with self administered adjuvant therapy. *Oncology Nursing Forum, 19,* 292.

Fisher, B., Sherman, B., Rockette, H., Redmond, C., Margolese, R., & Fisher, E. (1979). l-Phenylalanine mustard (L-Pam) in the management of premenopausal patients with primary breast cancer. *Cancer, 44,* 847–857.

Fisher, B., Costantino, J., Redmond, C., Poisson, R., Bowman, D., Coutre, J., Dimitrov, N. V., Wolmark, N., Wickerham, D. L., Fisher, E., Margolese, R., Robideoux, A., Shibati, H., Terz, J., Paterson, A. H., Feldman, M. I., Farrar, W., Evans, J., Lickley, H. L., & Ketner, M. (1989). A randomized clinical trial evaluating tamoxifen in the treatment of patients with node-negative breast cancer who have estrogen receptor positive tumors. *New England Journal of Medicine, 320,* 479–484.

Fogel, C. I., & Woods, N. F. (1995). *Women's Health Care,* Thousand Oaks, CA: Sage Publications.

Frey, F. (1981). Middle aged women's experiences and perceptions of menopause. *Women & Health, 6,* 25–36.

Gambrell, R. D. (1995). Hormone replacement therapy in patients with previous breast cancer. *Menopause 2(2),* 55–57.

Gershenson, D. M. (1988). Menstrual and reproductive function after treatment with combination chemotherapy for malignant ovarian germ cell tumors. *Journal of Clinical Oncology, 6,* 270–275.

Glazer, G., & Rozman, A. S. (1991). Marital adjustment, life stress, attitudes toward menopause and menopausal symptoms in premenopausal, menopausal and postmenopausal women. In D. L. Taylor, N. F. Woods (Eds.), *Menstruation, health and illness* (pp. 237–243). New York: Hemisphere Publishing.

Goldberg, R. M., Loprinzi, C. L., Gerstner, J., Miser, A., O'Fallon, J., Mailliard, J., Michalak, J., & Dose, A. M. (1992). Prospective trial of transdermal clonidine in breast cancer patients (pts) suffering from Tamoxifen-induced hot flashes (hf): A Mayo Clinic and North Central Cancer Treatment Group Trial. *Proceedings American Society Clinical Oncology, 11,* 378.

Goldhirsh, A., Gelber, R. D., & Castiglione, M. (1990). The magnitude of endocrine effects of adjuvant chemotherapy for premenopausal breast cancer patients. *Annals of Oncology, 1,* 183–188.

Goodman, M. J. (1982). A critique of menopause research. In A. M. Voda, M. Dinnerstein, & S. R. O'Donnell (Eds.), *Changing perspectives on menopause* (pp. 273–288). Austin: University of Texas Press.

Goodman, H. M. (1994). *Basic medical endocrinology,* 2nd ed. New York: Raven Press.

Greene, J. G. (1976). A factor analytic study of climacteric symptoms. *Journal of Psychosomatic Research, 20,* 425–430.

Greene, D., Nail, L., Fieler, V. K., Dudgen, D., & Jones, L. S. (1994). A comparison of patient reported side effects during three chemotherapy regimens for breast cancer. *Cancer Practice, 2,* 57–62.

Greenwood, S. (1984). *Menopause naturally.* San Francisco: Volcano Press.

Hatcher, R. A., Stewart, F., Trussell, J., Kowal, D., Guest, F., Stewart, G. K., & Cates, W. (1994). *Contraceptive technology,* 16th revised ed. New York: Irvington Publishers, Inc.

Headley, J. A. (1994). Chemotherapy-induced ovarian dysfunction in women with breast cancer. *Oncology Nursing Forum, 21,* 378 (abstract).

Holte, A., & Mikklesen, A. (1991). Psychosocial determinants of climacteric complaints. *Maturitas, 13,* 205–215.

Horning, S. J., et al. (1981). Female reproductive potential after treatment for Hodgkin's disease. *New England Journal of Medicine, 304,* 1377–1382.

Hull, M. (1993). Breast cancer experiences of premenopausal women. *Oncology Nursing Forum, 20,* 326 (abstract).

Huddleston, D. S., & McElmurray, B. J. (1990). The natural menopause. In C. J. Leppa (Ed.), *Women's health perspectives:An annual review* (Vol 3, pp 210–228). Phoenix, AZ: Oryx Press.

Hunter, M., Battersby, R., & Whitehead, M. (1986). Relationships between psychological symptoms, somatic complaints and menopausal status. *Maturitas, 8,* 217–228.

Jordan, V. C. (1990). Long term adjuvant tamoxifen therapy for breast cancer. *Breast Cancer Research & Treatment, 15,* 125–136.

Kaufert, P., & Syrotuik, P. (1981). Symptom reporting at the menopause. *Social Science & Medicine, 15E,* 173–184.

Knobf, M. T. (1986). Physical and psychological distress associated with adjuvant chemotherapy in women with breast cancer. *Journal of Clinical Oncology, 4,* 678–684.

Knobf, M. T. (1990). Symptoms and rehabilitation needs of patients with early stage breast cancer during primary therapy. *Cancer, 66,* 1392–1401.

Knobf, M. T., Sexton, D. S., Fox, J., Lenox, R., Miano, T., & Donlick, T. (1994). Quality of life in women with breast cancer receiving adjuvant therapy. New Haven, CT: Yale University. (Research in progress.)

Koyama, H., Wada, T., Nishizawa, Y., Iwanaga, T., Aoki, Y., Kosaki, G., Yamamoto, T., & Wada, A. (1977). Cyclophosphamide-induced ovarian failure and its therapeutic significance in patients with breast cancer. *Cancer, 39,* 1403–1409.

Kronenberg, F. (1990). Hot flashes: Epidemiology and physiology. *Annals of the New York Academy of Sciences, 592,* 156–161.

Kronenberg, F. (1995). Alternative therapies: New opportunities for menopausal research. *Menopause 2 (1),* 1–2.

Kronenberg, F., Hudson, T., & Lark, S. (1995). Alternative treatments for menopausal symptoms. Presented at the North American Menopause Society's 6th Annual Meeting, September 21–23, 1995, San Francisco.

Landau, C., Cyr, M. G. & Moulton, A. W. (1994). *The complete book of menopause.* New York: Grosset/Putnam Books.

Legha, S. S. (1988). Tamoxifen in the treatment of breast cancer. *Annals of Internal Medicine, 109,* 219–228.

La Rocca, S., & Polit, D. (1980). Women's knowledge about menopause. *Nursing Research, 29,* 10–13.

Loprinzi, C. L., Michalak, C., Quella, S. K., O'Fallon, J. R., Hatfield, A. K., & Oesterling, J. E. (1994). Placebo controlled clinical trial of megesterol acetate (MA) in ameliorating hot flashes in both men and women: A North Central Cancer Treatment Group Study. *Proceedings of the American Society of Clinical Oncology, 13,* 432.

Lorrain, J., Ravnikar, V. A., & Charest, N. (1994). Peri- and postmenopausal abnormal bleeding. In J. Lorrain, L. Plouffe, V. Ravnikar, L. Speroff, & N. Watts (Eds.), *Comprehensive management of menopause* (pp. 3–13). New York: Springer-Verlag.

Love, R. R., Leventhal, H., Easterling, D. V., & Nerenz, D. R. (1989). Side effects and emotional distress during cancer chemotherapy. *Cancer, 63,* 604–612.

Maddox, M. A. (1992). Women at midlife. Hormone replacement therapy. *Nursing Clinics of North America, 27,* 959–969.

Maguire, G. P., et al. (1980). Psychiatric morbidity and physical toxicity associated with adjuvant chemotherapy after mastectomy. *British Journal of Medicine, 281,* 1179–1180.

McElmurray, B. J., & Huddleston, D. S. (1991). Perimenopausal women: Using women's stories as a theoretical underpinning for women's health. In D. L. Taylor & N. F. Woods (Eds.), *Menstruation, health & illness* (pp. 213–222). New York: Hemisphere Publishing.

McKinlay, S. M., Brambilla, D. J., & Posner, J. G. (1992). The normal menopause transition. *Maturitas, 14,* 102–115.

Mehta, R. R., Beattie, C. W., & DasGupta, T. K. (1991). Endocrine profile in breast cancer patients receiving adjuvant chemotherapy. *Breast Cancer Research & Treatment, 20,* 125–134.

Mooney, K., Nail, L., Richtsmeier, J. & Ward, J. (1994). Symptom and symptom distress associated with taking Tamoxifen as chemoprevention for breast cancer. *Proceedings of the American Cancer Society Third Nursing Research Conference.* Atlanta: American Cancer Society.

Mortimer, J. E., Knapp, D., Fracasso, P. M., Rowland, J. H., & Kornblith, A. (1994). Assessment of sexual function in women on Tamoxifen. *Proceedings of the American Society of Clinical Oncology, 13,* 450.

Nachtigall, L. E. (1994). Comparative Study: Replens versus local estrogen in menopausal women. *Fertility Sterility, 61* (1), 178–180.

Nagamani, M., Kelver, M., & Smith, E. R. (1987). Treatment of menopausal hot flashes with transdermal administration of clonidine. *American Journal of Obstetrics & Gynecology, 156,* 581–565.

Nerenz, D. R., Leventhal, H., & Love, R. R. (1982). Factors contributing to emotional distress during cancer chemotherapy. *Cancer, 50,* 1020–1027.

Neugarten, B. L., & Kraines, R. J. (1965). "Menopausal symptoms" in women of various ages. *Psychosomatic Medicine, 27,* 266–273.

Plowman, P. N. (1988). Treatment of menopausal symptoms in breast cancer patients. *Lancet,* 164.

Polit, D. F., & La Rocca, S. A. (1980). Social and psychological correlates of menopausal symptoms. *Psychosomatic Medicine, 42,* 335–345.

Quinn, A. A. (1991). A theoretical model of the perimenopausal process. *Journal of Nurse-Midwifery, 36,* 25–29.

Ravdin, P. M., Fritz, N. F., Tormey, D. C., & Jordan, V. C. (1988). Endocrine status of premenopausal node-positive breast cancer patients following adjuvant chemotherapy and long term tamoxifen. *Cancer Research, 48,* 1026–1029.

Rausch, J. L. (1994). Psychobiological aspects of the menopause. In J. Lorrain, L. Plouffe, V. Ravnikar, I. Speroff, & N. Watts (Eds.), *Comprehensive management of menopause* (pp 318–326). New York: Springer-Verlag.

Reyno, L. M., Levine, M. N., Skingley, P., Arnold, A., & AbuZara, H. (1992) Chemotherapy induced amenorrhea in a randomised trial of adjuvant chemotherapy duration in breast cancer. *European Journal of Cancer, 29A,* 21–23.

Ringer, K. E. (1983). *Coping with chemotherapy.* Ann Arbor: UMI Research.

Rivkees, S. A., & Crawford, J. D. (1988). The relationship of gonadal activity and chemotherapy-induced gonadal damage. *Journal of the American Medical Association, 259,* 2123–2125.

Rose, D. P., & Davis, T. E. (1977). Ovarian function in patients receiving adjuvant chemotherapy for breast cancer. *Lancet, 1,* 174–176.

Rose, D. P., & Davis, T. E. (1980). Effects of adjuvant chemohormonal therapy on the ovarian and adrenal function of breast cancer patients. *Cancer Research, 40,* 4043–4047.

Roy, J. A., Pritchard, K. I., Sawka, C. A., & Franssen, E. (1994). A prospective cohort study to assess menopausal symptomatology and its impact on quality of life in women with breast cancer. *Proceedings of the American Society of Clinical Oncology, 13,* 81.

Samaan, N. A., et al. (1987). Pituitary-ovarian function in breast cancer patients on adjuvant chemoimmunotherapy. *Cancer, 41,* 2084–2087.

Sands, R., Boshoff, C., Jones, A., & Studd, J. (1995). Current opinion: Hormone replacement therapy after a diagnosis of breast cancer. *Menopause, 2* (2) 73–80.

Santen, R. J., Manni, A., & Harvey, H. (1986). Gonadotropin releasing hormone (GnRH) analogs for the treatment of breast and prostatic carcinoma. *Breast Cancer Research & Treatment, 7,* 129–145.

Santen, R. J., Manni, A., Harvey, H., & Redmond, C. (1990). Endocrine treatment of breast cancer in women. *Endocrine Reviews, 11,* 1–45.

Schilsky, R.L. Lewis, B. J., Sherins, M. D, Young, R. C. (1980) Gonadal dysfunction in patients receiving chemoth.erapy for cancer. *Annals of Internal Medicine, 93,* 109–114.

Schover, L. (1991). The impact of breast cancer on sexuality, body image and intimate relationships. *Ca-A Journal for Clinicians, 41,* 112–120.

Sherman, B. M., Wallace, R. B., Bean, J. A., Chang, Y., & Schalabaugh, L. (1981). The relationship of menopausal hot flashes to medical and reproductive experience. *Journal of Gerontology, 36,* 306–309.

Sinsheimer, L., & Holland, J. C. (1987). Psychological issues in breast cancer. *Seminars in Oncology, 14,* 75–82.

Speroff, L., Glass, R. H., & Kase, N. G. (1994). *Clinical gynecologic endocrinology and infertility,* 5th ed. Baltimore: Williams & Wilkins.

Tarpy, C., & Rothwell, S. (1983). Menses and related menopausal symptomatology of the breast cancer patient on chemotherapy. *Proceedings of the Oncology Nursing Society,* 50 (abstract).

Tormey, D. C., Taylor, S. G., Kalish, L. A., Olsen, J. E., Grage, T. & Gray, R. (1984). Adjuvant systemic therapy in premenopausal and postmenopausal women with node positive breast cancer. In S. E. Jones & S. E. Salmon (Eds.), *Adjuvant chemotherapy of cancer IV* (pp. 359–368). Orlando, FL: Grune & Stratton.

Treolar, A. E. (1982). Predicting the close of menstrual life. In A.M. Voda, M. Dennerstein, & S. R. O'Donnell (Eds.), *Changing perspectives on menopause* (pp. 289–306). Austin, TX: University of Texas Press.

Uphold, C. R., & Susman, E. J. (1981). Self-reported climacteric symptoms as a function of the relationship between marital adjustment and child rearing stage. *Nursing Research, 30,* 84–88.

Utian, W. H. (1980a). The etiology of menopause. In *Menopause in modern perspective. A guide to clinical practice* (pp. 11–23). New York: Appleton Century Crofts.

Utian, W. H. (1980b). Endocrinology of climacteric.In *Menopause in modern perspective. A guide to clinical practice* (pp. 25–33). New York: Appleton Century Crofts.

Utian, W. H. (1980c). Symptom formation. In *Menopause in modern perspective. A guide to clinical practice* (pp. 105–119). New York: Appleton Century Crofts.

Utian, W. H. (1980d). Target tissue response to ovarian failure. In *Menopause in modern perspective. A guide to clinical practice* (pp. 47–61). New York: Appleton Century Crofts.

Utian, W. H. (1990). The menopause in perspective. From potions to patches. *Annals of the New York Academy of Sciences, 592,* 1–7.

Varricchio, C. G., & Johnson K. A. (1993). The use of Tamoxifen in the prevention and treatment of breast cancer. In S. M. Hubbard, P. M. Greene, & M. T. Knobf (Eds.), *Current issues in cancer nursing practice* (pp. 1–10). Philadelphia: J. B. Lippincott.

Voda, A. M. (1981). Climacteric hot flash. *Maturitas, 3,* 73–90.

Voda, A. M., & George, T. (1986). Menopause. In H. H. Werley, J. J. Fitzpatrick, & R. L. Taunton (Eds.), *Annual review of nursing research* (pp. 55–75). New York: Springer-Verlag.

Walsh, B., & Schiff, I. (1990). Vasomotor flushes. *New York Academy of Sciences, 592,* 346–356.

Wingo, P. A., Tong, T., & Bolden, S. (1995). Cancer statistics 1995. *CA-A Journal for Clinicians, 45,* 8–30.

Woods, N. F. (1982). Menopausal distress. A model for epidemiologic investigation. In A. M. Voda, M. Dennerstein, & S. R. O'Donnell (Eds.), *Changing perspectives on menopause* (pp. 220–247). Austin, TX: University of Texas Press.

Woods, N. F. (1988). Women's health. In J. J. Fitzpatrick, R. L. Taunton, J. Q. Benoliel (Eds.), *Annual review of nursing research* (pp. 209–236). New York: Springer-Verlag.

Yanes, B., Ross, S., & Yanes, B. S. (1987). Treatment of hot flashes in patients with breast cancer. *Proceedings of the American Society of Clinical Oncology, 6,* 269.

Young, R. L., Kumar, N. S., & Goldzieher, J. W. (1990). Management of menopause when estrogen cannot be used. *Drugs, 40,* 220–230.

Young-McCaughan, S. (1995). Sexual functioning in women treated with chemoendocrine therapy for breast cancer. *Oncology Nursing Forum 22(2),* 371.

CHAPTER 8 | The Benefits of Exercise in Women with Breast Cancer

Victoria Mock, DNSc, RN, OCN

The sequelae of breast cancer treatment may be both distressful and long-lasting. Primary surgical treatment may lead to limited range of motion and lymphedema of the affected upper extremities. Radiation therapy following conservative surgical treatment is often accompanied by intense fatigue and may result in a slow, progressive tightening of the affected shoulder postradiation. Pneumonitis is a long-term complication of chest irradiation, which may involve respiratory compromise. Adjuvant cytotoxic chemotherapy commonly causes distressing side effects such as fatigue, nausea, vomiting, insomnia, weight gain, skin changes, and mucositis. With increasing acknowledgment of the therapeutic benefits of adjuvant chemotherapy in the early stages of breast cancer, this treatment is being recommended for larger numbers of patients. Furthermore, as chemotherapy protocols have become more intense, with combinations of high-dose toxic drugs, side effects have also become more intense.

Both the distressing side effects of treatments for breast cancer and inactivity secondary to treatment can impair functional status, decrease independence, and affect quality of life. Being able to maintain or resume usual roles and activities is an important aspect of a patient's quality of life. An individual's natural response to feeling fatigued or nauseated is to decrease physical activity. This consistent decrease in the level of activities of daily living over time reduces a patient's functional capacity and makes her less able to tolerate exercise and normal activity.

BENEFICIAL EFFECTS OF EXERCISE

Exercise is defined as deliberate physical activity or work of any type, intensity, or duration, undertaken to elicit a beneficial or therapeutic response. It involves muscle strength, flexibility, and endurance. Aerobic exercise uses large muscle groups in rhythmic, repetitive motions that promote cardiopulmonary endurance or fitness. Walking, jogging, swimming, and biking are some forms of aerobic exercise.

The physical and psychological benefits of exercise are well established. Indeed, physical activity can contribute significantly to the overall well-being and quality of life in midlife women (Gilliss & Perry, 1991). In older women, exercise may improve bone density, glucose tolerance, and balance (Topp, 1991). Meaningful improvements in fitness and disease risk profile are possible even with less than vigorous regular exercise in women (Duncan, Gordon, & Scott, 1991).

There is a potential psychosocial and physiological advantage in regular exercise that increases fitness. A review of 34 studies involving 1,449 subjects investigated the relationship between the aerobic fitness of subjects and their reactions to psychosocial stressors (Crews & Landers, 1987). Using meta-analytic techniques, the reviewers concluded that aerobically fit subjects had significantly reduced stress responses compared with either control groups or baseline measures for subjects.

In addition to the general benefits of increased endurance, lower heart rate and blood pressure, and greater muscle strength, exercise has other potential benefits for women with breast cancer. A walking exercise program has been shown to decrease fatigue and improve sleep patterns in women receiving adjuvant chemotherapy (Mock et al., 1994). Regular exercise may moderate the weight gain that often accompanies adjuvant chemotherapy.

For women with breast cancer, a fitness program that includes aerobic exercise offers the benefits of decreased risk of developing cardiovascular disease and osteoporosis, as well as providing rehabilitation for the effects of their disease and its treatment. Because treatment for breast cancer often results in a decrease in natural or exogenous sources of estrogen, these women face a greater risk of developing cardiovascular disease and osteoporosis.

Regular exercisers also report less nausea during chemotherapy (Mock et al., 1994; Winningham & MacVicar, 1988). For individuals experiencing the stress of a cancer diagnosis and treatment, an important benefit of exercise is an increased level of psychological well-being, with decreased anxiety and depression.

REVIEW OF RESEARCH ON EXERCISE IN WOMEN WITH BREAST CANCER

There is little published data on the effects of exercise on cancer patients. However, several of these studies involve women with breast cancer. A retrospective investigation of the relationship between aerobic exercise and quality of life in women with breast cancer compared 42 women who exercised with 29 matched controls who did not exercise (Young-McCaughan & Sexton, 1991). Women who exercised had a significantly higher quality of life. However, this sample included only three women receiving adjuvant chemotherapy and none receiving radiotherapy. The researchers concluded that regular exercise plays a role in physical and psychological rehabilitation from the effects of cancer.

An exercise rehabilitation program for women with breast cancer, described by the acronym STRETCH (Strength Through Recreation Exercise Togetherness Care Help), was evaluated. The 8-week program combined exercise to promote muscle strengthening with flexibility with group discussion (Gaskin, LoBuglio, Kelly, Doss, & Pizitz, 1989). Results indicated improved range of motion and posture as well as psychosocial benefits for the women in the program.

MacVicar, Winningham, and Nickel (1989) reported a 10-week rehabilitation program for 45 women with stage II breast cancer, who were on chemotherapy. In the experimental group, moderate aerobic activity on exercise bicycles increased functional capacity and moderated gains in body fat, compared with controls (Winningham, MacVicar, Bondoc,

Anderson, & Minton, 1989). Exercisers also had significantly less nausea (Winningham & MacVicar, 1988).

Johnson and Kelly (1990) implemented a multifaceted rehabilitation program for 12 women with breast cancer, which included a personal fitness plan, aerobic exercise classes, journal writing, and a 6-day wilderness experience. Evaluation of this pilot project by means of the subjects' journals revealed feelings of improved quality of life, fostered by the health-promoting behaviors included in the program and its positive orientation to living with cancer. No objective measurements of physiologic or psychosocial outcomes were reported.

The recent report of a preliminary study (Mock et al., 1994) evaluated the effects of regular walking, as part of a comprehensive rehabilitation program, on women with breast cancer receiving outpatient adjuvant chemotherapy. In an experimental design, nine women participated in the rehabilitation walking program and a support group, while five women in the control arm received the usual care with no structured exercise or support group.

The exercise component included a self-paced, progressive program of walking four to five times per week for 20 to 45 minutes in the subject's neighborhood. Physical performance increased over the program of chemotherapy in the rehabilitation group, while the control group reported a decrease in their usual level of physical activity. Distance walked on the posttest was significantly greater in the rehabilitation group, an important finding in such a small sample. In addition, comparison of the groups indicated significantly lower symptom intensity for the rehabilitation group on fatigue, nausea, depression, and insomnia. No walkers appeared to suffer any physical injury or bleeding episodes as a result of the walking program.

Continuing investigation by Mock and Dow (1994) of a walking exercise program for women with breast cancer includes subjects receiving radiation therapy following conservative surgery, as well as those on adjuvant chemotherapy. Although the research is still in progress, early indications show improved physical performance in the exercise group. This study evaluates the effects of exercise on these women's symptom intensity, quality of life, and adaptation to breast cancer.

The research reported to date on the effect of exercise on women with breast cancer is obviously limited, and the need for additional research is clear. However, the results of these studies indicate the important potential contribution of exercise to the rehabilitation of this population.

HELPING WOMEN TO DEVELOP AND MAINTAIN AN EXERCISE PROGRAM

For women with breast cancer, exercise carries great potential benefits and a few important risks. Health professionals can minimize the clearly identifiable hazards to patients by carefully following a few general guidelines.

Although it is not within the scope of this work to present all of the information needed by clinicians to conduct an exercise rehabilitation program for women with breast cancer, some guidelines are included. Many references on exercise are readily available—both those written for the education of health professionals and those written for exercisers themselves. A number of these have specific information on exercise for cancer patients—such as the chapter by Hicks in *Therapeutic Exercise* (1990). One helpful guide for walkers is the booklet *Rhythmic Walking—Exercise for People Living with Cancer* (Winningham, Glass, & MacVicar, 1990), used in the studies of rehabilitation exercise for women with breast cancer reported by Mock et al. (1994) and Mock and Dow (1994). The guidelines move beyond the traditional arm and shoulder exercises recommended for women recovering from surgery for breast cancer to present to these women a more comprehensive approach toward physical fitness as part of a healthy lifestyle.

Screening for Participation

It is essential to screen patients before recommending an exercise program and to tailor the exercise program to meet the individual's level of physical fitness, age, stage or extent of disease, current treatment type, and the presence of other alterations in general health. Women who are over 45, in current treatment for cancer, or who have other concurrent diseases—especially cardiovascular, respiratory, musculoskeletal, or renal—should be carefully evaluated by a physician before beginning an active exercise program. A heart rate-monitored exercise test may be indicated for those patients whose health profiles suggest possible risk.

The current fitness and activity level of the individual is also important. However, even patients with significant disability can benefit from muscle strengthening, range of motion, and flexibility exercises. Individuals with concommitant major health problems or significant functional limitations should be referred to a physical therapist or physician who specializes in rehabilitation medicine. These individuals should be in a carefully prescribed and supervised program.

Individualize the Program

Another important guideline for clinicians is to individualize the exercise program for each woman with breast cancer. Many women were regular exercisers before their breast cancer diagnosis and have a high fitness level. Others may have been relatively sedentary all their lives and require a more modest program that can be adjusted as their fitness level improves. It is essential to teach all cancer patients to monitor their bodies' responses to an exercise program and to consult with their nurse or physician if they experience any of the symptoms listed in Figure 8-1. All individuals, regardless of their current level of fitness, can benefit from an activity program tailored to meet their special needs, interests, and lifestyle.

The Exercise Prescription

A good general exercise program for cancer patients begins with range of motion (ROM)/flexibility exercises and muscle strengthening, to maximize joint ROM and muscle endurance. This is followed by submaximal aerobic exercise to enhance cardiopulmonary endurance (Hicks, 1990). Following surgery for breast cancer, it is important to address potential functional limitations in the affected shoulder girdle. Specific postoperative shoulder and upper extremity exercise programs vary according to the surgeon and hospital protocol. Some programs begin early in the postop period, and others are not implemented until the surgical wound is fully healed.

The three basic components of any exercise program are frequency, intensity, and duration. Frequency involves the number of exercises performed or number of walks per week. Beginning exercisers should be advised to exercise 4 to 6 days per week, not skipping more than 1 day in a row, and being certain to take 1 rest day every week. It is better to exercise for more frequent short time periods than to exercise for longer periods, but less frequently.

Intensity refers to how difficult the exercise is, difficulty being determined by the heart rate. Women in an exercise program should be taught to take their pulse for 60 seconds while resting, to assess rate and rhythm. During exercise, the peak pulse just before the cool-down period is best measured by counting the pulse for 6 seconds and multiplying by 10. Because the pulse drops quickly when the individual stops exercising to measure it, the 6-second monitoring check best captures the peak pulse rate. As an intensity guide, rating of perceived exertion is a helpful adjunct to heart rate. The Perceived Exertion Scale is valid in cases where the pa-

Figure 8-1   Exercise Prescription During Breast Cancer Treatment

Name:

Age: 50

Breast Cancer Stage: II

Medical History: moderately active; no major health problems

Treatment Protocol: lumpectomy, radiation therapy—6 weeks; CAF (cytoxan, adriamycin, 5-fluorouracil), 6 cycles

Exercise Program

Frequency: 4 times a week minimum; 6 times a week maximum

Intensity: 60% to 70% of target heart rate = 100–120 beats/minute

Duration: self-paced brisk walking 10–30 minutes, progressive as tolerated

Exercise Routine

1. 15 minutes—flexibility and strengthening exercises as prescribed
2. 5 minutes; slow walking warm-up
3. 10–30 minutes; brisk walking (training)
4. 5 minutes; slow walking cool-down

Stop exercises and seek medical advice if any of the following symptoms occur:

Bleeding from any source	Prolonged fatigue
Chest, arm, or jaw pain	Muscle weakness
Irregular heart beat	Muscle/joint pain or swelling
Nausea/vomiting during exercise	Dizziness or fainting
Fever	

tient is on beta-adrenergic drugs and the pulse is not appropriate as a guide.

Duration.   The length of the exercise period is initially determined by the usual activity level of the individual. For someone who has not been exercising because of illness, surgery, or other treatment, it is best to begin very gradually with a 5- or 10-minute brisk walk, always beginning and ending with several minutes of slow walking to warm up and to cool down.

A journal or exercise diary maintained by the patient can assist the clinician in monitoring responses to exercise and in adjusting the exercise prescription as needed. Figure 8-1 is an example of an individual exercise program prescribed for a woman with breast cancer in adjuvant treatment.

Precautions.   Attention to a few important precautions can help ensure a safe and comfortable exercise program. Walkers and joggers should wear comfortable, supportive shoes made specifically for walking or running and should exercise in safe areas. Carrying an emergency card and exercising with a partner are helpful precautions. Dehydration is a potential hazard in hot weather, and patients should be taught the importance of adequate fluid balance.

Patients receiving adjuvant cytotoxic chemotherapy need careful supervision during their therapy, especially if their drug regimen includes potentially cardiotoxic drugs such as doxorubicin (St. Pierre, Kasper, & Lindsey, 1992). Some degree of activity intolerance is a common side effect of cytotoxic chemotherapy. There is preliminary evidence that an exercise program may reduce or reverse this loss of function (MacVicar, Winningham, & Nickel, 1989; Mock et al., 1994).

Individual responses to similar chemotherapy regimens are highly variable. Some women respond to an intensive chemotherapy protocol with nausea, fatigue, anorexia, stomatitis, diarrhea, and episodic vomiting, while other women on the same protocol experience only noticeable fatigue for several hours following the infusion. Obviously, the former patient needs more supervision for symptom management, electrolyte imbalance, and hypovolemia. She also needs guidance in modifying her exercise program to be consistent with her health state, so that there is safe provision for minimal loss of function and for early restoration.

There are a few specific contraindications to exercise for cancer patients (Hicks, 1990):

1. Do not exercise on the days of intravenous chemotherapy administration.
2. Do not exercise before blood drawing to check laboratory values.
3. Do not exercise if any of the following laboratory values are present:
   - White blood cell count less than 3,000 mm³
   - Absolute granulocyte count less than 2,500 mm³
   - Hemoglobin/hematocrit less than 10g/dl/25%
   - Platelet count less than 25,000 mm³
4. Do not exercise if metastatic bone involvement of greater than 25% of cortex.

In addition to these situations, high-impact aerobics are contraindicated during chemotherapy and in recurrent disease. Patients should not exercise if they have a fever, and

should resume exercise carefully following illness, surgery, or new treatment protocols.

Encouraging Adherence. Adhering to an exercise regimen is a challenge for healthy individuals, and may be particularly difficult for those weakened by their disease and treatment. It is estimated that in most exercise programs, over 50% of exercisers drop out in the first 6 months (Allan, 1993).

Because exercise is a learned behavior, the first goal should be to establish the *habit* of exercise, even before efforts are directed toward a training effect. Because the ultimate goal is to produce a permanent lifestyle change, health care professionals should incorporate effective behavioral strategies to encourage adherence to a lifetime fitness program (Martin, 1989).

Some important considerations for improving a patient's adherence to an exercise program are motivation, scheduling, and the exercise program itself. Women with breast cancer are often highly motivated to do whatever they can to improve their health state, ease their course through therapy, and decrease the risk of recurrence. Health care professionals can take advantage of this high level of motivation to teach these women the benefits of a regular exercise program. Regular reinforcement by supportive friends and family members, as well as by members of the health care team, can help sustain the patient's commitment. An exercise diary offers a patient the reward of seeing her progress over time and may help reinforce the habit. Exercising with a committed friend or family member can help sustain her efforts. Some individuals prefer group exercise, and find that this enhances their adherence.

The form of exercise prescribed should be one the individual enjoys. Walking, jogging, swimming, and biking are all effective means of improving fitness.

Scheduling the exercise period as a part of a woman's daily activities, at a convenient time and location, often improves her adherence to the program and helps her to develop a life-long habit. Walking in her own neighborhood at a regularly scheduled time—before breakfast is a commonly preferred time—removes barriers to exercise such as travel time, parking problems, and expensive gymnasium fees. In very cold or hot, humid weather, walking in a shopping mall before the stores open can be a safe and comfortable alternative. Many malls encourage walkers, and even designate quarter mile markers on the walls.

The exercise program itself should be self-paced, to allow for periods of decreased performance due to effects of disease or treatment, and modest enough for the individual to feel successful. Nothing discourages continued efforts more than an intensive program that leaves an individual feeling sore and exhausted. How much better it is, physically and psychologically, for an individual to begin at a very modest level, to advance steadily as her strength and endurance improve, and to feel good about observable progress.

In summary, the most helpful rehabilitation program for women diagnosed with breast cancer is one that can be easily modified to meet changing needs during periods of surgery, radiation therapy, adjuvant treatment, and recurrent disease. Such a program is best developed and implemented by teams of experts in breast cancer treatment, exercise physiology, physical therapy, radiotherapy, and oncology nursing practice. Although this chapter has focused on physical exercise as important in rehabilitation, a *comprehensive* program might also offer support groups designed specifically for women with breast cancer; family and marital counseling; referrals for individual psychotherapy; and the program Reach to Recovery, to provide options for psychosocial rehabilitation as well.

SUMMARY

Current multimodal treatment regimens involving surgery, radiotherapy, and chemotherapy have resulted in increased survival for women with breast cancer. However, the intensity of these treatments may cause changes in functional status which threaten the quality of life of these patients. An exercise program that strengthens weakened muscles and increases endurance has the potential to improve functional status and quality of life.

Oncology nurses can facilitate the rehabilitation of women with breast cancer by encouraging exercise as a health-promoting lifestyle behavior.

References

Allan, J. D. (1993). Exercise program. In G. M. Bulechek & J. C. McCloskey (Eds.), *Nursing interventions—essential nursing treatments*, 2nd ed, pp. 406–424. Philadelphia: W. B. Saunders.

Crews, D. J., & Landers, D. M. (1987). A meta-analytic review of aerobic fitness and reactivity to psychosocial stressors. *Medicine and Science in Sports and Exercise, 19* (5), 5114–5120.

Dudas, S. (1984). Rehabilitation concepts of nursing. *Journal of Enterostomal Therapy, 11* (1), 6–18.

Dudas, S., & Carlson, C. E. (1988). Cancer rehabilitation. *Oncology Nursing Forum, 15*, 183–188.

Duncan, J. J., Gordon, N. F., & Scott, C. B. (1991). Women walking for health and fitness. How much is enough? *Journal of the American Medical Association, 266*, 23, 3295–3295.

Gaskin, T. A., LoBuglio, A., Kelly, P., Doss, M., & Pizitz, N. (1989). STRETCH: A rehabilitation program for patients with breast cancer. *Southern Medical Journal 82*, 467–469.

Gilliss, A. A., & Perry, A. (1991). The relationship between physical activity and health-promoting behaviors in mid-life women. *Journal of Advanced Nursing, 16*, 299–310.

Hicks, J. E. (1990). Exercise for cancer patients. In J. V. Basmajiian & S. L. Wolfe (Eds.)., *Therapeutic exercise*, 5th ed. Baltimore: Williams & Wilkins.

Johnson, J. B., & Kelly, A. W. (1990). A multifaceted rehabilitation program for women with cancer. *Oncology Nursing Forum, 17*, 691–695.

MacVicar, M. G., Winningham, M. L., & Nickel, J. L. (1989). Effects of aerobic interval training on cancer patients' functional capacity. *Nursing Research, 38*, 348–351.

Martin, J. E. (1989). Strategies to enhance patient exercise compliance. In B. A. Franklin, S. Gordon, & G. C. Timmis (Eds.). *Exercise in modern medicine*. Baltimore: Williams & Wilkins.

Mock, V., & Dow, K. H. (1994). An exercise rehabilitation program for women in treatment for breast cancer. *Oncology Nursing Forum, 22*, 370.

Mock, V., Burke, M. B., Sheehan, P., Creaton, E. M., Winningham, M. L., McKenney-Tedder, S., Schwager,

L. P., Liebman, M. (1994). A nursing rehabilitation program for women with breast cancer receiving adjuvant chemotherapy. *Oncology Nursing Forum, 21*, 899–908.

St. Pierre, B. A., Kasper, C. E., & Lindsey, A. M. (1992). Fatigue mechanisms in patients with cancer: Effects of tumor necrosis factor and exercise on skeletal muscle. *Oncology Nursing Forum, 19*, 419–425.

Topp, R. (1991). Development of an exercise program for older adults: Pre-exercise testing, exercise prescription, and program maintenance. *Nurse Practitioner 16* (10), 16–27.

Watson, P. G. (1992). The optimal functioning plan: A key element in cancer rehabilitation. *Cancer Nursing, 15*, 254–263.

Winningham, M. L. (1991). Walking program for people with cancer—getting started. *Cancer Nursing, 14*, 270–276.

Winningham, M. L., Glass, E. C., & MacVicar, M. G. (1990). *Rhythmic walking—exercise for people living with cancer.* Columbus, OH: James Cancer Hospital and Research Institute, Ohio State University.

Winningham, M. L., MacVicar, M. G., Bondoc, M., Anderson, J. I., & Minton, J. P. (1989). Effect of aerobic exercise on body weight and composition in patients with breast cancer on adjuvant chemotherapy. *Oncology Nursing Forum, 16*, 683–688.

Winningham, M. L., & MacVicar, M. G. (1988). The effects of aerobic exercise on patient reports of nausea. *Oncology Nursing Forum, 15*, 447–450.

Young-McCaughan, S., & Sexton, D. L. (1991). A retrospective investigation of the relationship between aerobic exercise and quality of life in women with breast cancer. *Oncology Nursing Forum, 18*, 751–757.

CHAPTER 9 | Depression in Women with Breast Cancer

Beverly Brandt, RN, MSN

A diagnosis of breast cancer commonly produces mild depressive symptoms in patients, caused by their fear of dying and anticipatory anxiety and grief. Sadness and grief are normal psychological responses for persons faced with either a threatened or an actual loss. Women with stable personalities, who have adapted well to previous life crises, usually adapt well to a diagnosis of breast cancer and are able to manage their distress. However, other women are not able to adjust well to the reality of their illness.

Depressive symptoms range from mild to severe, from normal states of sadness to clinical syndromes, such as an adjustment disorder with depressed mood, or a major depression. While this psychological phenomenon is certainly not unique to women with breast cancer, this chapter will examine depression within the context of the breast cancer experience. By learning to distinguish between normal, brief periods of sadness in patients and abnormal levels of depression, nurses allow for therapeutic interventions that promote quality of life for women with breast cancer.

PREVALENCE OF DEPRESSION IN WOMEN WITH BREAST CANCER

According to a National Institute of Mental Health study (Regier, et al., 1988), 5.8% of the general U. S. population will develop major depression at some point in their lives, and women are twice as likely as men to develop depression (Regier et al., 1988). Thus a small number of patients with cancer will experience depression during the course of the illness, due to a preexisting affective disorder.

Very little is known about the prevalence of clinically significant depression in women with breast cancer or its relationship to illness-related factors. In a study of 359 women with early-stage breast cancer, depression was observed in 6% of the participants 1 to 3 months after their diagnosis (Watson et al., 1991). Another study found that out of 205 women interviewed 18 months after first being diagnosed with breast cancer, 44 women had had symptoms of major depression in the preceding 2 weeks (Maunsell & Brisson, 1992). In a sample of 22 women with local recurrence, ten women (45%) experienced anxiety and depression (Jenkins, May, & Hughes, 1991). With advanced breast cancer, anxiety and depression are common symptoms, reported in 35 of 139 women (25%) in one series (Pinder, Ramirez, Black, Richards, Gregory, & Rubens, 1993) and 20 of 81 women (25%) in another study (Hopwood, Howell, & Maguire, 1991a). Anxiety and/or depression was reported in up to 25% of women with advanced breast cancer; one third of cases may be persistent (Hopwood, Howell, & Maguire, 1991b).

THE PROBLEM OF UNDERDIAGNOSIS OF DEPRESSION

There is evidence that clinicians underrate symptoms of major depression in patients with cancer. A number of factors in our contemporary health care delivery systems may increase the likelihood of overlooking the diagnosis of clinical depression in women with breast cancer. These factors are outlined in Table 9-1. The prevalence of early discharge after surgical treatment for breast cancer as well as outpatient chemotherapy regimens provide limited time for patient-caregiver interactions. It is common for positive results of breast biopsies that are performed in outpatient surgicenters to be conveyed to women who are discharged within an hour. Experiencing a void in support at the time when they need it most (i.e., at the time of diagnosis), women have described this time as "the darkest hour."

Results of the staging work-up and presentation of treatment options by the physician may not occur for several weeks, leaving women with unanswered questions about

Table 9-1 Factors Associated with Underdiagnosis of Depression

- Limited patient-clinician interactions
- Co-occurrence of cancer treatment side effects
- False assumption that individuals with serious depression will seek treatment
- Avoidance by health care professional
- Lack of training and assessment of risk factors for depression
- Lack of professional confidence

prognosis and treatment options until their follow-up visits. (Fortunately some of these issues are being addressed through the evolution of multidisciplinary breast cancer centers). It is increasingly common for patients with breast cancer to be discharged the same day or within 24 hours of modified radical mastectomy surgery, and for autologous bone marrow or peripheral stem cell transplantation to be performed as outpatient procedures. Health care professionals working in these settings require proficient psychosocial assessment skills in order to identify clinical depression in high-risk women within the time constraints imposed by the current health care environment.

A number of other factors may contribute to the underdiagnosis of depression. Clinical depression is often difficult to diagnose in women experiencing side effects of treatment. Likewise, with advanced disease, patients may experience a number of somatic symptoms attributable to both a cancer diagnosis and clinical depression.

Caregivers may assume incorrectly that women with depression serious enough to warrant intervention would request treatment. Clinicians may focus on physiologic treatment and symptom management, avoiding discussion of the patient's psychological adjustment, unless the patient makes it clear she is experiencing a problem. This may be due to the clinician's inadequate knowledge about the diagnosis and medical management of depression, lack of access to a psychiatric liaison team, or insufficient time to elicit and respond to patient expressions of the impact of the diagnosis and treatment. Unrecognized or untreated depression can have serious consequences on a patient's quality of life, affecting her physical well-being, social life, and her ability to fulfill her usual roles and activities. In addition, untreated depression may compromise a patient's compliance with treatment and increase the risk of suicide.

IMPACT OF DEPRESSION ON PATIENT/FAMILY/CAREGIVER RELATIONSHIPS

Depression can have a profound impact on the patient's relationships with family and friends. In an attempt to avoid further distressing loved ones, patients may be reluctant to share their fears related to survival or recurrence. Likewise, in an effort to avoid airing unpleasant issues that could upset the patient, friends and family may avoid inquiring about the patient's condition. The woman's depressive symptoms may cause the family to think that she has "given up" or that the disease is progressing.

With severe depression, friends and family express feelings of frustration, futility, and inadequacy in their attempts to improve the patient's mood. This may lead to withdrawal from the patient or the use of avoidance behavior. The resulting social isolation causes the patient to be further deprived of important emotional support and leads to feelings of emotional abandonment.

Nurses who are inexperienced (or lack confidence) in addressing the psychosocial needs of the clinically depressed patient may have similar feelings of ineffectiveness and frustration. Perceiving an inability to "reach" the clinically depressed patient, staff may find themselves avoiding the patient and focusing on the physical aspects of patient care. The fatigue commonly experienced by depressed patients may interfere with their motivation to perform self-care, or to cooperate with treatment. Health care professionals may misinterpret this behavior and label depressed patients as noncompliant or "difficult."

ETIOLOGY OF DEPRESSION

In an attempt to define the cause for major depression, researchers have established an association between depression and chemical disturbance in the central nervous system. Reduced levels of catecholamines and abnormal receptor activity reportedly play an important role in mood regulation (Guze & Gitlin, 1994). It is unclear whether these abnormalities are etiologic or pathogenic for clinical depression. During normal neurotransmission, catecholamines are released from their storage place in the presynaptic vesicles into the synaptic cleft. Postsynaptic receptors are activated by catecholamines, producing neuronal stimulation (Guze & Gitlin, 1994).

Catecholamine inactivation is caused by reuptake into the neuron from the synaptic cleft. Changes in the brain chemistry of depressed patients include alterations in serotonergic, adrenergic, and possibly dopaminergic and GABA systems. However, diagnostic tests for depression related to abnormalities in brain chemistry are currently not specific enough to be clinically useful. Identification of the clinical syndrome of depression in a patient depends on a clinician's recognition of clinical symptoms.

UNIQUE FEATURES OF THE BREAST CANCER EXPERIENCE AS PRECIPITATING FACTORS FOR DEPRESSION

What is it specifically about a diagnosis of breast cancer that places a woman at risk for depression? Understandably, women who undergo mastectomies may experience a negative reaction to the body image change that occurs with the loss of a breast. They also may experience a diminished sense of femininity and changes in sexual function, all of which may precipitate depression.

While treatment with breast-conserving procedures (i.e., limited resection and radiation therapy) reduces the negative impact on body image, psychological symptoms related to the threat of a painful, progressive, possibly fatal disease may persist in patients. For these women, the onset of reactive anxiety and depression often coincides with the fatigue experienced with daily radiation treatments and association with other ill patients in the radiation clinic (Rowland & Holland, 1990). Women patients are now aware that breast cancer recurrence may develop many years after the primary diagnosis. The number of treatment options has also grown in recent years. These factors contribute to the decision-making confusion and persistent fear of recurrence that these women face.

Information regarding the role of genetic factors in the development of breast cancer has left some women feeling responsible for increasing their daughters' risk of developing breast cancer. They describe feelings of guilt or anxiety about the possibility of passing breast cancer on to their daughters.

LIFE-STAGE VARIATIONS IN PREDISPOSING FACTORS FOR DEPRESSION

Recognition of the age of a patient when her breast cancer is first diagnosed, coupled with knowledge of the patient's career, family, and interpersonal goals that are interrupted or threatened, are critically important factors in anticipating problem areas and planning interventions. The meaning of breast cancer is often quite different for women, depending on their life cycle stage. Stressors imposed by a diagnosis of breast cancer, somewhat unique to the various life stages, serve as predisposing factors for the development of depression and other psychologic morbidity. These factors are shown in Table 9-2.

In the young adult woman (i.e., 20 to 30 years), disruption caused by illness may result in reluctance to begin or maintain an intimate

Table 9-2   Predisposing Factors for Depression Based on Life Stage

Young adult (20-30 years)
  Disruption of life, career, and educational goals
  Reluctance to start intimate relationship
  Fear of recurrence, death, and dying
  Major financial concerns
  Increased isolation from family and friends
  Threat to femininity, fertility, and self-esteem

Mature adult (31-45 years)
  Role reversal
  Major financial burden
  Care of aging parents

Older adult (45-65 years)
  Fear of increased dependence
  Resentment
  Forced early retirement
  Despair over unattained life goals

Aging adult (>65 years)
  Concurrent personal losses
  Loss of energy reserve
  Co-existing chronic illness
  Decreased sensorimotor, visual, and auditory senses
  Major financial burden

relationship with another person. Established relationships may become strained by the threat of disability and death. Young women with young children, especially single mothers, experience fears regarding guardianship and financial security of their children, should the woman die. Treatments (e.g., autologous bone marrow transplantation) may involve time away from children and family, resulting in feelings of guilt and isolation. The side effects of treatment (e.g., alopecia, nausea and vomiting, weight gain, menopausal symptoms) may be particularly pronounced and threatening to a patient's femininity, fertility, and self-esteem, disrupting the sexual and marital relationship. Disruption of a patient's educational and career goals are additional concerns. Anxiety related to job security, ability to meet job expectations during therapy, and financial concerns may precipitate a patient's premature return to work, allowing insufficient time for her adaptation to the diagnosis. Fear of recurrence and death threatens the childless woman's sense of continuity with future generations. Case Example 1 illustrates some experiences common to women in the young adult life stage.

Case Example 1.   Jennifer is a 30-year-old married woman, diagnosed with stage IV breast cancer while she was pregnant with her first child. Following the delivery, she had an autologous bone marrow transplant (BMT), during which time she experienced anxiety and symptoms of depression with extreme withdrawal. Cognitive psychotherapy was effective in treating the depression. Following disease recurrence 2 years later, Jennifer stated, "It's hard to be optimistic when you've failed a BMT. I'm so tired of having to go through Taxol treatments with no break every three weeks, with many problems in between treatments (e.g., cellulitis requiring repeated hospitalizations for antibiotics, constipation from narcotics, no energy). I never go anywhere anymore except the hospital. I feel safe when I'm here in the hospital—I feel like by taking chemotherapy, I'm doing something to control the cancer. So I don't really get depressed when I'm here. At home I'm more depressed. The nurses here understand what I'm going through. I doubt my mom and husband can understand. I'm fearful of anything that might interfere with my treatment schedule. I never go out—all our friends have young children—I'm afraid of getting an infection from them. (Crying) Right now for me it's like going through mourning or grieving. I know I won't be cured. Before I had hope that at least I would be able to have a remission. For at least 8 months now I've taken chemo[therapy] to control the pleural effusion. Mother is a great source of support with Catherine. She's very reality-oriented. She says, 'You do what you have to do.' For example, 'Your purpose today may be just to get bathed and dressed.' And I was afraid of going places and doing things because of what might happen. She encouraged me to go to the mall, taking medication and water with us in case a migraine starts. My husband says, 'It's like

we're just sitting around waiting for you to die.' We can't even make long-range plans, like planning a vacation. My husband can't live one day at a time—he needs something big to look forward to."

As in the preceding stage, the mature adult woman (i.e., 31 to 45 years) may experience fear of abandonment, as well as a sense of isolation due to real or perceived social stigmatization. Although friendships may be strengthened, some may falter when friends do not know what to say or do to support the patient, causing them to withdraw. Disease and treatment may at times necessitate role reversal, creating guilt, anger, and despair in the woman, her partner, and her children. The financial burden of the illness may threaten life goals and commitments. The care of aging parents may be a concern. Normal body image changes associated with aging are exacerbated by therapy that may result in alopecia, fatigue, nausea, vomiting, anorexia, infertility, weight gain, and menopausal symptoms.

The older adult woman (i.e., 46 to 65 years) may also have responsibility for the care of aging parents. She may experience fear of becoming dependent on others. She may experience resentment and guilt, depending on her partner or older children for care, being forced into early retirement, or feeling cheated out of an anticipated healthy retirement. Intensification of a chronically unhappy marriage, despair about unattained goals, and doubt as to the meaningfulness of life are other issues potentially contributing to depression.

The aging adult woman (i.e., 66 years and over) is likely to be experiencing a number of concurrent personal losses. She has less energy reserve than younger women. At this life stage, there is an increase in the prevalence of other chronic illnesses and a decrease in the sensorimotor, visual, and auditory senses. A number of adaptational changes and adjustments must be made, including retirement. Increasing limitations on physical energy, income, and mobility lead to restrictions in a woman's social life. Meager social support, due to frequent personal losses such as death of spouse, siblings, and friends, contribute to increased risk for depressive symptoms. A diagnosis of breast cancer added to multiple personal losses places the aging woman at risk for major psychological disruption. Stress caused by unfamiliar treatments and health care settings and the fear of being a burden to others, especially to her children, are not uncommon reactions. On occasion, the patient may become inappropriately dependent, "giving up" upon diagnosis. The aging woman is more susceptible to complications of the illness and treatment side effects, and may have difficulty comprehending complex information about the therapy. A diagnosis of breast cancer has an additive effect on the multiple losses of the elderly woman, leading to the potential for bereavement overload. Case Example 2 illustrates some of the issues faced by the aging woman with breast cancer.

Case Example 2. Margaret is a 65-year-old widowed woman with breast cancer, initially diagnosed at age 40. She had a history of recurrent episodes of endogenous depression, precipitated by a diagnosis of breast cancer and the death of her husband. These events placed her at high risk for major depression when recurrent local disease was diagnosed at the old mastectomy site. She had responded well to tricyclic antidepressants during previous depressive episodes. Astute nurses elicited this information at the time of Margaret's physician visit for treatment planning for the recurrent disease. Identifying Margaret's high risk for depression, the nurses arranged for telephone follow-up to determine her state of coping. Two weeks after Margaret learned of her recurrent disease, she complained of insomnia, loss of ability to enjoy family visits, loss of interest in her usual daily activities, lack of energy, difficulty making decisions, and feelings of worthlessness and "being a burden" to her family. These symptoms persisted and a referral was made for psychiatric intervention. Supportive psychotherapy and antidepressant therapy were initiated. In view of Margaret's history of a myocardial infarction

(MI) one year earlier, the physician was concerned about the potential for cardiac conduction disturbances and orthostatic hypotension, associated with tricyclic antidepressants. He prescribed an SSRI. Within several weeks, Margaret's mood and sleeping pattern improved, she became interested in her usual activities, "perked up" when her family visited, and reported "feeling like myself" again.

Dismay at family dreams not realized and financial disruption; fear of the potential for disability, dependence, or abandonment; adjustment to an altered appearance and changed body function; feelings of guilt and of being "different"; and fear of a painful death are universal concerns shared by women with breast cancer. Regardless of age, the breast cancer experience may challenge one's religious faith. Some women relate that if their faith were stronger, it wouldn't be as hard to handle. The disease is viewed by some patients as a punishment. For others, religious faith is viewed as a major source of support (Mahon, Cella, & Donovan, 1990). Individual perceptions cause the woman to search for meaning in life and death in the cancer experience.

INFLUENCE OF THE ILLNESS TRAJECTORY ON DEPRESSION

Certain crisis or transition points in the breast cancer disease trajectory may influence the degree of psychosocial morbidity. For some women, anxiety and depression may be more prevalent at the time of diagnosis, and at the beginning and end of primary therapy. Anticipation of chemotherapy may serve to produce fears of potential side effects, with reactive anxiety and depression. Fears of recurrence may peak at the completion of adjuvant chemotherapy or radiation, possibly precipitating anxiety and depression (Rowland & Holland, 1990). Critical events such as recurrence or treatment failure may be more traumatic than the initial diagnosis, because the prognosis is guarded. With recurrence, many of the fears experienced at the time of initial diagnosis are

Table 9-3   Diagnosis of Major Depression

Criteria for Major Depressive Episode (DSM IV)

A. Five (or more) of the following symptoms have been present for the same 2-week period and represent a change from previous functioning; at least one of the symptoms is either (1) depressed mood or (2) loss of interest or pleasure.

1. Depressed mood most of the day, nearly every day, as indicated by either subjective report (eg. feels sad or empty) or observation made by others (e.g. appears tearful).
2. Markedly diminished interest or pleasure in all, or almost all, activities most of the day, nearly every day.
3. Significant weight loss when not dieting or weight gain, or decrease or increase in appetite nearly every day.
4. Insomnia or hypersomnia nearly every day.
5. Psychomotor agitation or retardation nearly every day.
6. Fatigue or loss of energy nearly every day.
7. Feelings of worthlessness or excessive or inappropriate guilt nearly every day.
8. Diminished ability to think or concentrate, or indecisiveness nearly every day.
9. Recurrent thoughts of death (not just fear of dying), recurrent suicidal ideation without a specific plan, or a suicide attempt or a specific plan for commmitting suicide.

B. The symptoms cause clinically significant distress or impairment in social, occupational, or other important areas of functioning.

C. The symptoms are not due to the direct physiological effects of a substance or a general medical condition.

D. The symptoms are not better accounted for by bereavement, i.e. after the loss of a loved one, the symptoms persist for longer than 2 months or are characterized by marked functional impairment, morbid preoccupation with worthlessness, suicidal ideation, psychotic symptoms, or psychomotor retardation.

Note. From American Psychiatric Association: *Diagnostic and Statistical Manual of Mental Disorders, Fourth Edition.* Washington DC, American Psychiatric Association, 1994. Reprinted with permission.

revived. When the treatment goal is changed from curative to supportive care, and during the advanced and terminal stages of the disease, anxiety and depression may recur with greater severity.

HALLMARK SYMPTOMS OF DEPRESSION AND THE DIAGNOSTIC CHALLENGE WITH BREAST CANCER

Greater familiarity with the clinical syndrome of depression can help oncological clinicians make a more timely diagnosis of depression. Identifying factors related to clinical depression may be useful indicators of women at high risk for this disorder.

Physically healthy patients with major depression frequently exhibit only somatic complaints, denying affective or cognitive symptoms. Certain physical complaints are so commonly associated with depression that they constitute the hallmark of the syndrome: fatigue that persists despite rest; pain that is usually undifferentiated; sleep disturbances in the form of insomnia or hypersomnia; anxiety or irritability; gastrointestinal complaints. According to the American Psychiatric Association DSM IV criteria (Table 9-3), diagnosis of major clinical depression is based on the intensity and duration of certain core symptoms, which must be present daily for at least 2 weeks.

Clinical depression may be especially difficult to diagnose in medically ill patients. As with other oncology patients, the diagnostic challenge in evaluating depression in women with breast cancer is differentiating symptoms of disease and treatment side effects from symptoms of true clinical depression. Somatic symptoms of depression, such as anorexia, fatigue, and sleep disturbance, are commonly experienced in patients with advanced disease, making it difficult to clearly differentiate medical and psychological symptoms. Diagnosis cannot depend on these vegetative signs, but must depend on the qualitative aspects of the clinical profile of depression.

Among patients with cancer, a variety of medical disorders that produce the same symptoms as depression must be ruled out, to make a diagnosis of true depression (Massie, 1990; Massie & Holland, 1990). Conditions that can cause the same symptoms as depression include: metabolic encephalopathies, secondary to hypokalemia, hypoglycemia, and hypercalcemia; and endocrine disturbances, such as hypothyroidism, hyperparathyroidism, adrenal insufficiency, brain metastasis, and nutritional deficiencies. Various pharmacologic agents (e.g., psychotrophics, barbiturates, diazepam, and certain chemotherapy agents) can cause depressive side effects. Steroids can cause mood disturbances, including depression, sometimes accompanied by suicidal ideation. Folate or Vitamin B-12 deficiency and anemia may cause the patient to appear depressed.

In patients with cancer, cognitive or mood symptoms (e.g., feelings of sadness, hopelessness, helplessness, decreased self-esteem, guilt, suicidal thoughts, anorexia, insomnia, isolation) are more reliable indicators for diagnosis of major depression (Holland, 1987; Massie & Holland, 1990).

Endogenous (biologically determined) depression unrelated to a precipitating event is seen in certain individuals. However, a crisis such as a diagnosis of breast cancer may serve to exacerbate endogenous depression. This type of depression tends to be a recurring illness in certain patients. The condition may be chronic, in which the depression never resolves completely, although the vegetative signs may diminish.

DISTINGUISHING NORMAL REACTIONS FROM MAJOR DEPRESSION

There is a strong reactive component related to most depressions seen in patients with cancer. Thus, it's often difficult to differentiate between the dysphoria or depressed mood that is a normal response to loss or a life-threatening event and major clinical depression in which dysphoria is accompanied by multiple somatic and cognitive symptoms. A period of initial disbelief, denial, and despair is common at the time of diagnosis and commonly lasts for several days. Dysphoric mood generally continues 1 to 2 weeks, during which time patients report anxiety, depressed mood, anorexia, insomnia, and irritability. Patients may find it difficult to concentrate. Intrusive thoughts about the diagnosis and uncertainty about the future may be present. At this time, a patient frequently experiences anxiety and depression concurrently. The transitional sadness or bereavement about loss of health and anticipated losses including death is common and tends to be transient, rarely persisting beyond a couple of weeks. Normally, adaptation begins within a few weeks.

Adjustment disorder with depressed mood is diagnosed when symptoms become more severe and persistent, interfering with daily functioning. It is difficult to distinguish adjustment disorder with depressed mood from a major depressive episode. When the reactive state evolves to more severe symptoms, the diagnosis of a major depression is made (Massie & Holland, 1990).

CHARACTERISTICS OF WOMEN AT HIGH RISK

In the general population, women at risk for major clinical depression include those with a personal or family history of depression, substance abuse, and hypochondriasis, with persistent and frequent somatic, psychosomatic, or pain complaints. Common predisposing factors include severe or unanticipated stress (e.g., death of a loved one, divorce, loss of employment, family or marital problems, financial problems, relocation, parenthood), inadequate social support, and impaired body image. Additional concurrent chronic illness may precipitate major depression. Women who already have a considerable amount of stress in their lives may be particularly vulnerable when faced with the additional stressor imposed by breast cancer and treatment.

A history of depression before a diagnosis of breast cancer and experience of a number of stressful life events (e.g., serious physical illness or injury for patient or significant other, death of family member or friend, change of residence, children leaving home) are reported as strong indicators for high psychologic distress, including depression in the 18-month period after initial treatment for breast cancer (Maunsell & Brisson, 1992). Advanced stage of disease, deteriorating physical function, inadequately controlled pain, and the experiencing of treatment side effects are additional high-risk factors for depression in oncology patients (Valente, Saunders, & Cohen, 1994).

Because there appears to be a genetic link for depression, women with a relative who had clinical depression may be at greater risk than those with a depression-free family history. The memory of a close friend or relative's death from breast cancer may make the diagnosis more ominous for some patients. Assessing these risk factors during the initial evaluation at the time of diagnosis may permit concentration of psychosocial resources on women in whom clinical depression is more likely to develop.

BARRIERS/FUTURE CHALLENGES TO DIAGNOSIS AND INTERVENTION

Recognizing the vulnerability of high-risk women should lead to prompt referral for psychosocial intervention. A number of reasons for the lack of referrals for psychiatric intervention in patients with cancer have been identified (Pasacretta & Massie, 1990). Under-referral

may arise from clinician and/or patient concerns that psychiatric referrals are stigmatizing or that psychiatric intervention will make the patient feel worse by "unleashing" negative emotions. The belief that depression is an expected response to a diagnosis of cancer and that there is no effective treatment, or that depressive symptoms are self-limiting, are additional clinician barriers to intervention. Clinician education about indicators for depression in women with breast cancer, knowledge of the availability of resources, and the efficacy of therapeutic interventions to manage depression may serve to overcome these barriers to treatment of depression.

CLINICAL EVALUATION OF DEPRESSION

Oncology nurses can learn to recognize symptoms of clinical depression and can initiate referral of a patient to an appropriate mental health care professional. These nurses must learn and master certain essential interviewing skills to improve their ability to identify women exhibiting signs of depression.

Clinical evaluation for depression includes assessment of the patient's symptoms, mental and physical status, laboratory data and current medication regime, as well as what the patient feels and believes about the experience of disease and cancer treatment effects. The patient's personal and family history of depression or suicide should be obtained, including her responses to previous treatment for depression, concurrent life stresses, and the degree of social support she has. Consideration should be given to incorporating the use of an assessment guide for major depression into the initial evaluation of each new patient diagnosed with breast cancer. Table 9-4 may be used as an assessment guide to evaluate major depression in women.

The diagnosis of depression is based on clusters of symptoms, which persist over time and are associated with distress, dysfunction, or risk for suicide. The areas of thought, mood, behavior, and somatic symptoms are assessed to make a determination of the clinical syndrome of depression. Assessment of the patient's thought processes, to determine presence of suicidal ideation or negative self-evaluation, may be accomplished by asking: "What do you think about your future?" or "Have you thought about not waking up tomorrow morning?"

To determine a patient's mood state, it may be helpful to determine if she has lost the ability to experience pleasure when her family visits. Asking questions like, "What do you see for yourself for the next 6 or 12 months?" or "Have you given up anything you enjoy as a result of your diagnosis?" can glean helpful information. Responses such as "I feel terrible now and am unlikely to improve" serve as red flags warranting intervention. Behavior can be evaluated by assessing if there is a decrease in self care or if the patient "perks up" when her family visits. The presence of somatic symptoms related to sleep, energy, appetite, and libido frequently overlaps with disease symptoms and must be evaluated within the context of the patient's physical condition.

MANAGEMENT OF DEPRESSION

Treatment of depression is a complex task requiring considerable skill and knowledge. Depression is usually treated with a combination of antidepressant therapy and supportive interventions. Mental health care professionals have utilized a variety of approaches to address the psychosocial needs of oncology patients experiencing depression. The clinician is faced with the dilemma of how to decide among the numerous interventions. Support groups, group therapy, individual counseling, and psychotherapy are used as vehicles to assist women with their adjustment to breast cancer. Because there is a lack of consensus on the best form of therapeutic intervention, clinicians must be guided by information gleaned from individualized patient assessment. Table 9-5 outlines the various categories of interventions for depression.

Table 9-4   Assessment Guide for Major Depression

Risk Factors (past/present):
   Affective disorder
   Chemical dependency
   Physical abuse/self-injury
   Poor control of pain/symptoms
   Advanced stages of cancer
   Medications with depressive side effects
   Inadequate social support
   Impaired body image
   Changed work/family roles

Precipitants Stress from:
   Meaning of cancer
   Unmet needs
   Pain/symptom distress
   Anxiety/fears
   Financial concerns
   Automatic negative thinking
   Drugs causing depression

Symptoms
   Sad facial expression/mood
   Decreased interest in self
   No enjoyment of pleasurable activities
   Social withdrawal
   Somatic symptoms: anorexia, insomnia, fatigue
   Slow thought, concentration
   Thoughts of suicide

Note. From "Evaluating Depressions Among Patients with Cancer" by S. M. Valente, J. M. Saunders, and M. Z. Cohen, 1994, *Cancer Practice*, January/February. Copyright 1994 by J. B. Lippincott Company. Reprinted with permission

SUPPORTIVE INTERVENTIONS

For women experiencing situational stress with mild depressive symptoms, oncology nurses can use counseling as a vehicle to promote adaptation. Women experiencing feelings of sadness should receive validation that this is a normal reaction to diagnosis and at various phases of the illness trajectory. Supportive understanding of the multiple personal and physical losses should be provided. This may involve a focus on grief associated with the patient's loss of health and anticipated goals. Therapeutic interventions may include an emphasis on past strengths, support for previous effective coping strategies, and encouragement to mobilize inner resources. Assisting patients to explore and identify their purpose in life, and the role of spiritual meaning, and to determine effective coping strategies may be beneficial. In women experiencing disease- and treatment-related physical discomfort, every effort must be made to achieve optimal pain control and symptom management.

Exercise programs and behavioral methods, such as relaxation combined with visual imagery suggesting a peaceful scene of the patient's choice, may be beneficial in decreasing the anxiety that frequently accompanies depression. These methods are generally not indicated in the management of severe depression.

Cognitive behavioral therapy, often managed by clinical psychologists, is aimed at controlling target symptoms (i.e., anxiety and depression) (Massie, Holland, & Straker, 1990). This therapy may be beneficial for those women for whom illness has connotations of punishment or weakness, who hold unrealistic and distorted fears and expectations, or who have an exaggerated pathologic response to losses associated with the diagnosis. Assisting a depressed patient to derive meaning and purpose in her breast cancer experience, and focusing on positive rather than negative changes that have occurred since diagnosis, may serve to improve her self-esteem and mood.

Psychotherapy interventions are best provided by social workers, psychiatric clinical nurse specialists, and psychologists and psychiatrists with knowledge of the specialty of oncology (Massie et al., 1990). However, early intervention by the nurse may prevent more serious symptoms of depression. Goals of individual psychotherapy are to maintain a primary focus on the illness and its implications, explore issues that affect the adjustment to illness, and reinforce the patient's past coping strategies. Patients are encouraged to express feelings and fears about their disease and

Table 9-5   Types of Interventions for Depression

Supportive
  Managed by nurses and social workers
  Individual counseling
  Support groups

Behavioral
  Generally under guidance of nurses and social
    workers
  Exercise programs
  Relaxation and visual imagery

Cognitive
  Generally managed by clinical psychologists
  Control of target symptoms
  Focusing on positive strengths
  Deriving meaning in life

Psychotherapy
  Referral to psychologists, psychiatrists, social
    workers, psychiatric clinical nurse specialists
  Goal is to maintain focus on illness
  Explore issues affecting adjustment
  Reinforce past coping strategies

its outcome. Supportive psychotherapy generally uses weekly outpatient visits, which are tapered off as adjustment occurs.

Support groups may meet the needs of women who are in treatment or adjusting to life after cancer. The newly diagnosed woman may require focused support and information to manage depression. A peer counselor (i.e., breast cancer survivor) can more effectively facilitate coping and adjustment to cancer in newly diagnosed women. For some women experiencing depressive symptoms, group therapy may foster a sense of belonging and sharing.

WHEN TO REFER/LEVELS OF REFERRAL

Oncology nurses provide much of the psychological support in many clinical oncology settings. Giving full recognition for the vital part oncology nurses play in providing psycho-

Table 9-6   Classes of Pharmacologic Agents Used in the Treatment of Depression

Type	Side Effects

Tricyclic antidepressants
  amitriptyline, imipramine,
  desipramine, nortriptyline
	Anticholinergic effects
	Antihistaminic effects
	Cardiovascular effects
	Weight gain
	Sexual dysfunction

Second-generation antidepressants trazadone, maprotiline	Drowsiness, fatigue, dizziness, orthostatic hypotension

Selective serotonin re-uptake
inhibitors (SSRIs)
  paroxetin, sertraline,
  fluoxetine, fluvoxamine
	Mild nausea, nervousness

logical support, it is important to be aware of personal strengths and limitations and recognize when it is appropriate to refer patients to another discipline. One reason for referral is in situations where added expertise is needed (e.g., patients experiencing symptoms of major depression requiring antidepressant therapy). Nurse-to-nurse consultation with the oncology or psychiatric clinical nurse specialist may be especially helpful in providing support and offering additional suggestions for effective psychosocial care of depressed patients. The decision to refer begins with the nursing assessment. Mild depressive symptoms generally respond well to supportive psychosocial intervention by oncology staff nurses, oncology and psychiatric clinical nurse specialists, and oncology social workers. When depressive symptoms last longer than a week, worsen, or interfere with a patient's daily activities or her ability to cooperate with treatment, psychiatric consultation is indicated. Expression of suicidal thoughts, hopelessness, withdrawal, insomnia, or dysphoria signal a major depression requiring psychiatric evaluation and treatment. Depressed patients who verbalize plans for suicide or exhibit self-destructive behavior must be considered for immediate psychiatric referral. In desperation, patients suffering depres-

sion from intractable pain and inadequate symptom management may consider suicide. It is important to assess how long the patient has felt this way, and to ask if they have thought out a plan to commit suicide. Definitive, prompt intervention is required.

For women with religious beliefs, referral to clergy for spiritual counseling may provide an important source of support. Spiritual counseling provides the patient with a forum for expressing and understanding painful emotions associated with the breast cancer experience.

PHARMACOLOGIC THERAPY

Pharmacotherapy is the mainstay of treatment for moderate to severe depression (Guze & Gitlin, 1994). Oncology patients experiencing severe reactive and major depression have benefitted from antidepressant medications (Lederberg & Massie, 1993). The choice of an antidepressant agent for a particular patient depends on the nature of her depressive symptoms, the side effects of the drug, and concurrent physical problems that would be adversely affected by these side effects. Table 9-6 shows the different types of antidepressants and their related side effects.

Until recently, the most consistently prescribed antidepressants were the tricyclic antidepressants, including amitriptyline (Elavil, Zeneca Pharmaceutical), imipramine (Tofranil, Geigy Pharmaceuticals), desipramine (Norpramin, Merrell Dow), and nortriptyline (Pamelor, Sandoz Pharmaceuticals) (Massie & Lesko, 1990). Mood improvement may not occur for 2 to 3 weeks after the tricyclic is started. Concerns about the anticholinergic (e.g., xerostomia, constipation, urinary hesitancy, blurred vision, delirium), antihistaminic (e.g., drowsiness, sedation), and cardiovascular (e.g., cardiac conduction disturbance, orthostatic hypotension) side effects of many tricyclic medications, as well as weight gain and sexual dysfunction, may contribute to the underprescribing or underdosing of antidepressants by physicians. Second-generation antidepressants such as trazadone (Desyrel, Apothecon) and maprotiline (Ludiomil, Ciba) are commonly prescribed when a therapeutic response is not seen with tricyclic agents. The undesirable effects associated with second-generation antidepressants are drowsiness, fatigue, dizziness, and orthostatic hypotension. The benzodiazepine, alprazolam (Xanax, Upjohn Co.), has been shown to decrease anxiety and depressive symptoms in patients with cancer (Massie & Lesko, 1990). However, it is not recommended for long-term treatment.

Today, a new class of antidepressant drugs, the selective serotonin re-uptake inhibitors (SSRIs), is available: paroxetin (Paxil, Smith-Kline Beecham Pharmaceuticals), sertraline (Zolof, Roertig), fluoxetine (Prozac, Dista Products Co.), and fluvoxamine (Luvox, Solvay). The selective blockade of the re-uptake of serotonin into the presynaptic neuron increases the availability of serotonin at the synaptic cleft, enhancing its effectiveness. These drugs are more easily tolerated and have fewer undesirable side effects than traditional antidepressants, making patient management easier. Primary SSRI side effects include mild nausea and nervousness, which usually abates within a few weeks. A major advantage of this drug class is safety with regard to medication overdose, a primary con-

cern for all patients with depression. The SSRIs are not noted to affect cardiac function. The use of SSRIs in the management of depression in the oncology population looks promising, but further study is needed.

CONCLUSION

Concern with quality of life in women with breast cancer supports the need to identify women at high risk for psychosocial morbidity. Depression and anxiety are common sequelae of the diagnosis and treatment of breast cancer and may occur at varying stages of the illness trajectory. The diagnosis of depression may be overlooked unless clinical indicators for women at high risk are integrated into a systematic assessment. Consideration should be given to incorporating assessment of factors that appear predictive of depression into the initial evaluation of women newly diagnosed with breast cancer. Constraints on resource utilization imposed by the current health care environment support the prioritization of psychosocial services. The detection of subtle signs of depression and the monitoring women at high risk allow targeting of interventions that reduce depression and improve quality of life.

References

American Psychiatric Association. (1994). *Diagnostic criteria from DSM-IV.* (pp. 161–172). Washington, DC: American Psychiatric Association.

Guze B. H., & Gitlin M. (1994). New antidepressants and the treatment of depression. *Journal of Family Practice, 38,* 49–57.

Holland J. C. (1987). Managing depression in the patient with cancer. *Cancer, 37* (6), 366–371.

Hopwood P., Howell A., & Maguire P. (1991a). Screening for psychiatric morbidity in patients with advanced breast cancer: Validation of two self-report questionnaires. *British Journal of Cancer, 64,* 353–356.

Hopwood P., Howell A., & Maguire P. (1991b). Psychiatric morbidity in patients with advanced cancer of the breast: Prevalence measured by two self-rating questionnaires. *British Journal of Cancer, 64,* 349–352.

Jenkins P. L., May V. E., & Hughes L. E. (1991) Psychological morbidity associated with local recurrence of breast cancer. *International Journal of Psychiatry in Medicine, 21*, 149–155.

Lederberg M. S., & Massie M. S. (1993). Psychosocial and ethical issues in the care of cancer patients. In V. T. De Vita, S. Hellman, & S. A. Rosenberg (Eds.), *Cancer principles and practice of oncology,* 4th Ed. (pp. 2448–2463). Philadelphia: J. B. Lippincott.

Mahon S. M., Cella D. F., & Donovan M. I. (1990). Psychosocial adjustment to recurrent cancer. *Oncology Nursing Forum, 17* (Suppl. 3), 47–54 .

Massie M. J. (1990). Depression. In J. C. Holland, & J. H. Rowland (Eds.), *Handbook of psychooncology: Psychological care of the patient with cancer.* (pp. 283–290). New York: Oxford University Press.

Massie M. J., & Holland J. C. (1990). Depression and the cancer patient. *Journal of Clinical Psychiatry, 51,* (7, Suppl), 12–17.

Massie M. J., Holland J. C., & Straker N. (1990) Psychotherapeutic interventions. In J. C. Holland, & J. H. Rowland (Eds.), *Handbook of psychooncology: Psychological care of the patient with cancer.* (pp. 455–469). New York: Oxford University Press.

Massie M. J., & Lesko L. M. (1990). Psychopharmacological management. In J. C. Holland, J. H. Rowland, (Eds.), *Handbook of psychooncology: Psychological care of the patient with cancer.* (pp. 470–491). New York: Oxford University Press.

Maunsell E., & Brisson J. (1992). Psychological distress after initial treatment of breast cancer. *Cancer, 70,* 120–125.

Pasacretta, J. V., & Massie M. J. (1990). Nurses' reports of psychiatric complications in patients with cancer. *Oncology Nursing Forum 17* (3), 347–353.

Pinder K. L., Ramirez A. J., Black, M. E., Richards, M. A. Greggory, W. M., & Rubens, R. D. (1993). Psychiatric disorder in patients with advanced breast cancer: Prevalence and associated factors. *European Journal of Cancer, 29A* (4), 524–527.

Regier, D. A. et al. (1988). The NIMH depression awareness, recognition and treatment program: Structure, aims and scientific basis. *American Journal of Psychiatry, 145,* 1351–1357.

Rowland J. H., & Holland J. C. (1990). Breast cancer. In J. C. Holland, & J. H. Rowland (Eds.), *Handbook of psychooncology: Psychological care of the patient with cancer.* (pp. 188–207). New York: Oxford University Press.

Valente S. M., Saunders J. M., & Cohen M. Z. (1994). Evaluating depression among patients with cancer. *Cancer Practice, 2* (1), 65–71.

Watson M., Greer S., Rowden L., Gorman C., Robertson B., Bliss J., & Tunmore R. (1991). Relationships between emotional control, adjustment to cancer and depression and anxiety in breast cancer patients. *Psychological Medicine, 21,* 51–57.

CHAPTER 10 | Social Support in Breast Cancer

Nelda Samarel, EdD, RN

A BRIEF OVERVIEW

Shumaker and Brownell (1984, p. 13) define social support as an "exchange of resources between two individuals [which is] perceived by the provider or recipient to be intended to enhance the well-being of the recipient." Social support has been shown to help patients, particularly women with breast cancer (Bloom & Spiegel, 1984; Northouse, 1988; Samarel & Fawcett, 1992; Spiegel, Kraemer, Bloom, & Gottheil, 1989), adapt to the stresses of illness and its treatment (Cassileth, Lusk, Strouse, Miller, Brown & Cross, 1985; Ell, Nishimoto, Morvay, Mantell, & Hamovitch, 1989; Friedland & McColl, 1987).

Forms of Social Support

Social support is a multidimensional concept, encompassing psychosocial and instrumental dimensions. *Psychosocial support* addresses the affective aspects of breast cancer diagnosis, treatment, and survival, and is primarily involved with emotional sustenance. *Instrumental support* addresses problem-solving with regard to specific biopsychosocial aspects of breast cancer diagnosis, treatment, and survival. Instrumental support may include goods, services, or information; it is tangible assistance. Table 10-1 provides examples of psychosocial and instrumental social support that may be of particular interest to women with breast cancer.

The Need for Social Support in Breast Cancer

Inadequate social support is associated with declining psychological adaptation following breast cancer diagnosis (Ell et al., 1989). In contrast, the social support literature clearly demonstrates that informal support from fellow patients, family members, and the health care team can influence adaptation to cancer

Table 10-1   Examples of Psychosocial and Instrumental Social Support

Psychosocial Support	Instrumental Support
Listening to fears related to the diagnosis and treatment of breast cancer	Providing information about the diagnosis and treatment of breast cancer
Encouraging verbalization about fears of recurrence	Teaching and reinforcing importance of regular breast self-examination
Offering understanding of feelings of separation at conclusion of adjuvant therapy	Providing an opportunity for networking with other breast cancer survivors
Discussing the importance of understanding emotions and needs	Informing of the availability of local support groups
Exploring the relationship between cancer and stress, particularly, cancer as a cause of stress	Teaching stress management strategies
Exploring sexuality as a broad concept, as well as specific sexual issues, from both physical and psychological perspectives	Teaching strategies to deal with specific physiologic sexual problems, such as vaginal dryness resulting from chemically induced menopause
Normalizing the experience of common problems associated with the treatment of breast cancer, such as anxiety, insomnia, anorexia, fatigue, and discomfort	Suggesting strategies to deal with common problems associated with breast cancer treatment
Exploring the effects of cancer on self-image	Suggesting specific strategies to improve self-image
Emphasizing how utilization of community resources may assist with the adaptation to breast cancer	Providing a list of available community resources

(Dunkel-Schetter, 1984; Willey & Silliman, 1990), and especially to breast cancer (Bloom & Spiegel, 1984; Levy & Schain, 1988; Neuling & Winefield, 1988; Northouse, 1988). According to Oakes and Teasdale (1992), professional social support provided by nurses, specially trained volunteers, and support groups can help reduce the high incidence of anxiety and depression immediately following the diagnosis of breast cancer. Indeed, social support and, in particular, support groups may be the most powerful influences on adaptation to breast cancer diagnosis and treatment (Sparks, 1988), resulting in reduced psychological distress, increased self-concept, and a sense of power through enhancement of coping responses (Bloom, 1982). A balance between structured educational programs and group discussion has been found to be effective (Pillon & Joannides, 1991). The combination of social support, information seeking, and use of problem-solving skills also is useful in decreasing patients' feelings of helplessness and cancer-related worrying (Hilton, 1989).

Individual support, both in person and via telephone, as well as group support, have been shown to be effective in reducing depression, anxiety, and worry, leading to increased feelings of control in patients with breast cancer (Edgar, Rosberger, & Nowlis, 1992). Although one study examining the effects of nurse telephone support revealed no significant differences in physiological and psychological variables between those radiation therapy patients who received the support and those who did not, subjects receiving the support reported greater satisfaction with their health care professionals (Hagopian & Rubenstein, 1990). In addition, patients with advanced cancer who participated in an automated telephone outreach program reported fewer unmet needs than the controls (Siegel, Mesagno, Karus, & Christ, 1992). One report, showing the therapeutic results of psychotherapy by telephone for cancer patients, specifically highlights the beneficial aspects of telephone communication with regard to increased accessibility to support (Mermelstein & Holland, 1991).

Social support in the form of social relationships with other women, professional support, and education help women with breast cancer to adapt.

SOCIAL SUPPORT AS AN INTERVENTION: THE RESEARCH

Social Support and Adaptation

Research has clearly indicated that there is a relationship between social support and adaptation to breast cancer. Bloom (1982) describes the adjustment to breast cancer as an interactional process that involves psychosocial and behavioral components. In a study exploring the effects of social support on adjustment to breast cancer, she studied 133 women from a period of 1 week postsurgery to 30 months postsurgery. Results indicated that a woman's perception of social support was the strongest predictor of her adjustment to breast cancer. Specifically, the results suggested that women having greater perceived social support had a higher self-concept, experienced greater feelings of empowerment regarding their illness, and experienced less psychological distress than women with less perceived social support.

Cancer Support Groups

A specific social support intervention is the cancer support group. It has long been recognized that cancer support groups help patients with cancer to adapt. The support groups are based on the premise that patients with cancer benefit from contact with other cancer patients through mutual social support.

Informal patient-to-patient dyadic social support has had a positive influence on arm mobility following mastectomy, perception of health and body image, and reduction in negative feelings (Van den Borne, Pruyn, & Van Dam de May, 1986). In a study begun in the 1970s, Spiegel, Bloom, and Yalom (1981) found that women with metastatic breast cancer who participated in therapeutic group support had significantly less mood disturbance, fewer maladaptive coping responses, and less pain than women in the control group (who did not participate in support groups).

Despite the general perception that cancer support groups are beneficial, few studies have evaluated the effectiveness of formal support groups for women with breast cancer. Spiegel et al. (1989) studied 86 women with metastatic breast cancer, 50 of whom participated in weekly group therapy sessions. Results indicated that those women participating in the sessions survived significantly longer than those who did not. In another study, Pritzker (1988) combined the use of a facilitator manual with the development of a psychoeducational support group for post-mastectomy women (n=7). Although the findings of this study demonstrated that participants showed significant gains in knowledge of the disease process, perceived assertiveness, coping with isolation, and dealing with negative behaviors, there were several methodological flaws in the study, such as no control group, a small sample, and use of instruments with no reported validity or reliability.

Johnson and Kelly (1990) recognized the unmet needs of women with breast cancer and developed a rehabilitation program for this population based on the Outward Bound program. The program included a week-long wilderness trip that involved carrying heavy packs, paddling canoes, hiking through forests, traversing ropes rigged in treetops, and sharing in camp chores. All 12 study subjects completed the program, suggesting a high level of commitment to a structured program of support.

Coaching as Social Support

Research findings indicate that support of a significant other, including physicial presence, willingness to listen, assistance with household tasks, and caring attitudes, was of critical importance to women following diagnosis of and surgery for breast cancer (Shaw, 1989). Coaching as social support has been explored by Samarel and Fawcett (1992) and Samarel, Fawcett, & Tulman (1993). In their work, coaches were identified as partners or spouses, relatives, or close friends. The role of the coach was to assist the woman with breast cancer to adapt by providing social support, monitoring return to daily living, being present and available physically and emotionally, and offering the patient access to sympathetic dialogue. In this role, it was expected that the coach would positively influence adaptation.

The support group leaders' roles in this study were similar to those in other support groups: facilitator, change agent, consumer advocate, and consultant. As group facilitators and change agents, the leaders provide information to patients and coaches and teach strategies that facilitate adaptation to breast cancer. As consumer advocates, they inform and support patients, enabling them to make and/or participate in decisions affecting their health and adaptation. As consultants, the leaders help patients to deal with the problems that may confront them.

Although the interim quantitative data for the first 158 subjects completing study participation in Samarel and Fawcett's larger randomized controlled clinical trial examining the effects of short-term (8 weeks) group social support and education, both with and without coaching, did not support the study hypothesis that the experimental group with coaching would experience higher levels of adaptation, analyses did indicate that women over 50 years of age participating in groups, both with and without coaching, had less emotional distress

than their counterparts who did not participate in any group. Moreover, participation in groups, both with and without coaching, had a significant effect on the quality of the participants' relationships with significant other, especially for women under 50 years of age. However, group participation, with or without coaching, had no significant effects on symptom distress or functional status.

Content analysis of qualitative data obtained from semi-structured interviews with these subjects revealed differences between those who participated in group support and those who did not. In particular, subjects who participated in support groups stated that they experienced more positive attitudes, greater stress reduction, and less confusion due to their increased understanding of their cancer diagnosis and treatment; greater feelings of normalization and control; less social isolation; greater acceptance of changes in appearance; and less concern related to their physical symptoms than the subjects who did not participate in group support. Moreover, support group subjects overwhelmingly indicated the need for earlier postoperative support and continuing support following the termination of the group meetings. More specifically, they suggested that support that began within a few weeks of surgery and lasting for 1 year would have been even more helpful. Although subjects indicated that weekly group support helped them to adapt, they also indicated that continuing support could be less intense than the weekly group meetings. In second interviews conducted 1 year following surgery, many subjects indicated that individual telephone support would have been appropriate following termination of the group support, because their needs were less acute at this time.

Social Support and Survival

Research examining the effects of social support on survival of women with metastatic breast cancer has yielded fascinating and unexpected results. In 1989 Spiegel et al. published the results of a 10-year follow-up of their original (1981) subjects, and reported a remarkable and significant difference in survival between the experimental and control subjects. At 48 months after entry into the original study, one third of the experimental sample were still alive, whereas all the control subjects had died. Mean survival at the 10-year follow-up was 18.9 months for the control group, compared with 36.6 months for the experimental group. These results were both statistically and clinically significant. Spiegel (1991) further reports that an exhaustive analysis of the prognostic variables revealed no other differences between the two groups that could account for the difference in longevity. Contrary to initial expectations, the conclusion was that something about the experience of the support group participation contributed to the length of survival of these women. Inasmuch as the study was designed to test the effects of psychotherapeutic support groups on subjective well-being and quality of life of women with metastatic breast cancer, the impact of this intervention on survival was of secondary interest and, therefore, unexpected.

In attempting to explain the theoretical rationale for the conclusions that psychotherapeutic support groups have a positive influence on survival, Spiegel (1991) suggests a model that purports that social support is a buffer against the effects of stress, referring to the literature on social support and immune function. In addition to implying that neuroendocrine and immune systems play a role in the extension of survival, he contends that social support in the form of group participation may extend survival time by producing improvements in sleep, diet, activity, and treatment compliance. Dr. Spiegel and his colleagues are currently conducting a randomized controlled clinical trial to study the effects of psychotherapeutic group support on survival of women with early-stage breast cancer.

FUTURE DIRECTIONS

Anecdotal and empirical data support the clinical significance of social support as an in-

tervention to enhance adaptation to breast cancer. Clearly, social support interventions are needed to help women adjust to the diagnosis and treatment of breast cancer. In fact, such interventions should be considered *essential* services of any comprehensive breast cancer diagnosis/treatment center. To meet the needs of those women receiving treatment outside these centers, additional social support interventions need to be offered through community-based programs. Across the United States, such services are offered by hospitals and local American Cancer Society units. In many areas, however, particularly the underserved rural regions, programs of social support are not consistently available.

To more fully support efforts to ensure the availability of social support programs for all women with breast cancer, additional research is needed to answer four questions, outlined below.

The first question to be addressed is related to the description of those women who would receive greatest benefit from social support interventions. Would all women benefit from such interventions, or would only certain populations derive benefit? For example, are there differences in benefits derived for women who live alone? Do socioecomically disadvantaged women require more intense social supports? Are there ethnic and/or racial differences in social support needs?

The second research question addresses who receives and benefits from social support interventions. Should social support be offered only to patients with breast cancer? Do family members also require such interventions? If family members benefit from social support, what are the most effective ways to provide this support? These questions are fully discussed by Northouse in Chapter 14.

The third area of research relates to the identification of the particular women, and possibly families, in need of social support interventions. How can we best identify and target those individuals and families that will derive benefit from their participation in these interventions?

Finally, the fourth area relates to fiscal limitations. Our limited health care resources require that available resources be used judiciously. What is the cost-benefit ratio for social support interventions? Do the benefits of such interventions merit their costs? Samarel and colleagues are currently piloting a randomized controlled clinical trial that includes a cost-benefit analysis of a 13-month social support intervention for women with early-stage breast cancer. If the beneficial effects of social support interventions result in less concern with somatic symptoms, less health care intervention may be required. That is, the presence of social support may result in decreased use of health care resources, meaning fewer health care dollars spent.

SUMMARY

In summary, social support is a multidimensional concept encompassing psychosocial and instrumental dimensions. Social support may be one of the most powerful influences on adaptation to breast cancer. Empirical evidence indicates that cancer support groups, one form of social support, have a beneficial effect on adaptation to breast cancer. Coaching, another form of social support, may also be a positive influence on adaptation. There is also limited empirical evidence supporting the effects of social support on survival of women with metastatic breast cancer.

In determining the future use of social support interventions to help women adapt to the diagnosis and treatment of breast cancer, additional research is needed.

References

Bloom, J. R. (1982). Social support, accommodation to stress and adjustment to breast cancer. *Social Science and Medicine, 16,* 1329–1338.

Bloom, J. R., & Spiegel, D. (1984). The relationship of two dimensions of social support to the psychological well-being and social functioning of women with advanced breast cancer. *Social Science & Medicine, 19,* 831–837.

Cassileth, B. R., Lusk, E. J., Strouse, T. B., Miller, D. S.,

Brown, L. L., & Cross, P. A. (1985). A psychological analysis of cancer patients and their next of kin. *Cancer, 55,* 72–76.

Dunkel-Schetter, C. (1984). Social support and cancer: Findings based on patient interviews and their implications. *Journal of Social Issues, 40,* 77–98.

Edgar, L., Rosberger, Z., & Nowlis, D. (1992). Coping with cancer during the first year after diagnosis. *Cancer, 69,* 817–828.

Ell, K., Nishimoto, R., Morvay, T., Mantell, J., & Hamovitch, M. (1989). A longitudinal analysis of psychological adaptation among survivors of cancer. *Cancer, 63,* 406–413.

Friedland, J., & McColl, M. (1987). Social support and psychosocial dysfunction after stroke: Buffering effects in a community sample. *Archives of Physical Medicine and Rehabilitation, 68,* 475–480.

Hagopian, G. A., & Rubenstein, J. H. (1990). Effects of telephone call interventions on patients' well-being in a radiation therapy department. *Cancer Nursing, 13,* 339–344.

Hilton, B. A. (1989). The relationship of uncertainty, control, commitment, and threat of recurrence to coping strategies used by women diagnosed with breast cancer. *Journal of Behavioral Medicine, 1,* 39–54.

Johnson, J. B., & Kelly, A. W. (1990). A multifaceted rehabilitation program for women with cancer. *Oncology Nursing Forum, 17,* 691–695.

Levy, S. M., & Schain, W. S. (1988). Psychologic response to breast cancer: Direct and indirect contributors to treatment outcome. In M. E. Lippman (Ed.), *Diagnosis and management of breast cancer.* (pp 439–56). Philadelphia: W. B. Saunders.

Mermelstein, H. T., & Holland, J. C. (1991). Psychotherapy by telephone: A therapeutic tool for cancer patients. *Psychosomatics, 32,* 407–412.

Neuling, S. J., & Winefield, H. R. (1988). Social support and recovery after surgery for breast cancer: Frequency and correlates of supportive behaviors by family friends and surgeon. *Social Science & Medicine, 27,* 385–392.

Northouse, L. L. (1988). Social support in patients' and husbands' adjustment to breast cancer. *Nursing Research, 37,* 91–95.

Oakes, J., & Teasdale, K. (1992). Emotional support can precipitate recovery: Setting up a counseling service for breast cancer patients. *Professional Nurse, 7,* 780, 778–783.

Pillon, L. R., & Joannides, G. (1991). An 11-year evaluation of a Living with Cancer program. *Oncology Nursing Forum, 18,* 707–711.

Pritzker, J. K. (1988). The development and formative evaluation of a psychoeducationally based program for post-mastectomy women. (Doctoral dissertation, University of Georgia). *Dissertation Abstracts International, 49,* 2547A.

Samarel, N., & Fawcett, J. (1992). Enhancing adaptation to breast cancer: The addition of coaching to support groups. *Oncology Nursing Forum, 19,* 591–596.

Samarel, N., Fawcett, F., & Tulman, L. (1993). The effects of coaching in breast cancer support groups: A pilot study. *Oncology Nursing Forum, 20,* 795–798.

Shaw, C. R. A. (1989). Exploration of experiences of women during the initial treatment for breast cancer. (Doctoral dissertation, University of Wisconsin-Milwaukee). *Dissertation Abstracts International, 50,* 1327B.

Shumaker, S. A., & Brownell, A. (1984). Toward a theory of social support: Closing conceptual gaps. *Journal of Social Issues, 40,* 11–36.

Siegel, K., Mesagno, P., Karus, D. G., & Christ, G. (1992). Reducing the prevalence of unmet needs for concrete services of patients with cancer. *Cancer, 69,* 1873–1883.

Sparks, T. F. (1988). Coping with the psychosocial stresses of oncology care. *Journal of Psychosocial Oncology, 6,* 165–179.

Spiegel, D. (1991). Mind matters: Effects of group support of cancer patients. *The Journal of NIH Research, 3,* 61–63.

Spiegel, D., Bloom, J., & Yalom, I. (1981). Group support for patients with metastatic cancer. *Archives of General Psychiatry, 38,* 527–533.

Spiegel, D., Kraemer, H. C., Bloom, J. R., & Gottheil, E. (1989). Effect of psychosocial treatment on survival of patients with metastatic breast cancer. *Lancet, 2,* 888–891.

Van den Borne, H., Pruyn, J. F., & Van Dam de May, K. (1986). Self help in cancer patients: A review of studies on the effects of contacts between fellow patients. *Patient Education & Counseling, 8,* 367–385.

Willey, C., & Silliman, R. A. (1990). The impact of disease on the social support experiences of cancer patients. *Journal of Psychosocial Oncology, 8,* 79–95.

PART 4 | Personal Experiences with Breast Cancer

CHAPTER 11	# The Breast Cancer Journey and Emotional Resolution
	## A Perspective from Those Who Have Been There

Kathy LaTour, MFA

BREAST CANCER SURVIVORS: THE EMOTIONAL JOURNEY

When I was diagnosed with breast cancer in 1986 at the age of 37, my friends immediately asked if I would be keeping a journal of my experience. They asked not only because I was a journalist, but also because they knew writing was my way of expressing my feelings about issues that affected me most. They knew that I had written and published my first book, *For Those Who Live: Helping Children Cope With the Death of a Brother or Sister,* in which I resolved my feelings about the death of my brother in a helicopter crash. In *For Those Who Live,* I had used my journalistic skills to gather information about what happens to the other children in a family when a child dies. It had been my resolution of the loss of, and a tribute to, my brother.

But this was different. This was *cancer.* And every time I thought about writing the word *cancer,* I was immobilized. I know now

that this was part of my denial. If I wrote the word *cancer,* it would be real. And I couldn't face it. At the time I just told friends I was too busy. When I was diagnosed, I had a 13-month-old toddler at home, as well as free-lance assignments that I was struggling to find the energy to finish while undergoing chemotherapy.

It was not until almost 3 years after my diagnosis that I began to feel the urge to write about breast cancer. Until then, I wasn't ready, or in enough emotional pain, to look at what had happened to me and deal with it. Even after I had begun writing, the working title for my book *The Breast Cancer Companion* was *Life Goes On.* That's how resistant I was at the time to look at the reality of this disease and what it has done to the lives of many American women.

When I finally started writing about breast cancer, it became my obsession. At this point I was beyond the medical aspect of my treatment. I had had reconstructive surgery, and physically, I was well. But I had started to realize that there was more to healing than scars and surviving the side effects of chemotherapy. I needed help with the emotional issues that still lingered, some of which had begun to seriously affect my life. After finally joining a support group, I realized that the most valuable information about emotional recovery from breast cancer comes from other women with the disease. As a journalist, I could rely on my "writing" to show me answers that I may not have been willing to see for myself. In addition to the support group, I sought out women who were further along in their recovery than I was. I wanted their insights into the disease and what they had experienced. The strongest voices in my book are those of the women survivors, with medical professionals and other health care providers serving in a supporting role.

After interviewing more than 120 women, their husbands, and some of their children, I learned that breast cancer must be fought on two fronts: medical and emotional. While all breast cancer patients undergo fairly standard medical procedures, each woman's emotional recovery from the disease—or lack of it—is a distinctly individualized journey. The women in the book and my support group gave names to what were very distinct emotional stages, but *when* a woman arrived at each of the stages was determined by her own individual journey, how strong her denial was, and whether she found a supportive place to express her feelings.

What most of the women agreed on was that the emotional issues related to breast cancer did not really begin until treatment ended and they were sent home to get back to "normal," when in fact the "normal" that was life before breast cancer no longer existed.

When I was diagnosed with breast cancer, no one discussed with me the emotional process of living with cancer, or life after cancer. Nor was there any mention of how I might explore my feelings about my disease. My medical team had as their goal whether I would live, not how I would come to terms with and

resolve a life-threatening illness and become the new person who emerges from the cancer experience.

Ironically, the mid-1980s marked the beginning of a number of explorations into the emotional ramifications of cancer. In the last 100 years, there have been tremendous advances in cancer treatment, meaning more and more patients are surviving the experience. A new field of medicine, psychooncology, focuses on the emotional reaction to cancer. Dr. Jimmie Holland, Chief of Psychiatry Service at Memorial Sloan-Kettering Cancer Center, and her colleagues Dr. Mary Jane Massie and Dr. Julia Rowland were pioneers in the psychooncology field.

At the same time, cancer survivors were beginning to find each other. Support groups were forming, and those who had had cancer were sharing their experiences—only to find that many of them had the same issues and fears. Models for survivorship began emerging as the new survivor community began connecting. In fact, the week I underwent surgery, a group met in Albuquerque, New Mexico, to discuss the issues of "survivorship" and form the nucleus for the National Coalition for Cancer Survivorship, which today represents thousands of survivors from its office in Silver Spring, Maryland. This exploration of who we are as cancer survivors is reflected in the terminology that has emerged to describe the stages we experience and the universal feeling that there is a need to look at our "new way of living" that is life after a cancer diagnosis.

To heal emotionally from breast cancer, a woman must assimilate the experience into her life. Indeed, some researchers have observed a definite connection between medical and emotional recovery and believe the emotional healing could actually impact the physical. In 1989, Dr. David Spiegel's study of women with metastatic breast cancer showed, to everyone's surprise, that the women in a breast cancer support group lived twice as long as those who did not attend. And Spiegel points out, in his book *Living Beyond Limits,* that it wasn't the "smile and you will live" kind of talk that helped these women. It was the darker discussions, about fears, pain, and death, that extended their lives. Indeed, in exploring a number of mind/body studies, Spiegel says,

> ". . .these studies provide evidence that the type of intervention that seems to be most helpful is one which focuses on facing directly the threat posed by the illness and increasing social support, rather than positive mental imagery. Facing bad possibilities does not, according to these studies, convert them into bad probabilities. *Living Beyond Limits*, p. 86.)

The message I received from the women I interviewed is that medical and emotional healing are inextricably intertwined. We *will* be different people after a breast cancer diagnosis. We *should* be different people. Our disease, its treatment, and our assimilation of these enormous changes are great challenges. We need intervention and education from our medical professionals to bring about emotional healing, just as we need surgery and chemotherapy.

Stages of Healing

The model for emotional resolution that emerged from my support group and the women in my book had distinct stages. Some women began the process and moved very clearly through the stages. Others would take three steps forward and two backward, moving a little more into the next stage with every leap. (See Table 11-1).

We affectionately called the first stage *The rabbit caught in the headlights* phase. We have just heard the word *cancer* and we wait, frozen with fear, while the monster comes toward us. Even those of us who are empowered are immobile—death is at the door. We are dying, no ifs, ands, or buts.

Then we meet with the oncologist or surgeon about our options and begin to realize that we may not be at death's door. We also have moved to the next stage, which we called *doctor bonding*. Now we have a plan that will

Table 11-1   Stages of Healing

1. Rabbit caught in the headlights —being immobilized by cancer
2. Doctor bonding on the "Fine, fine" stage
3. Crash and burn
4. Resolution

save us, and we develop a strong bond with the person presenting this plan. (I also call this the "Fine, fine" stage. When a woman is asked how she is doing, she says very quickly, "Fine, fine.") At this stage, we begin to function again in that lovely state of denial that allows us to continue functioning in most of our usual roles in life, while undergoing surgery and treatment. "Automatic pilot" takes over, getting us to the grocery store, work, and school. Our friends are amazed at how well we are handling everything. We are reading the "keep a positive attitude" books that well-meaning friends have given us.

Unfortunately, we *aren't* fine, and we shouldn't be encouraged to be, but we won't know that for a while.

A woman knows she is doctor bonding when she knows where to park at the massive centers where cancer is usually treated nowadays. This is also the point where she begins to understand "medispeak." In this strange language, a *port*, which used to be where ships dock, is something that goes under the skin, and a wig becomes a *cranial prosthesis*.

Doctor bonding usually lasts until treatment is over. A woman puts her life and her complete trust in this person, who is usually optimistic about her chances. And then comes the time when the doctor tells the woman patient that it is time for her to go home and resume her normal life.

What life? The one she had before she heard the word *cancer*? All of a sudden that person she once was seems a little blurry. The woman patient will try to find her again, to get back her goals and plans for the future.

At this point, as breast cancer survivors, *we begin to realize that we are all alone now.*

The next stage we arrived at in my support group was affectionately called *crash and burn,* which usually comes sometime after treatment is over. Our doctors have sent us home, friends and family cheering, "Aren't you glad that's over?"

But in reality, we come to understand at this stage that what we must do now is wait. And all women with this capricious disease soon learn that breast cancer can recur, even when we have done everything right in terms of treatment. Women only have to absorb a small amount of information to understand that they are not home free—and most never will be.

I asked my oncologist at my 3-month checkup when I would be considered cured. I had heard about the "magic" 5-year mark. He looked at me and said, "Not with breast cancer. You are considered cured when you die of something else."

Those women who join a support group immediately after diagnosis will see women recur. Observing this either will cause them to fall away from the group, or will crack their denial and take them to crash and burn.

Because I was a journalist and a very verbal person, I first sought out a support group for young adults with cancer. I went four times and then found excuses not to return. Three of the participants had already had recurrence. I just couldn't handle it yet. I wasn't ready. My denial was still too strong.

What we should all strive for is the final stage, *resolution,* when the cancer experience has been integrated into our lives in a healthy realistic manner. But in order to do this, we must accept that at some point we will have to experience crash and burn, and this isn't easy. Beyond our comprehension of the pain of surgery or chemotherapy is the pain of reality. I have come to like crash and burn as an image, because it represents what we are really going through. It is a violent image, because what happens to our bodies and our psyches is violent. Both our bodies and our souls are rearranged. But the positive outcome of this violence is that like the phoenix that rises from the flames of the experience, we are wiser from and tempered by pain.

I found women who were truly traumatized, as they struggled not to enter the crash and burn phase, myself included. We spend incredible time and energy trying desperately to keep a lid on the fear consuming us. Any number of little things send us scurrying to the oncologist for a check up, or into a panic attack. We are terrified over any unusual pain, a well-publicized diagnosis, a friend's diagnosis or recurrence, or an upcoming checkup (by now we know that quarterly blood work is a search for recurrence.)

My oldest stepdaughter Kari is a costume designer, and was working in Los Angeles on her first big movie when a strong earthquake hit in January 1994. She told me that when the initial quake hit, it took her a minute to figure out she might be in danger. She had been in Los Angeles only a few days, and because she had never experienced an earthquake before, she lay on the bed and thought, "Oh, this must be an earthquake." It was not until she heard shouting and screaming that she realized it wasn't a small one.

Because she had never had the experience, she had nothing to compare it with. But as soon as she understood the magnitude of the quake, she was more frightened than she has ever been in her life. For a few minutes she thought she was going to die. I told her, "Now you know what it's like to hear you have cancer."

Kari further explained that after that quake, every time there was an aftershock, she felt the same impending doom all over. Now she knew *exactly* what was happening as soon as the shaking began, and every time she wondered if this would be the "big one" that would kill her.

That, I explained, is what it's like to live after breast cancer. Our aftershocks come in the little aches and pains, or the strange lump we find. Even the little reminders like checkups take us again to that moment when we thought we would die. And in reality, when we have a checkup or feel an ache, it *could* be the beginning of the end. We have seen it happen too often with friends, and know too well how capricious this disease is.

This understanding leaves us with two choices:

1. We can live in denial, using our energy to keep our feelings locked up tight. But we must understand that keeping fear locked up destroys our ability to experience many other feelings— including passion. I defy any woman to enjoy healthy sex while trying to keep the lid on her fears. I wondered why I cried so often during this time of my resolution. I cried during sex. I cried in the car. I cried when I felt anything remotely resembling a strong emotion. And I had no idea why.

2. We can look at the reality of this disease, accepting the hard truth that it might return, and move on with that resolution. The Valley of the Shadow of Death is a real place for us—and understanding that can be incredibly liberating. In order to truly resolve a breast cancer diagnosis, a woman has to face the fact that she might die.

A woman facing breast cancer must make many medical choices, about who will care for her and what kind of surgery and treatment she wants. After diagnosis, her doctor is prompting her, and these decisions must be made.

A woman must also choose to begin the emotional treatment for breast cancer, which is often more painful than surgery. It can be more complicated and time-consuming, because every woman brings to the diagnosis a unique set of coping skills and support. And often, a woman in crash and burn won't even understand what is happening.

For example, one of the interviews that appears early in my book was with Cindy. Diagnosed at 33 with three tumors that totaled six centimeters, she had undergone preoperative chemotherapy, and then had a mastectomy and additional chemo. We met for lunch about 6 months after she had finished chemo. Her short black curly hair was stylish and she was incredibly bubbly. I was amazed at her good spirits. She felt that the experience was behind her, that she was feeling better, and she couldn't wait to get on with her life. She and her fiancée of 5 years had set a wedding date and she couldn't have been more excited about the future.

Our interview took place before I understood the cycle, but when I did some months later, I called her back. I wanted to see how she was and interview her fiancée.

She was a completely different person. She didn't understand what had happened and was depressed much of the time. She thought her fears were stupid, but try as she might, she couldn't control them. I told her what I had seen from other women and explained that she had hit crash and burn. Just the news that she wasn't the only one to experience this made a tremendous difference. Like many of the women I interviewed, she thought she was crazy and unreasonable.

Since then, she has begun a new life. She has broken off her engagement with her fiancée and found her own house.

Undergoing the process of assimilation of breast cancer gives us tremendous gifts. We have more depth, more dimension. I like images for my resolution, and this year I found another that I think clearly demonstrates this growth.

Imagine, if you will, two clay pots. One is perfect, every curve symmetrical. The other has been broken and then put back together. But now this pot has bits of color in the clay, and the cement between the pieces has glitter in it. (One of the nice things about reinventing yourself is that you can give yourself more color and dimension.) Cancer survivors are like clay pots that have been shattered. We have been put back together and now are much more interesting to look at and have more dimension than the perfect pot.

But in order to be put back together, we have to risk falling apart, and we need to know that we will have help finding the pieces and putting ourselves back together again.

BARRIERS TO EMOTIONAL RESOLUTION

The barriers to healthy resolution of breast cancer come from both internal and external sources. While a woman may have overcome one barrier, another may emerge (Table 11-2).

Our Denial

The day I received the call that my mammogram was "highly suspicious," I was watching my daughter try to take her first steps. All I could think was, "It took me two years to get pregnant, and now I am going to die, and she won't even remember me." It was a thought too overwhelming to sustain for more than an instant. The thought that I might leave my child was my worst fear. It controlled what I was able to hear, comprehend, and accept, and defined my emotional work for 2 years. I think I stayed in denial longer than most women because of my young child. Other young mothers with breast cancer have confirmed my feelings. The idea that we might die and leave our child is incomprehensible, and leaves us unable to move beyond this fear.

Some women have already faced mortality issues when they are diagnosed. Older women have seen friends receive a cancer diagnosis, and some almost expect one. How strongly a woman will hang onto the denial that protects her truly depends on the woman and where she is in her life work. My denial at diagnosis was necessary for me to continue to function. Had I been told that day I was dying, I would have rejected it as impossible. Denial allows us to absorb what we can at the time, and select out what we need to hear.

A woman in denial is hard to help. She won't hear what has to happen because it is too painful. But as time goes on, she may be more willing.

Table 11-2   Barriers to Emotional Healing

1. Denial
2. Family denial
3. Physician misunderstanding

Our Family's Denial

Denial, which is a woman's friend and defender at the beginning, helps us appear composed to the outsider. It prompts family, friends, and our health care providers to comment on how well we are doing, how well we are handling everything. Before the emotional work can begin, denial must be cracked. This becomes more complicated when the woman recognizes she is in emotional pain, but her community is encouraging her to be "fine, fine," which one woman described as an acronym for "Frustrated, Insecure, Neglected, and Emotional." The second "fine" should be defined as "Fragile, Isolated, Nauseated, and Exhausted."

After my surgery, a church friend called me "an inspiration." I was functioning like an automaton and doing what I call my "I Am Woman" routine. What I really needed was a padded room, where I could scream, *feel*, and express what had happened to me. But it was very hard to give up being "an inspiration" in order to be crazy. Cancer survivors often are not supported to do the emotional work we need to deal with life crises. We are encouraged to be "fine, fine."

Family and friends also reinforce an attitude of "aren't you glad that's over" after chemo. They think the worst is behind you. Consistently, the women I interviewed told me they were in worse shape emotionally a year after their diagnosis than when they were going through treatment—when they felt they were *doing* something to fight the disease.

They want to be the person they were before diagnosis, but they can't. Friends and family are telling them it's over, so they have lost that outlet for expressing their fears—and they are left isolated.

Our Physician Misunderstanding

Most physicians still don't discuss emotional issues with patients, during or after treatment, because it is so hard to assess individual women. When they do, they usually just ask, "How are you?" To which we repond, "Fine, fine." Where we are is a complicated emotional issue, and we aren't all at the same place. Most surgeons and oncologists don't have the necessary training or time to interpret correctly where we are emotionally.

Those physicians who do strive to get their patients to open up about their feelings often find resistance that is related to the issue of doctor bonding. Women feel that they are failing their doctors if they are well physically, but having a difficult time emotionally. One woman even told me, "I owe him my life, and I am going to complain about a little depression?"

Communication between doctor and patient is even more difficult when this reluctance to talk is compounded with the fact that most of these discussions take place in the examination room. This room is where we came when we were sick. We sat there waiting for the blood work numbers that would tell us if we were going to live for the next 6 months. Why would we want to hang around here for a chat?

I watched this phenomenon with my mother, who was diagnosed with breast cancer in October 1991 at the age of 72, almost exactly 5 years after I was diagnosed. She became a different person as soon as our oncologist entered the exam room. She would have had a number of painful emotional issues that she would clearly express to me on the way to her appointment, *issues that she was willing to discuss with the female study nurse.* But the minute our oncologist walked through the door, mother was a little girl trying to please. He was not asking her to assume that attitude. In fact, during my 5-year relationship with

him, he had always been open to questions and feelings. I know that I didn't share mine with him because my denial was so intense, but here was my mother with acute depression that she would not express to him. She was fulfilling what she saw as her role as the *good patient.* Good patients make doctors like them. Doctors who like their patients keep them alive. This is not a logical attitude, but it is a very real one. It is too frightening to risk disappointing the person who holds your life in his or her hands.

RESOLUTION: WHAT IT LOOKS LIKE

I had closed the door on my feelings on the day of my diagnosis, when I denied my worst fear, the fear of leaving my daughter. It was as if I had locked that fear, along with most of my other feelings, away in a dark room and thrown away the key. No one was telling me to open it. In fact, I was being told, "Aren't you over this yet?" I kept thinking I was crazy that I had all these fears.

When it became clear that there were a few feelings I wanted back from that locked room—passion, love, joy—I began to open the door. More than 2 years after my surgery, I began to look at what had happened to me.

I did this in a support group begun by my surgeon at her office and facilitated by an oncology nurse who also had earned a PhD in grief counseling. In the summer of 1989, when I told my surgeon about my emotional pain, she said a number of her patients were going through the same thing and she had hired a counselor to work with them. At the time, it was a revolutionary idea. But by 1994, most breast centers and breast surgeons had psychologists, social workers, or oncology nurses on staff to assist with emotional issues.

When I joined the support group in August 1989, I was the furthest out from surgery. I had hit crash and burn while the rest of the group was still in doctor bonding. I talked about suffering back spasms when a friend told me her cancer had metastasized to her back. They looked at me like I was crazy. I envied their attitudes of "It will all be over soon and I can get back to normal." Still, I sensed even then that we were all on the same journey, and that they would soon share my emotional state, instead of the other way around.

But as I talked of my fears and expressed my pain, they began to share theirs, and soon we truly loved each other. Then I learned that one of the women had had fourteen positive nodes. I knew what that meant, although no one else did, yet. At that point, I had to decide whether or not to stay in the group, knowing that I would have to face her future.

I stayed. Soon after that, one other member of the group hit crash and burn and suddenly I saw in her a familiar friend. My journey was affirmed, and she had a role model who could validate her feelings. I remember her asking me before the group meeting that night, "Do you ever lie in bed and cry and think about your own funeral?" I replied, "Welcome to crash and burn."

In our group, we could laugh about panic attacks and the sure feeling that you are dying when your arm hurts. We laughed as much as we cried.

This was not a smile-and-you-will-live group, and we couldn't attract the large numbers of women that other breast cancer support groups could, with their games and chit-chat. We were working through the dark emotional issues. We soon also became known as "the group," among our doctors. We were known for asking hard questions and demanding information from our health care providers.

We also became what I would call a "closed group" —visitors would sense the intensity and, with few exceptions, beat a hasty retreat. This was when it became clear to me why I had run from my first group. It also made it clear that breast cancer support groups have to come in many shades and degrees for where a woman is at the moment.

We had one visitor who sat and smiled all night during one of our sessions. When it came time for her to talk, she said she was fine

and ready to get back to her life, and that she really didn't understand what all the fuss was about. The look the rest of us exchanged said, "Bye for now. We'll see you in a year or so." And we did.

When Carolyn, a member of the group from the start, recurred, my worst fear was realized. She was going to die. Do I stay or go? Do I shut down, or face my worst fear? I stayed, and faced Carolyn's death with her and the group.

And then the tears came. All the intellectualizing was gone, and all that was left was tremendous emotion. I cried for a month—for myself, for my daughter should I die, for my husband, for my stepchildren, for my mother, for myself. I cried for my past and for my future, my future that had become so uncertain. I cried tears of anger and joy. Then I cried for Carolyn.

Another group member, Marilyn, was coping with recurrence at the same time that Carolyn died. She knew that breast cancer would take her life, and, because I had finally opened the door to the pain, she became my guide. We talked about living and dying, and two weeks before she died, Marilyn said, "You know Kathy, there are worse things than dying. Live until you die."

I decided she was right. I thought about what I wanted for my daughter and put friends in charge of different aspects of her upbringing should I die. I talked to my husband about dying. I went into that locked room full of my feelings and fairly flung open the doors and windows.

What I learned from the women in that group was that by *naming* a fear it becomes manageable, a fear I could control. And by *naming and facing* my worst fear, I could be free to feel again, at a new level.

SPECIFICS TO ASSIST WOMEN WITH RESOLUTION

1. Accept that emotional resolution is a part of healing. Be committed to helping your patients with education about their disease and the need for emotional intervention. Explore models for intervention and how best to present information.

In the fall of 1993, I attended the Annual Breast Symposium in San Antonio, to promote my book. A number of doctors scanned the book and earnestly engaged me in conversation about how to help their patients ask questions and be actively engaged in their treatment.

Cancer patients ask questions when we have information that makes us think. My first impulse was to ask these doctors what kind of reading material they had for their patients in their waiting rooms. In most offices, there is some combination of magazines such as *People, Field and Stream,* and *Architectural Digest,* magazines the doctors order for themselves and then pass on. Why aren't the waiting room walls covered with book cases filled with leading books on cancer? I know that I could have read a good portion of the Library of Congress in the amount of time I waited, because my oncologist takes time to answer questions and doesn't make his patients feel rushed.

Information helps break down the barriers. Doctors must risk the misinformation and additional questions and give their patients the freedom and encouragement to read all the books from Siegel to Spiegel, and then ask questions. There are many wonderful books about breast cancer, and cancer in general. Most of these books languish in warehouses, however, because they are not promoted to be immediate best sellers, and book stores won't allow the time for word-of-mouth recommendations to bring in sales.

I suggest physicians buy three of the books listed at the end of this chapter as a start. Have copies of these books in exam rooms, and work out a lending policy. Ask one local bookstore to stock these books, and let them know you will be referring people.

It makes me ill to see women reading pocket romance novels or staring into space when they could be informed, moved, and motivated by another woman's story of her breast cancer experience. Yes, some patients have such strong denial that they won't read such books, but most women will begin to absorb information that the nurses and physicians can explain and expand upon.

An ideal situation would be a room away from the exam room and the waiting room, and away from the chemo room (the smell can bring on panic attacks), where there are books and a patient educator. This room should be small and cozy enough to encourage patients to talk with each other.

Women need information about both the medical and emotional issues on *every visit* to the surgeon or oncologist. Studies show women hear 10% of what is told to them in the first meeting when they learn they have cancer.

Physicians need to address the emotional resolution issue as more than a passing suggestion. A physician doesn't *suggest* chemotherapy; he or she picks up the phone and makes the appointment. If emotional healing is treated as a part of standard medical care, then there needs to be a program or a person a physician can access on the day that surgery is planned. This can be an individual therapist, such as the one I saw, or a small group where information can be exchanged and emotional issues shared. If each oncologist would designate one nurse educator in the office to act as a liaison to other resources, it would greatly assist the physician and the patient. At the time of diagnosis or surgery, women may want medical information more than emotional support, but that resource may be one they can return to when the issues become more emotional.

Certainly there are women who will resist any notion that they are on an emotional journey. For some women, a breast cancer diagnosis is just another life crisis to be gotten through with a minimum of fuss. They will ignore the feelings and pain associated with it, just as they have minimized other trauma in their lives. If the doctor does succeed in providing one of these women with some emotional intervention, the cancer experience will probably have to get in line behind other unresolved issues in her life.

But most women will welcome their physician's concern, and while they may not take you up on offers for emotional support immediately, the seed will be planted—to be nurtured at each visit from that point forward until the last treatment. Indeed, some women will demand such interventions be in place as a part of their care. Today's women are more assertive, educated, and demanding of her physicians.

2. Establish an exit interview at the end of chemotherapy or radiation to prepare a woman for the next phase. This phase involves emotional issues that they may experience and how to access programs to begin the next phase. Address it as emotional resolution and what they may experience. This is a chance for the nurses to refer to survivorship groups or individuals for support.

Consistently, I have heard from women that their strongest need for support and intervention was 1 to 1½ years after surgery. So many of them told me, "I was so ready for the last chemo, but then I went home and depression set in. I thought I was crazy."

As the medical care is terminated, the woman is cut loose from her medical team. And if she has been educated at all about her disease, she knows that she has to go home and wait to see if the cancer recurs.

The medical team must prepare women for "after treatment" and the emotional crises that may be ahead of them. How wonderful it would have been if someone had just said to me at this time, "You know, I know you are excited that treatment is over, but some women tell us that the emotional issues really overwhelm them after they go home. They tell us that they worry excessively about little aches and pains." My oncologist would have saved a few extra hours that he ended up spending with me on the phone if someone had told me that one little bit of information. And, I would have taken the issue where it belonged—to my support group—instead of ordering a bone scan.

Some oncologists have a special ritual for the last chemo—a red rose on the chemo chair, a gift certificate for a manicure, or just a hug goodbye, for completing what is often the most difficult thing many of us ever go through.

There should be a time line to guide the nurse on the presentation of emotional information to the cancer survivor. At the first 3-month posttreatment checkup, asking a few questions may give the nurse a sense of whether the woman should be referred to a support group. The nurse may recommend my book or others that address emotional issues, or the name of a former patient she could talk to. The nurse should then follow up with a phone call. If the woman is resistant, don't give up. Accept that issues may change for her in the coming months, and if she has your phone number and a warm word from you, she may be willing to call.

3. Enhance and develop the role of nurse specialist in a comprehensive breast health center. Today, many women are seeking out a Breast Center for their care when they are diagnosed. These specialized centers offer under one roof all the services related to breast cancer, and often have an oncology nurse who is a key player in the education and psychological concerns of patients.

This oncology nurse specialist is an important liaison for the patient and the busy physician. She explains, educates, and cares, which results in more productive discussions between the doctor and the patient and helps the patient feel happier and more willing to comply with her treatment.

Among the nurse's responsibilities could be to meet with the patient before the exam, to answer questions and help her formulate questions for the doctor. The nurse can assess the patient's emotional state before the exam and then pass this information on to the physician before she meets with the patient.

This nurse can provide educational material for the patient and her family, oversee a lending library, and serve as a resource/liaison to existing therapists and survivor groups. This nurse should have the special training required to assess whether a woman needs an individual therapist or a group support network. The oncology nurse should be the expert on programs already in operation, and can help with other stressors not related to the disease, such as sexual issues, financial issues, nutritional information, home health, and chaplains. The oncology nurse should be easily accessible by phone, and should be able to offer unlimited time to be asked questions and clarify misconceptions about the disease, in an unhurried and trusting environment. All of the patient's questions and reactions can be reported to her physicians.

The role of the oncology nurse specialist must evolve, just as has every other support person in the physician's office. Although these suggestions appear costly to the physician, it is the physician who now pays for unnecessary phone calls and appointments that have been brought on by a patient's panic attacks, which can only be resolved emotionally, not medically.

If emotional treatment is accepted as a part of standard care, it should be funded in the same way as are treatments such as chemotherapy, radiation therapy, or any other medical treatment. Just as specialists in these fields have emerged, so too must members of the health care team whose focus is education and emotional support for the women recovering from breast cancer.

RECOMMENDED READING

The Breast Cancer Companion, Kathy LaTour (William Morrow)

The Breast Cancer Journal, Juliet Wittman (Fulcrum)

Charting the Journey (available through NCCS. Call 301–650–8868 for purchase information.)

Fighting Cancer, Richard Bloch (free, call 816–932–8453)

Gentle Closings, Ted Menten (Running Press)

Healing and the Mind, Bill Moyers (Doubleday)

Healing Into Life and Death, Stephen Levine (Anchor Books)

Healing Words, Larry Dossey, MD (Bantam)

Living Beyond Limits, Dr. David Spiegel (Simon and Schuster)

Medicine and Meaning, Larry Dossey, MD (Bantam)

Recovering the Soul, Larry Dossey, MD (Bantam)

Spinning Straw into Gold, Ronnie Kaye (Fireside, a division of Simon and Schuster)

Susan Love's Breast Book, Dr. Susan Love (Addison Wesley)

Who Dies?, Stephen Levine (Anchor Books)

References

Spiegel, D. (1993) *Living beyond limits*, New York: Times Books.

Spiegel, D., Bloom, J. R., Kraemer, H. C., & Toggheil, E. (1989). Effect of psychosocial treatment on survival of patients with metastatic breast cancer. *Lancet ii:*, 888–891.

CHAPTER 12 | Choice and Decision Making for Women with Breast Cancer

Susan A. Leigh, RN, BSN

"At every turn there are bewildering arrays of choices, and often there is no adequate external guidance that you can count on. So when all the information is before you, consider turning inward to discover from as deep a source as possible what *makes sense to you.*" (Lerner, 1994)

When you are first told that enemy cancer cells have invaded your body and are threatening your future, it is difficult, if not impossible, to calmly make decisions that will affect your very existence. Fear, panic, and uncertainty are common initial responses to a cancer diagnosis, yet it is introspection that truly helps us make the best decisions for ourselves at this time. But before a decision can be made, all the possible options must be understood.

We have choices and make decisions every day of our lives. We decide to get out of bed, and then decide what we eat, what to wear, and what we will say and do during the day. "Making a choice" is a process of selecting from our options. This process assumes that there is more than one option, and implies that an opportunity to choose is available. It can be purely automatic activity or a highly complicated process. Building on experiences from the past, we make decisions in the present, with varying degrees of concern about the future.

As Frank (1991) notes in his book *At the Will of the Body*, "the future disappeared" at the moment his malignancy was diagnosed. Like Frank, most people feel almost paralyzed with fear when they hear the word *cancer*, a word describing one of the most dreaded diseases of our (or any) time. Yet few people diagnosed with cancer have the luxury of remaining immobile for very long. Once the shock of the situation has registered, the issue of choice and decision making takes on utmost importance.

ISSUE OF CHOICE

Within the arena of breast cancer, *choice* has simultaneously become encouraging and discouraging. While women appreciate the greater selection of therapeutic modalities, they can also be overwhelmed by the sheer magnitude of their options. Physicians from different specialty areas offer different types of therapy. Within each of these specialties or sub-specialties—surgery, chemotherapy, radiation therapy, bone marrow transplantion, gene therapy—numerous options are offered. The media also add to the options by informing the public of great scientific breakthroughs, even though opportunities to utilize new treatments are often unavailable, rationed, or controversial. The encouraging news with breast cancer is that improvements in early detection and treatments offer many more choices that can help optimize our chances for survival. The discouraging news is that these increased options are often not offered, are not understood enough to allow patients to make informed decisions, are subject to the biases of individual physicians, are limited by payors, or simply are not available to everyone.

The following statements from "Words That Harm, Words That Heal," a paper prepared by Clark in 1995 after surveying members of the National Coalition for Cancer Survivorship (NCCS), illustrate some of the difficulties that women face when attempting to make personal decisions related to their individual care.

When a patient asked her surgeon about alternative therapies:

"I'm not going to discuss your questions. Do it my way or don't do it at all."

From a radiation oncologist:

"You should have seen me first and the surgery would not have been necessary."

Also:

"I don't know why we're doing this radiation protocol. There isn't that much hope!"

And in trying to make a decision about reconstruction, a physician offered:

"You should have reconstructive surgery because you have a nice breast, and you would be more attractive to men if you had two breasts."

Insensitive interchanges do nothing to assist decision making, except possibly motivate patients to change doctors. Yet the impact can be devastating, and these *word wounds*, as described by Clark, simply compound already existing stress.

Even though increasing amounts of information are available, decisions surounding cancer therapy are usually made when women are most vulnerable. The language of medicine is foreign, the care providers can be intimidating, and the current health care or *disease-repair* system is challenging at best.

CHANGING SOCIAL TRENDS

As social trends change, the once passive patient is frequently encouraged to be an active partner in decision making and treatment planning. Some women who wish to take on some of this responsibility experience resistance from physicians who feel that only they can make medical decisions.

"I remember the surgeon doing the biopsy telling me: 'I don't know why you want to be cut on. You are much too young to have breast cancer.' She then told me that I was asking way too many questions and should just wait until she decided if I needed any further assistance."

This young woman subsequently found out the biopsy was positive and fired her surgeon, who continued to think the diagnosis was a mistake (Ferrell, Dow, & Leigh, 1995).

Alternately, the decision making can be handed over to the patient, who may be feeling overpowered by fear and confusion. She may feel totally unprepared, intellectually or emotionally, to make such decisions. Or the patient might demand that this decision be solely her responsibility.

> *"I'd . . . question the almost universal recommendation to take the decision-making process into your own hands—at least in one respect. It's fine to prowl medical libraries and talk to everyone you've ever known who might have a smidgen of useful information, but you cannot find out enough to save your own life in two or three frantic weeks of searching."* (Wittman, 1993).

Neither extreme is satisfactory. Women diagnosed with breast cancer need guidance through the selection process and support for the decisions they make. Also from "Words That Heal, Words That Harm," a patient described the following positive encounter with her gynecologist:

> *"As the doctor pushed aside the charts and papers on his desk, he said, 'You must be devastated by your diagnosis. Let's talk. You can cry or scream or whatever you want and I will listen.' It showed he cared about me and what I had to say, and that he had time for me."* (Clark, 1995).

Health care providers, whether physicians, nurses, or social workers, need to be advocates in the agenda-setting process, and many cancer survivors have called their oncology nurses their best and most consistent allies.

WHO SETS THE AGENDA

The question of *who* sets the agenda for choice and decision making for women facing breast cancer is a major concern within the current consumer-driven survivorship movement. As this movement represents the voices of the people who are actually living through the experience, the semantics of survival are being defined, and the stages experienced by cancer survivors are being extended to reflect the needs of the survivors themselves. Quality of life has become a major concern. And the range of survival issues has been extended far beyond the initial diagnosis and treatment, into long-term survival.

At the same time, there is considerable confusion surrounding the meaning of survivorship, and its place within the overall context of cancer care. Is it defined by a time frame, by a stage of survival, or by clinical parameters? Does it have any impact at all on early-stage decision making? Should survivorship only focus on non-medical issues and decisions that are made after treatment is completed?

SURVIVORSHIP DEFINED

When viewed from a purely clinical perspective, i.e., a medical model, survivorship has been described in a number of ways: as the period of time that begins when patients complete therapy, are in remission, are free of disease for 5 years, or are considered cured. While some care providers see survivorship as a later stage along the survival continuum, others simply separate patients who are receiving therapy, from survivors who have completed their treatment. This perspective does not take into account the differences in disease and illness, the biologic chronicity of some cancers, or the lingering psychosocial effects that can continue after therapy. It does, however, offer an understandable way to define two separate populations of people—those who are currently receiving therapy versus those who are not.

Historically, the medical model put health care providers in a paternalistic role, in which they were making decisions *for* the patient. This viewpoint is currently being challenged by a growing grassroots movement, especially with the founding of the NCCS, which defines the concept of survivorship and its related issues from the perspective of the consumer. By combining the definitions of Mullan and Hoffman (1990) and Carter (1989), survivorship can be seen as a *dynamic process* rather than a *stage of survival*, a process that includes living with, through, and beyond cancer (Leigh, 1991). When defined in this context, the survivor's role of choice and decision making is critical to the survival process, and this role must be supported from the moment of diagnosis, continuing indefinitely.

Historical Shift

It was not too many decades ago that choices were simple, staightforward, and limited. A lump was discovered, the woman was hospitalized, and she underwent surgery not knowing if she would wake up with or without her breast. Psychological concerns were given little if any consideration, and the treatment options were mainly surgical. Besides mastectomy, surgeons could recommend oophorectomy, adrenalectomy, and hypophysectomy, depending on the stage of the disease and the patient's menopausal status. Neither admission to the hospital nor length of stay was a problem, and money did not primarily determine the type or quality of care. The physician was seen as the primary decision maker, and decisions were relatively easy because there were so few choices.

How different the cancer world is today! Just as biomedical miracles have increased our chances for being cured of cancer, or living longer with a chronic illness, they have also elevated our expectations for *beating the disease*. The current challenge facing women diagnosed with breast cancer is clearly summarized in Kabat-Zinn's foreword for *Choices in Healing* (Lerner, 1994):

> "...the message of the entire book is aimed just where it ought to be, namely, at making realistic, hopeful, and uniquely personal choices under time pressure and on the basis of incomplete evidence and partial understanding of an extremely complex disease, where nobody has the last word or a magic bullet, and many approaches can be complementary to one another."

No cancer typifies this scenario better than breast cancer. It has become an arena for increasing awareness about changing decision-making patterns, to challenge assump-

tions about informed consent, to advocate for supportive consumer services and networks, and to rally behind activism for *social change*, such as access to treatment and employment and insurance discrimination.

CHANGING DECISION-MAKING PATTERNS

The ability to make effective decisions has become a critical survival skill for patients in today's health care arena, and women must first realize that the ultimate responsibility for making decisions belongs to them. This does not mean that all women will make the same choices or use the same decision-making process. Oncology nurses must recognize these differences, and support the individual styles of their patients.

In describing decision-making behaviors, Pierce (1993) recognizes individual differences and identifies three separate styles: the deferrer, the delayer, and the deliberator. In addition to defining decision-making styles, Newfeld, Degner, and Dick (1993) encourage patient involvement in the decision-making process and delineate role preferences: the passive role, the collaborative role, and the active role.

The deferrer tends to be an older patient, who grew up in a time when physicians made all the decisions. It is not as if she has no choice, but rather that she *chooses* a passive role and defers decision-making to the individual whom she sees as the expert. Her decisions are made rather quickly and with minimal conflict, because she is more likely to accept the option favored by her physician.

The delayer, on the other hand, tends to be younger than the deferrer, and wants more options for comparison. This person vacillates when trying to make a decision and changes her mind repeatedly, until one option appears to be the best. Her role is more collaborative, as she seeks to share decision-making responsibility with her doctor or health care team.

The third defined role is that of the deliberator, who takes charge of and feels personally responsible for making the decision that feels right. By choosing an active role, the deliberator controls her circumstances as much as possible. She tends to develop a strategy or plan of action. She carefully considers all treatment risks and attempts to minimize those risks by gathering information. She is confident in her ability to make decisions, yet is unsure about long-term outcomes, often doubting her choices (Cederberg et al., 1994). This category of decision maker experiences the greatest amount of psychological distress and exerts a tremendous amount of energy to come to a conclusion that she can accept.

None of these varying types of decison makers is better or worse than the others. They simply need to be recognized as different role preferences.

Informed Consent

When there are multiple options available, even the most informed women need guidance to clarify the issues and their choices. There is a huge difference between having information provided and actually comprehending that information. Only when a patient comprehends diagnosis and treatment information can she make a truly informed choice.

Hughes (1993) suggests "that a patient's recall of information conveyed around the time of diagnosis is exceedingly poor." Although this study did not measure comprehension of information that was critical to decision making, the lack of retention raises doubts as to how much conveyed information is understood by a patient when anxiety levels are high. Hughes asks whether it is realistic "to assume that an extremely anxious patient with cancer can adequately assess treatment risks and benefits—an assumption on which the doctrine of informed consent is predicated.". And Gray and Doan (1993) caution us to not make assumptions about the type and amount of information patients want, as some people may actually be hampered by certain information.

Furthermore, few physicians are without a bias toward certain treatment options, especially with breast cancer: lumpectomy versus mastectomy; adjuvant therapy versus watchful waiting; immediate versus delayed reconstruction; clinical trial versus standard therapy. Because physician preference and recommendation can greatly influence a patient's decisions (Hughes, 1993), the process of informed consent can easily be swayed by the subtle coercion of a skilled practitioner. Paternalism of this sort—a physician feels more qualified to make medical decisions than the patient—is less accepted in this day and age. Partnership in decision making is gaining acceptance in this era of patient autonomy (Kodish, Lantos, & Siegler, 1991). Or as Lerner (1990) wrote in *Wrestling With the Angel*:

> *"the idea of 'doctor-patient partnership'... made considerable sense, since it recognized the need for pooling the resources of both agents in the illness-healing process."*

Availability of Resources

Supportive networks and resources abound for women with breast cancer. Can anyone actually remember when Reach to Recovery, the American Cancer Society (ACS) support program, did not exist? Over the past few decades, women have formed or joined breast cancer support groups and worked with oncology nurses and social workers to create different models of support and educational programs. They have published numerous books on their personal experiences and have show-and-tell sessions with make-up, prosthetics, and breast reconstruction techniques. Online computer services for support and information are available, and interactive videos are being produced to educate women about the subtle differences in treatment options. Complementary or alternative therapies are an integral part of many women's treatment plans. Women with breast cancer can also lay claim to a powerful national network that voices their concerns better than any other cancer-specific group.

Helping each other along their cancer journey is an important task for both the newly diagnosed patient and the seasoned survivor. In the words of one newly diagnosed patient (Mullan and Hoffman, 1990):

"I needed to find someone immediately who knew my terror; someone I could talk with on a personal —rather than clinical—level; someone who had `been there.' I needed to find a survivor."

Wittman (1993) believes that although medical knowledge is best gathered from professional journals and interpreted by health care professionals," . . . a different, and nourishing, kind of information comes from other cancer patients."

Long-term survivors often have a need to *give back,* and are one of the greatest resources for women just beginning their cancer journeys. An example of this need to be heard and give back was evident in a recent Quality-of-Life Survivor's Project, which sent questionnaires to the NCCS constituency. The authors found that almost half of the respondents had histories of breast cancer, and many decribed the need to find meaning in their experiences by helping others (Ferrell et al., 1995).

"Since my treatment, I've counciled new patients —sharing my experiences. I truly feel that since I've `survived', I must give back so that others may find the strength in themselves to overcome the disease."

ACTIVISM

An interesting trend for women with breast cancer over the past decade has been the rise of consumer activism. No longer willing to stand by as passive recipients of care, women diagnosed with breast cancer have joined forces to voice their concerns. They are asking health care providers, policy makers, insurers and payors to stop making unilateral assumptions as to what choices are best for women with breast cancer, and to include them in the decision-making process. This is especially important for ethnic minorities and medically underserved populations, whose needs often dramatically differ from mainstream groups. Providers of care can no longer treat all cancer patients as a uniform group. They must attempt to understand the individuality of people—their cultures, their values, and their goals.

But this shift away from the conventional, paternalistic model of care has been such a dramatic change, many breast cancer activists are viewed as adversaries by the very people for whom they care. Activists, in fact, are *vigorous* in their efforts to effect change. Leaders of the Breast Cancer Coalition (BCC) describe themselves not as survivors, but as activists, and have highly sophisticated workshops to teach women how to be effective in changing governmental policy. These are women using aggressive tactics, not only to raise awareness about their disease, but also to demand action. Even though they have been highly successful in earmarking funds for breast cancer research, they have been subject to much criticism due to their style and agenda. I suspect that if this were a group of men with prostate or testicular cancer, their efforts would be applauded without hesitation.

"Consumers belong at every level of the research process, from advisory boards and study sections at the agency level, to steering committees, data monitoring committees and IRBs at the institutional and study level." (National Breast Cancer Coalition, 1994)

But this is far from the only agenda of breast cancer groups. Other breast cancer organizations want to target the pharmaceutical industry and to have input into the development and delivery of new therapies. Others have hotline numbers and act as information and referral sources to women around the country, or facilitate support groups for diverse populations. Some pride themselves in working *with* providers and payors, while others feel more effective *challenging* the system.

It often appears that the only thing these groups all have in common is breast cancer. Their views on the tamoxifen prevention trials differ, as do their views on experimental therapies, on the need for educational and supportive services, and on methods to effect change. Clearly, there is no automatic consensus on issues relating to breast cancer. But what these groups do have in common is the desire to advocate for women who are traumatized by what seems to be an epidemic.

Levels of Advocacy

Advocacy is not just about activism, and is not only for those who are energetic, vocal, and assertive: it begins at a very personal level. Self-advocacy includes the ability to access and understand information, to find appropriate resources and therapy, to get second and third opinions, and to make informed choices about treatment, including choosing *no* treatment. There is also advocacy on an interpersonal level. In this situation, survivors advocate for each other, such as in local networking and support group sessions, or they advocate for services and support for family members, partners, and other caregivers. There is also the level of community or national advocacy, as described above, where survivors strategize, educate, collaborate, and testify as consumer representatives and political activists. There seems to be something for everyone's style and desire for involvement.

I feel that all of us, both providers and consumers of cancer care, require greater understanding of advocacy issues, better communication, and more earnest collaboration. Most women with breast cancer want mutually respectful relationships with their physicians and nurses, so that the decisions impacting their cancer journeys are right for them. Whether survivors are seen as knocking *on* doors or knocking *down* doors, they simply want assurance that their voices will be recognized as part of the debate and decision making surrounding current and future cancer care.

FINAL THOUGHTS

To oncology nurses everywhere—you who are our caregivers, our allies, our advocates, our friends—I invite you to:

1. view each of your patients as an individual with a different sets of needs;
2. acknowledge patients' vulnerabilities and difficulties in decision making;
3. recognize the value of *time* in order to support and educate patients and family members about options;
4. help to translate confusing information, especially consent forms, in ways that individual patients can understand;
5. encourage questions, no matter how simplistic they might seem;
6. avoid being judgmental when choices are made that differ from the ones offered;
7. not put conditions on continuing treatment or support;
8. support the expression of feelings, even if they make you uncomfortable;
9. know what resources are available locally and nationally, and share them selectively as patients are ready for them;
10. realize that decision making does not stop when treatment ends, and offer continued support to long-term survivors;
11. remember that choices must make sense to the person affected by them;
12. advocate for women with breast cancer.

Living with, through, and beyond cancer is a balancing act. In the words of one of our earliest activists, Natalie Davis Spingarn (1982), from *Hanging In There: Living Well on Borrowed Time*:

> *"It is a world where I trade precious time for treatment and risk treatment for precious time."*

References

Carter, B. J. (1989). Cancer survivorship: A topic for nursing research. *Oncology Nursing Forum, 16*, 435–437.

Cederberg, et al. (1994). *Breast cancer? Let me check my schedule!* Vancouver, WA: Innovative Medical Education Consortium, Inc.

Clark, E. J. (1995). Words that harm, words that heal. Available through the National Coalition for Cancer Survivorship, 1010 Wayne Ave, 5th Floor, Silver Spring, MD 20910.

Ferrell, B. R., Dow, K. H., & Leigh, S. A. (1995). Quality of life in cancer survivors. (Unpublished data).

Frank, A. W. (1991). *At the Will of the Body*. Boston: Houghton Mifflin.

Gray, R. E., & Doan, B. D. (1990). Empowerment and persons with cancer: Politics in cancer medicine. *Journal of Palliative Care, 6*, 33–45.

Hughes, K. K. (1993). Decision making by patients with breast cancer: The role of information in treatment selection. *Oncology Nursing Forum, 20*, 623–628.

Kodish, E., Lantos, J. D., & Siegler, M. (1991). The ethics of randomization. *CA-A Cancer Journal for Clinicians, 41*, 180–186.

Leigh, S. A. (1991). The cancer survivorship movement. *Cancer Investigation, 9*, 571–579.

Lerner, M. (1990). *Wresting With the Angel*. New York, NY: Simon & Schuster.

Lerner, M. (1994). *Choices in healing: Integrating the best of conventional and complementary approaches to cancer*. Cambridge, MA: The MIT Press.

Mullan, F., & Hoffman, J. D. (Eds.). (1990). *Charting the journey: An almanac of practical resources for cancer survivors*. Mt. Vernon, NY: Consumers Union.

National Breast Cancer Coalition. (1994). *Call to action: The Quarterly Newsletter of the National Breast Cancer Coalition, 1*, 8.

Newfeld, K. R., Degner, L. F., & Dick, J. A. M. (1993). A nursing intervention strategy to foster patient involvement in treatment decisions. *Oncology Nursing Forum, 20*, 631–635.

Pierce, P. (1993). Deciding on breast cancer treatment: A description of decision behavior. *Nursing Research, 42*, 22–28.

Spingarn, N.D. (1982). *Hanging in there: Living well on borrowed time*. New York: Stein and Day.

Wittman, J. (1993). *Breast cancer journal: A century of petals*. Golden, CO: Fulcrum Publishing.

CHAPTER 13

Understanding the Experiences of Long-Term Survivors of Breast Cancer

Story as a Way of Knowing

Barbara J. Carter, DNSc, RN, CS

Having slumbered
She rose and shook
Victorian shadows from her hair.

Rita Mae Brown, *The Hand That Cradles the Rock*

THE SURVIVORSHIP MOVEMENT

In recent years, breast cancer has become an everyday household topic and major concern of women. This heightened awareness was achieved largely through the efforts of the National Cancer Institute, the American Cancer Society, and patient advocacy groups such as Y Me, the National Association of Breast Cancer Organizations, the National Breast Cancer Coalition, and the National Coalition for Cancer Survivorship. Increased social dialogue about breast cancer runs parallel with the feminist, women's health, and self-care movements. Breast cancer activists have emerged as an unparalleled force in the women's health move-

ment, and have changed the emphasis of breast cancer treatment. After initially advocating the two-step surgical procedure, these activists then campaigned for more informed decision-making, which included options such as breast conservative surgery, radiation therapy, and reconstruction. Most recently they have worked for increased funds for breast cancer research and the involvement of patient advocates in the design and implementation of breast cancer research studies. At no time in women's history have women been more involved in directing their own health care. And at no time in women's history have women been more fearful of contracting this disease.

It has been a pleasure for me to be involved in the cancer survivorship movement since the mid-1980s, serving both as a member of the Board of Directors of the National Coalition for Cancer Survivorship (NCCS), and as Chair of the Research Committee. During the early years of NCCS, advocacy efforts were aimed at raising the consciousness of breast cancer survivors, health care professionals, policy makers, and others about survivorship issues. A national network emerged and continues to emerge, linking organizations and individuals through hotlines, education and information materials, assemblies, support groups, and research ideas. The NCCS is now based in Silver Spring, Maryland, and 10 years after its inception ranks among the most influential patient advocacy organizations in the country.

Background

Research Inquiry.   I began studying cancer survivorship formally during doctoral study in psychosocial oncology at the University of California at San Francisco in the mid to late 1980s, and concurrent to advocacy involvement with NCCS. A review of the current literature showed that little was known about long-term breast cancer survivors (Carter, 1989). Most oncology nursing research in the late 1970s and early 1980s focused on symptom management and early psychosocial outcomes of treatment (Carter, 1989, 1990; Fernsler, Holcombe, & Pulliam, 1984; Grant & Padilla, 1983; Scott, 1985). Only one study, Woods and Earp (1978), investigated psychosocial adjustment in long-term breast cancer survivors. This study documented the coexistence of physical complications and psychosocial distress in 4-year survivors who were cured of breast cancer.

For my dissertation research, I embarked on a qualitative investigation of the stories of long-term breast cancer survivors. (Carter, 1990, 1993). The study was the first to explore the realm of breast cancer survivors' experience 5 years after treatment and beyond. The study generated over 3,000 pages of interview text and took nearly 3 years to complete. Twenty-five women, all of whom had survived breast cancer for at least 5 years and suffered no recurrences, shared their stories. Study participants had survived from 5 to 26 years, with a mean survival time of 10.56 years. Participants described "going through"

a common process theme that involved the following phases: interpreting the diagnosis, confronting mortality, reprioritizing, coming to terms, moving on, and flashing back.

Survivors described the phases as overlapping, and described their experience of surviving as moving back and forth between the phases, sometimes simultaneously. For example, when interpreting the diagnosis, survivors interpreted the meaning of the diagnosis, considered the types of treatment available, and the impact of cancer on their lives. When confronting mortality, survivors experienced themselves existentially as mortal, and confronted the possibility that their cancer could lead to death. By reprioritizing, survivors reorganized their lives in order to meet the demands of cancer treatment, and in order to survive cancer. By coming to terms, survivors accepted and integrated the fact of having cancer into their lives. Moving on involved survivors putting the cancer experience into the past, and into the background, and getting on with life. Flashing back, recalling and reliving aspects of the cancer experience, allowed survivors to experience their former experience sometimes all at once (Carter, 1990; 1993).

Surviving as Phenomenologic Experience.   In general, survivors experienced cancer phenomenologically as a traumatic, life-threatening event. Initially, the event required social distance and withdrawal from social life during the treatment and convalescent stages. The initial primary concerns of long-term survivors are focused on their biological survival. Early on in the survivorship trajectory, survivors were concerned with making the right choices about treatment, with mortality, with managing their symptoms, and with prioritizing their lives in order to undergo treatment successfully (Carter, 1990, 1993). Described retrospectively by participants, the primary concerns of survivors at the time of treatment and during early convalescence differed qualitatively in intensity and focus from their concerns after successful treatment and convalescence.

Survivors' concerns at later stages of treatment were more psychosocial in nature than at the start. After the end of treatment, survivors were most focused on living with the impact of cancer on their lives. Their concerns included managing an altered body image, maintaining relationships, managing the negative reactions of others, coping with infertility, maintaining a balance in their lives, maintaining their jobs and health insurance, and managing their fear of cancer recurrence. With increased survival time, most survivors' concerns about their biological survival became less intense.

Having cancer, exploring the "why me," searching for meaning in the experience, and achieving an inward resolve, helped survivors adjust to changes in their lifestyles, perspectives, and social world after cancer. After completing treatment, survivors in the "coming to terms" phase continued to be concerned about their biological survival and social reintegration, as they both accepted and integrated cancer into their lives, with varying degrees of success (Carter, 1990, 1993). Some survivors experienced long-term physical and emotional complications of treatment, e.g., lymphedema, chronic back pain, infertility, anxiety, and depression, that made social adjustment after cancer treatment problematic.

Maher (1982) eloquently described the negative emotions that survivors experience, including ambivalence, when they are faced with demands and limitations on social reentry after cancer treatment. The attempt to return to "normal" is problematic, because their interpreted world is a changed world, where both survivors and others are aware of their cancer diagnosis and the life-threatening nature of cancer.

Sense of Self.   The sense of Self is most vulnerable for many survivors during social reentry after cancer treatment. The process of acceptance and integration, integral to a survivor's "coming to terms" with her cancer experience, may require years of endeavor, depending on the survivor's personal and so-cial resources, and experiences (Carter, 1990, 1993).

Potentially, the validation of the survivor as a person may confirm the Self, buffer the loss of Self (Charmaz, 1983, 1987), assist in the struggle to regain a sense of Self, and provide a pivotal relationship for an ongoing reinterpretation of the Self over time as a survivor adjusts to life after cancer. It has been said that it is as important to know what *type of person* has a disease as it is to know what *type of disease* a person has (Siegel, 1986).

As one survivor's story profoundly depicted, the sense of Self mediates bodily concerns and psychosocial consequences of cancer. In her 5-year trajectory of surviving breast cancer, the Self was interpreted as mortal, diminished, vulnerable, primary, and as surviving (Carter, 1994). This teacher's story of cancer-based discrimination in the workplace portrays the confounding impact of conflicting goals (returning to work vs. staying at home) and medical complications (lymphedema and pericarditis) on lived experience in an unrelenting social world characterized by stigma.

From the latter study, it was learned that the Self, as the principal agent or perspectival lens of the person, reflects biological, personal, and social integration. The sense of Self is thereby constituted by the cancer experience and is subject to ongoing interpretation throughout the cancer survivor's lifetime. It is the concept of the Self, the sense of Self and in particular the phase of "coming to terms" (Carter, 1990, 1993), that requires ongoing work for many long-term cancer survivors. Wyatt's (1994) research concurs that integration of the cancer experience is an ongoing, long-term task.

Integrating Trauma.   Bettelheim (1980), one of the first authors to use the term *survivorship*, discussed the lifelong aftereffects of trauma suffered by concentration camp survivors. Holocaust survivors were faced with a life-threatening situation and extreme social isolation, followed by the aftereffects of such trauma. Like concentration camp survivors, cancer survivors are faced with an existential predicament—they must integrate trauma into their lives and make sense out of their experience.

Surviving breast cancer involves living with the ongoing fear of cancer recurrence and uncertainty about the future. Fear of cancer recurrence is constituted by the lived memory of cancer (Carter, 1989, 1990, 1993), and is a common concern of survivors of other types of cancer as well (Welch-McCaffrey, Hoffman, Leigh, Loescher, & Meyskens, 1989). Fear motivated some survivors to undergo medical follow-up throughout their lives and to seek and maintain "healthy" lifestyle choices. Fear caused others to avoid medical follow-up and to assume an ambivalent stance toward survivorship in general. Beliefs about cancer and the causes of breast cancer influenced the lifestyle choices of survivors (Carter, 1990). For most long-term breast cancer survivors, fear of cancer recurrence subsided with increased survival time. However, survivors reported that as many as 26 years after treatment, fear of recurrence could be easily activated by treatment anniversaries, awareness of symptoms, and knowledge of others who were diagnosed, treated, or had died of cancer. Survivors could, in effect, "flash back" and relive the cancer experience many years after successful treatment (Carter, 1990, 1993).

Story as a Way of Knowing

Processes of Integration.   Although much is written about the "why me" and the cancer survivors' search for the meaning of their disease, little is understood about the processes by which survivors achieve healthy integration and move on with their lives. As survivors integrate trauma, loss, and change into the larger context of their lives, they connect life before cancer with life after cancer, and weave the past with the future with varying degrees of success. Close family ties, stable spousal relationships, and hearty support networks keep many survivors afloat during the trials and tribulations of cancer recovery. Survivors who experience physical and emotional

complications, and those with limited support networks, may experience greater difficulty during social reintegration.

Therapy is one formal means of providing support and promoting integration, but therapy has not been sufficiently studied. Therapy offers a safe place for patients to tell their stories and work through issues, and thereby know themselves more intimately, revealing themselves to the others. Therapy may not be available to survivors with limited financial resources and for those who do not have health insurance. Many insurance companies do not provide mental health benefits to cancer survivors and fail to cover the total cost of mental health counseling even when coverage is provided.

Alternatively, support groups, cancer clubs, wellness houses, and communities offer networks of support to survivors sharing common experiences. Stories of illness experience abound in these types of social settings. However, a scarcity of research has investigated the benefits of participating in social support groups. Spiegel, Kramer, Bloom, and Gottheil's research in 1989 documented the improved quality of life and increased survival time enjoyed by women with advanced metastatic breast disease who participated in support groups. More research is needed to explore the effectiveness of group interventions for women recovering from early-stage disease, and longitudinally for long-term breast cancer survivors.

Why Stories?   As both a clinician and a researcher, I have found that the best way to understand a survivor's experience is to listen to her stories. Stories convey an interpretation of biographical disruption (Denzin, 1989; Riessman, 1990), as well as an interpretation of the Self, revealing the discontinuities and contradictions with which people live (Riessman, 1990). Telling stories is one of the most important processes people use to make sense out of their life experience, and to convey that experience to others. Berry (1993), for example, in researching patients' experiences at work, discovered that patients tell stories selectively in order to mobilize social support when returning to work after cancer treatment.

Patients' stories are always purposive, and are a way of expressing concerns, asking for help, providing diversion, or establishing relationships with others. Through stories, patients identify with and befriend one another. Attendees at the NCCS assemblies, for example, are often intrigued by the "characters" they have gotten to know through the storytelling and camaraderie that goes on in that setting. Stories provide patients with a sense of connection with others (Brody, 1987), with inspiration, with an appreciation of tragedy and of suffering, and with a model of transcendence. The spirit of survival is commonly conveyed through story.

A patient's narratives can help nurses understand change in a patient's health status. Both the theme and the direction of a story convey perceptions. Patients may let us know about their fears and anticipated outcomes through stories. Stories may provide clues about the meaning of illness (Siegel, 1986) and the meaning of symptoms (Good & Del Vecchio Good, 1980).

Illness narratives place the nature of illness in the temporal context of an individual life (Robinson, 1990). Patients may use storytelling as a way of collecting their inner life drama (Sacks, 1987) or of describing their social worlds of illness (Kleinman, 1988, 1992; Kirmayer, 1992). Narrative knowing (Sandelowski, 1991) through stories can be transformed by researchers into descriptions and theories of lives people live. Lives can be revealed and transformed in stories and by the act of storytelling itself (Sandelowski, 1991). Stories provide images that inspire hope and transform suffering. Stories of care providers and caregivers enhance our understanding of the meaning of collaboration in healing (Baker & Diekelmann, 1994) and of the knowledge inherent in nursing practice (Benner & Wrubel, 1982).

Stories ultimately transcend mortality, in that stories outlive situations and may transcend the lifetimes of both the storyteller(s) and the community of listeners. Good stories capture the essence and universal nature of human experience. They evoke our sentiments and may result in action to correct circumstances.

The Nurse in Storytelling

Active Listening.   Out of the team of cancer care providers, it is often the nurse who listens to the patient's story, knows the patient as a person, and provides the person with psychosocial care. Because nurses spend quality time with patients, nurses have multiple opportunities to listen to a patient's stories. Frequent lines of nursing inquiry, such as "Why are you here?" and "How can I help?," evoke stories. Patients are often eager to tell their stories and to share their illness experiences. Many patients want only to have their personhood and concerns validated—to be heard. It is the connectedness with the "other" that makes the story a powerful tool of relatedness and the nurse a predominant source of healing.

As a nurse, I believe that presence and active listening are central to the practice of healing. Interactions that confirm and validate a patient's concerns are powerful antidotes that may mitigate the effects of depersonalization and social isolation that cancer patients and survivors often suffer. Drew (1986), in a phenomenology of patients' experiences with care providers, identified confirming behaviors of care providers as listening, taking time, touching, using positive eye contact, and being warm. Exclusion behaviors were identified as being abrupt or impersonal, avoiding eye contact, hurrying through interactions, and being cold. Patients experienced fear, anger, and shame as a result of the negative disregard shown by exclusion behaviors.

The potential long-term impact of care providers' exclusion behaviors on a survivor's changing sense of Self after cancer can be profound. We must all work to correct the factors that contribute to exclusion behaviors. These factors may include short staffing, overwork, burnout, insensitivity, and unresolved issues and unhappiness in our own lives.

Nurse–Patient Relationships.   Morse (1991) described "connected relationships" as a type of nurse–patient relationship that I believe is most healing for persons with cancer. According to Morse, connected relationships are close and lengthy and feature a nurse who "goes the extra mile" for the patient. This type of nurse treats the patient first as a person, and places a higher priority on the patient's concerns than on treatment concerns. Through the connected relationship, the nurse enters into the patient's world of suffering and eases that suffering through his or her presence and concern over time. The connected relationship bridges the past with the future.

In order to know patients, nurses must become involved with them. Getting to know a patient and his or her typical pattern of responses encourages skilled clinical judgment and sets the stage for possible patient advocacy (Tanner, Benner, Chesla, & Gordon, 1993).

Swanson (1993) outlined the structure of caring nurse–patient relationships as follows: caring is "maintaining belief" that a patient will get through a situation; "knowing" the meaning of an event in the life of the patient; "being with," meaning being actively present for the patient; "doing for" the patient that which she cannot do for herself; and "enabling," or facilitating, the person's long-term well-being. As nurses, the beliefs, perceptions, actions, and the patient's outcome are factors in the interpretive interactions that occur within the context of caring nurse–patient relationships. These factors are also central to our work as nurses. For a full account on how to be fully present for others, see Travelbee's seminal text (1971) on interpersonal nursing.

Especially now, with health care reforms being considered by government, we must ensure that oncology nurses are placed strategically so that they may hear patient's stories, know patients as people, and provide compassionate care across the continuum of cancer care. Currently, oncology nurses practice in acute care settings, in follow-up outpatient clinics, cancer centers, and doctors' offices. Oncology nurses serve as staff nurses, clinical nurse specialists, primary case managers, counselors, therapists, support group leaders, consultants, educators, fellow cancer survivors, and mentors in the survivorship community. Nurse oncologists link patients and families with appropriate specialists, groups, organizations, agencies, and other survivors, providing connections to the medical community and to the survivorship community at large. Support groups, patient hotlines, and advocacy organizations are today a frenzy of activity, largely through the advocacy efforts of nurses.

Facilitating Integration.   Nurses must be aware that the needs and capacities of long-term survivors change over time. In order for survivors to heal emotionally, and to integrate the cancer experience into their lives, energy is required that initially may be used for biological survival. Suffering emerges periodically as patients endure the experience of cancer (Morse, in review; Stanley, Morse, & Carter, 1994). Commonly during the cancer treatment phase, as patients are interpreting the diagnosis, confronting mortality, and reprioritizing, a high level of existential anxiety is experienced, and emotions are often repressed. Anxiety that first surfaces during the time of interpreting the diagnosis resurfaces when treatment ends. Repressed emotions, such as depression and anger, may be experienced at a deep level when treatment is over. Patients should be encouraged to tell their stories, and to talk or write about their feelings, whenever feelings begin to surface (Freund, 1990). The idea is to provide an opportunity to "debrief" and thereby assist patients in tieing the past with the future by integrating their experiences emotionally in the present.

The experience of loss often emerges as survivors attempt to integrate the effects of cancer into the context of their lives without the support of the treatment team. Reentry into the social world may be problematic as survivors face "what is" compared with "what used to be." Talking or writing about the losses caused by cancer or attending a support group may be helpful to survivors during this time.

Social reentry may be fraught with rejection, stigma, and discrimination. Support groups and work reentry groups are especially helpful to survivors dealing with these issues. (Cella & Yellen, 1993; Clark & Landis, 1990). Hoffman (1989) reported that about 25% of cancer survivors experience discrimination in the workplace. Other common psychosocial problems include difficulties with intimacy, communication and relationships, fear of cancer recurrence, and job and insurance discrimination (Welch-McCaffrey, et al., 1989).

Nurses can encourage survivors to tell their stories. I have found that patients freely share their experiences with care providers, support group participants, and others that are willing to listen. The telling of the story in and of itself may be healing. Other benefits for patients include expressing emotions, connecting with others, and alleviating social isolation. It may be helpful for some patients to write about their experiences in journals or diaries, discussing events, expressing feelings, and recording progress over time. Some patients may benefit from writing about their experiences to pen pals, or in articles, books, letters to editors, or newsletters. Some people find reading books, articles, stories, and poetry written by other survivors instructive and supportive. Writers such as Brinker and Harris (1990), Dow (1990), Kahane (1990), Kaye (1991), Kushner (1982), LaTour (1993), Lifshitz (1988), Lorde (1980), Metzger (1983), Rollin (1976), Spingarn (1982), Steinem (1992), Wear (1993), and others reverberate the lived experiences of surviving breast cancer. Survivors who want their experiences to be known should be encouraged to tell their stories at conferences, advocacy meetings, panel discussions, survivors' day celebrations, and congressional hearings. Additionally, the essence of surviving may be expressed through other forms of art, such as movies, plays, music, paintings, drawings, and sculptures.

Successes and failures in the social world shape survivors' experiences, goals, and feelings about themselves. Whether survivors successfully integrate cancer into their lives and move on with life depends largely on their own motivation, the availability of resources, and the responses of others in the social setting.

FUTURE DIRECTIONS

To better understand the realities and problematic experiences of long-term survivors, we need to hear survivors' stories. Stories are needed that bear witness to the trauma caused by cancer, to heal the lives of those affected by cancer and to guide the way for survivors who follow. Survivors themselves can best address the barriers to well-being and the possibilities that are inherent in survivorship. Multiple accounts are needed from the survivorship community to record the wide range of human experience. Stories should be recorded both through the formal means of qualitative research and through the popular lay literature. Research describing the terrain of survivorship will guide our lives well into the twenty-first century (Carter, 1989; Dow, 1992; Mooney, Ferrell, Nail, Benedict, & Haberman, 1991). Wisdom that is handed down from survivor to survivor is invaluable. The time has come to break the silence about long-term cancer survival. Story offers an exciting and challenging means.

SUMMARY

The chapter addressed the overall aim of the survivorship movement—to provide long-term compassionate care to cancer survivors. Research on long-term breast cancer survivors and the concerns of long-term survivors were presented. It was argued that story offers a useful means of understanding the experiences of cancer survivors and of healing the wounds of survivorship. Nurses are viewed as key listeners to survivors' stories and as influential in encouraging survivors to share their stories with others. Researching the lived experiences of long-term breast cancer survivors is encouraged.

ACKNOWLEDGMENTS

Research for this chapter was supported in part by a grant from the American Cancer Society; the research was completed at the University of California, San Francisco.

I thank the following for sharing story: Virginia Woolf, Margaret Mead, Gloria Steinem, my mother, a long-term breast cancer survivor, Mary Peck, Etta K. Owens, Marilyn Crist Umphrey, Jennifer Wengler, Patricia Benner, Diane Scott-Dorsett, Bert Dreyfus, Marylin Dodd, Jeanne Hallburg, Holly Wilson, James Jarrett, Bernie Siegel, Larry LeShan, Catherine Logan, Ruth McCorkle, Janice Morse, Karyn Holm, and Karen Hassey Dow.

References

Baker, C., & Diekelmann, N. (1994). Connecting conversations of caring: Recalling the narrative to clinical practice. *Nursing Outlook, 42*, 65–70.

Benner, P., & Wrubel, J. (1982). Clinical knowledge development: The value of perceptual awareness. *Nurse Educator, 7*, 11–17.

Berry, D. L. (1993). Return to work experiences of people with cancer. *Oncology Nursing Forum, 20*, 905–911.

Bettelheim, B. (1980). *Surviving and other essays.* New York: Vintage Books.

Brinker, N., & Harris, C. M. (1990). *The race is run one step at a time: My personal struggle and everywoman's guide to taking charge of breast cancer.* New York: Simon & Schuster.

Brody, H. (1987). *Stories of sickness.* New Haven: Yale University Press.

Brown, R. M. (1971). *The hand that cradles the rock.* Oakland, CA: Diana Press.

Carter, B. J. (1989). Cancer survivorship: A topic for nursing research. *Oncology Nursing Forum, 16*, 435–437.

Carter, B. J. (1990). A phenomenological study of long-term survivors of adult cancer. *Dissertation Abstracts International (50)*, 3395.

Carter, B. J. (1993). Long-term survivors of breast cancer: A qualitative descriptive study. *Cancer Nursing, 16*, 354–361.

Carter, B. J. (1994). Surviving breast cancer: A problematic work reentry. *Cancer Practice 2*, 135–140.

Cella, D. F., & Yellen, S. B. (1993). Cancer support groups: The state of the art. *Cancer Practice, 1*, 56–61.

Charmaz, K. (1983). Loss of self: A fundamental form of suffering of the chronically ill. *Sociology of Health & Illness, 5*, 168–195.

Charmaz, K. (1987). In J. Roth & P. Conrad (Eds.), Struggling for a self: Identity levels of the chronically ill. *Research in the Sociology of Health Care* (pp. 283–321). Greenwich, CT: JAI Press.

Clark, J. C., & Landis, L. L. (1990). *Reintegration and maintenance of employees with breast cancer in the workplace.* Atlanta: American Cancer Society.

Denzin, N. K. (1989). *Interpretive interactionism.* Newbury Park, CA: Sage Publications.

Dow, K. H. (1990). The enduring seasons in survival. *Oncology Nursing Forum, 17*, 511–516.

Dow, K. H. (1992). Cancer survivorship in the 1990s. *Proceedings of the Sixth National Conference on Cancer Nursing, Surviving Cancer.* Atlanta: American Cancer Society, 1–8.

Drew, N. (1986). Exclusion and confirmation: A phenomenology of patient's experiences with caregivers. *Image: Journal of Nursing Scholarship, 18*, 39–43.

Fernsler, J., Holcombe, J, & Pulliam, L. (1984). A survey of cancer nursing research, January 1975–June 1982. *Oncology Nursing Forum, 11*, 46–52.

Freund. P. E. S. (1990). The expressive body: A common ground for the sociology of emotions and health and illness. *Sociology of Health & Illness, 12*, 452–477.

Good, B. J., & Del Vecchio Good, M. J. (1980). The meaning of symptoms: A cultural hermeneutical model for clinical practice. In L. Eisenberg, & A. Kleinman (Eds.), *The relevance of social science for medicine* (pp. 165–196). Boston: D. Reidel Publishing.

Grant, M. M., & Padilla, G. V. (1983). An overview of cancer nursing research. *Oncology Nursing Forum, 10*, 58–69.

Hoffman, B. (1989). Cancer survivors at work: Job problems and illegal discrimination. *Oncology Nursing Forum, 16*, 39–43.

Kahane, D. H. (1990). *No less a woman: Ten women shatter the myths about breast cancer.* New York: Prentice Hall.

Kaye, R. (1991). *Spinning straw into gold: Your emotional recovery from breast cancer.* New York: Simon & Schuster.

Kirmayer, L. J. (1992). The body's insistence on meaning: Metaphor as presentation and representation in illness experience. *Medical Anthropology Quarterly, 6*, 323–346.

Kleinman, A. (1988). *Illness narratives: Suffering and the human condition.* New York: Basic Books.

Kleinman, A. (1992). Local worlds of suffering: An interpersonal focus for ethnographies of illness experience. *Qualitative Health Research, 2*, 127–134.

Kushner, R. (1982). *Why me?* New York: W. B. Saunders.

LaTour, K. (1993). *The breast cancer companion: From diagnosis through treatment to recovery, everything you need to know for every step along the way.* New York: William Morrow & Company.

Lifshitz, L. (Ed.). (1988) *Her soul beneath the bone: Women's poetry on breast cancer.* Urbana: University of Illinois Press.

Lorde, A. (1980). *The cancer journals.* San Francisco: Spinster/Aunt Lute Press.

Maher, E. (1982). Anomic aspects of recovery from cancer. *Social Science and Medicine, 16*, 907–912.

Metzger, D. (1983). *The woman who slept with men to take the war out of them & Tree.* Berkeley: Wingbow Press.

Mooney, K. H., Ferrell, B. R. Nail, L. M., Benedict, S. C., & Haberman, M. R., (1991). 1991 Oncology Nursing Society research priorities survey. *Oncology Nursing Forum, 18,* 1381–1388.

Morse, J. (1991). Negotiating commitment and involvement in the nurse-patient relationship. *Journal of Advanced Nursing, 16,* 455–468.

Morse, J., & Carter, B. J. (in press).

Riessman, C. K. (1990). Strategic uses of narrative in the presentation of self and illness: A research note. *Social Science & Medicine, 30,* 1195–1200.

Robinson, I. (1990). Personal narratives, social careers and medical courses: Analyzing life trajectories in autobiographies of people with multiple sclerosis. *Social Science & Medicine, 30,* 1173–1186.

Rollin, B. (1976) *First you cry.* New York: New American Library.

Sacks, O. (1987). *The man who mistook his wife for a hat: And other clinical tales.* New York: Harper & Row.

Sandelowski, M. (1991). Telling stories: Narrative approaches in qualitative research. *Image: Journal of Nursing Scholarship, 23,* 161–166.

Scott, D. W. (1985). The research connection, practice, research and theory. *The American Cancer Society Fourth Cancer Nursing Research Conference Proceedings,* pp. 19-47.

Siegel, B. (1986). *Love, medicine and miracles: Lessons learned about self-healing from a surgeon's experience with exceptional patients.* New York: Harper & Row.

Spiegel, D., Kraemer, H. C., Bloom, J. R., & Gottheil, E. G. (1989). Effects of psychosocial treatment on survival of patients with metastatic breast cancer. *Lancet, 2,* 888–891.

Spingarn, N. D. (1982). *Hanging in there: Living well on borrowed time.* New York: Stein & Day Publishers.

Stanley, K. (Moderator & Speaker), Morse, J. (Speaker), & Carter, B. J. (Speaker). (1994). *Understanding the experiences of enduring and suffering* (Cassette Recording No. IS 25). Denver, CO: National Nursing Network.

Steinem, G. (1992). *Revolution from within: A book on self-esteem.* Boston: Little Brown & Company.

Swanson, K. M. (1993). Nursing as informed caring for the well-being of others. *Image: Journal of Nursing Scholarship 25,* 352–357.

Tanner, C. A., Benner, P., Chesla, C., & Gordon, D. R. (1993). The phenomenology of knowing the patient. *Image: Journal of Nursing Scholarship, 25,* 273–280.

Travelbee, J. (1971). *Interpersonal aspects of nursing.* Philadelphia: F. A. Davis.

Wear, D. (1993). "Your breasts/sliced off": Literary images of breast cancer. *Women and Health, 20,* 81–100.

Welch-McCaffrey, D., Hoffman, B., Leigh, S. A., Loescher, L. J., & Meyskens, F. (1989). Surviving adult cancers. *Annals of Internal Medicine, 111,* 517–524.

Woods, N., & Earp, J. L. (1978). Women with cured breast cancer: A study of mastectomy patients in North Carolina. *Nursing Research, 27,* 279–285.

Wyatt, G. (1994). Quality of life of long-term female cancer survivors. *Oncology Nursing Forum, 21,* 382.

PART 5 | Breast Cancer as a Family Issue

CHAPTER 14 | Spouse and Family Issues in Breast Cancer

Laurel L. Northouse, PhD, RN, FAAN

Over the past two decades, research has documented that breast cancer is a family affair and that spouses and other family members play a major role in helping women adjust to the impact of the disease (Baider & Kaplan De-Nour, 1988a). Family members are frequently identified as the primary source of emotional support and as the primary providers of physical care to women with breast cancer (Northouse, 1988). Given the close, interdependent relationship between breast cancer patients and their family members, it is no surprise that breast cancer impinges on the lives of family members as well as on the lives of the women with the disease.

To assist both breast cancer patients and their family members to cope effectively with the stressful impact of the illness, nurses and other health professionals need to maintain an up-to-date understanding of how the illness affects women as well as their family members. This chapter reviews prior research as well as the most recent findings on the impact

of breast cancer on the family. The chapter begins by comparing the perceptions of illness held by women with that of their spouses. Next, the demands that breast cancer puts on family members are discussed. Various factors that influence the ability of family members to adapt to the illness are reviewed, and the chapter concludes with some general guidelines for clinical practice.

PERCEPTIONS OF ILLNESS

Recent research indicates that the perceptions of illness held by cancer patients and their spouses are not always the same. Although little research has compared the perceptions of breast cancer patients with that of their family members, differing perceptions have been reported by couples coping with other types of cancer. Clipp and George (1992), for example, interviewed patients with lung or colon cancer and interviewed their spouses; they found differences in the perceptions of how well the patient was managing with the cancer. For the most part, spouses rated patients as having more pain, more symptoms, more fear, more discouragement, and less ability to cope with the illness than the patients' own self-ratings. The investigators found higher levels of agreement between partners and patients in the more observable and more "objective" aspects of adjustment, such as their ratings of the patient's ability to carry out activities of daily living (i.e., dressing self, ability to use the toilet). There were more differences between partners and patients in subjective areas involving patients' feelings and emotional adjustments. According to Clipp and George (1992), these internal, more private feelings of patients may be more difficult for spouses to assess or to accurately interpret.

Other investigators have also found differences in partners' perceptions of the illness experience. Gotay (1984) found that women with gynecological or breast cancer and their partners ranked several areas of concern differently. Women reported more worry about side effects of treatment and restrictions of activities, while their spouses reported more worry about their wives' emotional state and their wives' ability to survive the disease.

In a recent study, investigators interviewed women and their partners prior to a breast biopsy and found that the amount of distress they experienced differed significantly during the diagnostic period (Northouse, Jeffs, Cracchiolo-Caraway, Lampman, & Dorris, 1995b). Women reported more distress than their husbands, due, in part, to their differing perceptions of the significance of the breast biopsy. Women tended to view the biopsy procedure as a more threatening procedure that would determine whether or not they had breast cancer. Husbands, on the other hand, viewed the biopsy as a routine diagnostic procedure, with less associated threat. This research, along with the research of the previous investigators, underscores the importance of assessing the perceptions of both patients and their spouses. Partners' perceptions can differ

at times, and their perceptions can influence their reactions to the illness.

Although partners' perceptions may differ when asked *individually* about their concerns, there is some research that suggests that when the family unit is interviewed as a whole, a fairly high consensus emerges about the most pressing aspects of the patient's cancer. Halliburton, Larson, Dibble, and Dodd (1992) interviewed family members together with patients with recurrent cancer. Family units came to a relatively rapid consensus about which cancer-related problems were the most difficult for them. Family members were uniformly concerned about disease progression and treatment effectiveness. It is worth noting that many of the families said that the research interview, conducted with the family as a whole, was the first opportunity that many of them had to talk with one another about the cancer experience. This suggests that an open dialogue among family members may be a particularly useful means of enabling family members to clarify their individual perceptions and come to a consensus about the most important issues that the family needs to address.

DEMANDS OF ILLNESS ON SPOUSE AND FAMILY

Breast cancer creates a number of demands on spouses and other family members. These demands have been grouped into three categories: emotional demands, physical demands, and social demands.

Emotional Demands

Of the many demands placed on family members, dealing with the emotional demands of breast cancer are among the most challenging. Zahlis and Shands (1991) interviewed husbands of breast cancer patients and found that husbands reported feelings of shock, fear, sadness, and remorse, as well as symptoms of physical illness, in response to their wives' breast cancer diagnosis. One of the most difficult parts of the cancer experience for husbands was watching their wives suffer and not knowing how to help. Many husbands said that they were not used to seeing their wives experiencing pain, losing hair, or even crying in front of their children. Many husbands expressed frustration at their inability to "fix" the situation or to alleviate their wives' suffering.

Family members, especially spouses, repeatedly say that they feel unprepared to assist their wives with the emotional issues that accompany breast cancer (Lewis, Ellison, & Woods, 1985; Sabo, 1990). Although husbands try to help in various ways, such as being more supportive, tolerant, and understanding, many husbands are often critical of their own efforts to help (Zahlis & Shands, 1991). Some husbands try to help by maintaining a strong front around their wives (Sabo, 1990), assuming that if they do not appear worried, their wives will not worry either. Unfortunately, this strategy has many drawbacks; it prevents partners from being honest with one another and limits their opportunity to provide each other with support.

Given the tremendous emotional impact that cancer has on spouses and other family members, some investigators have questioned who is the "real" patient during the cancer experience—the woman or her partner (Baider & Kaplan De-Nour, 1988b)? This question is especially relevant in light of research indicating that spouses of breast cancer patients report as much distress as their wives (Northouse & Swain, 1987), and in some cases even more distress than their wives (Given & Given, 1992). Although these findings are not consistent across all studies, most family researchers agree that both the woman with breast cancer and her partner/family are affected by the illness; both have legitimate needs for support and information from health professionals.

In past research, most of the emphasis has been on the woman with breast cancer and how her adjustment may affect her family. However, recent research suggests that we also need to look at the adjustment of family members and determine how their reactions may affect the patient. In a recent study of couples' adjustment to recurrent breast cancer, investigators found that the level of emotional distress reported by spouses was a significant predictor of the amount of distress reported by breast cancer patients (Northouse, Dorris, & Charron-Moore, 1995a). Husbands who were adjusting well to their wives' breast cancer had a positive influence on their wives' adjustment, while husbands who were adjusting poorly had a negative impact. This study suggests that it is important to assist spouses of breast cancer patients not only because they have legitimate needs for support, but also because their adjustment may have a significant impact on the well-being of their wives.

Physical Demands

There are a number of physical demands that confront spouses and other family members when a woman is diagnosed with breast cancer. While most women with breast cancer are able to carry out their usual routines with few, if any, physical limitations, there appears to be a subgroup of women who experience physical difficulties. These are women who are either on chemotherapy, have advanced disease, or have had a recurrence of their breast cancer. Furthermore, as women's levels of physical disability increase, the physical demands made on spouses or family caregivers also increase, as they must provide additional care for her and do more chores around the house.

Wilson and Morse (1991) studied the experiences of husbands whose wives were undergoing chemotherapy (the majority of the women had breast cancer). The investigators identified a number of strategies, such as "softening the blow," "resisting disruptions," and "preserving the self," that husbands used to assist their wives with the day-to-day stresses associated with chemotherapy. Husbands tried to soften the blow caused by the treatments by being available to their wives, helping without hovering, or assisting them with bathing or walking. Husbands also attempted to resist disruptions that treatment caused in the life of the family by exerting a great deal of self-control in the face of their wives' mood swings or physical sickness. Husbands also tried preserving their own selves or engaging in activities that maintained their own energy and health (i.e., power naps, exercise) so that they would be able to continue to help and support their wives. Throughout the months of chemotherapy, many husbands assumed the "doer" role, in which they tried to meet their wives' physical and emotional needs, maintain household functioning, and provide care for the children.

Stetz (1987) studied the caregiving demands reported by spouses of patients with advanced cancer (some of whom had breast cancer), and found that managing the physical aspects of the women's illness was the most frequently reported demand. Patients in this study were experiencing high levels of physical disability and required constant assistance from their spouses. One fourth of the spouses said that they experienced some alteration in their own pattern of living and a deterioration in their own health as a result of being a caregiver.

When cancer returns after a remission, the physical demands of breast cancer on the spouse and family caregivers also increase. Given and Given (1992) compared the amount of burden reported by caregivers of patients newly diagnosed with breast cancer versus the burden of caring for patients with recurrent breast cancer. Not surprisingly, family caregivers of women with recurrent disease reported considerably more burden than caregivers of women newly diagnosed with breast cancer. Women with recurrent disease had more symptom distress and more dependencies, which continued to increase over time. Caregivers of patients with recurrent disease reported higher levels of depression and a greater impact of the illness on their own health than did caregivers of women newly diagnosed with the disease.

The research suggests that breast cancer creates certain physical demands on patients *and* on their family members. Nurses and other health professionals need to assist family caregivers with these demands and, at the very least, should provide them with support and information to carry out their important caregiving roles. Caregivers may also need help in obtaining outside resources, such as home care services, if the patient's condition starts to deteriorate. Finally, the caregiver's emotional and physical ability to carry out the caregiving role should also be assessed, especially in light of the reports that the caregiver's health can deteriorate over time.

Social Demands

Breast cancer also creates social demands. For the purpose of this discussion, social demands refer to the added interpersonal or role demands that arise within the family or that occur between the family and others as a result of the women's illness. Packard, Haberman, Woods, and Yates (1991) studied the demands of illness experienced by women with various chronic diseases, including breast cancer, and found that one third of the women reported difficulty in their social roles and interpersonal relationships with others. Among the specific problems women reported were adapting to role changes in the family, dealing with the responses of others, and interacting with health care providers.

Spouses and other family members are also affected by the social demands created by breast cancer. Husbands of breast cancer patients interviewed by Zahlis and Shands (1991) discussed the changes that occurred in their social roles and lifestyles as a result of the cancer. The majority of husbands had to make changes in their work schedules to accommodate new responsibilities in household management and child care. Husbands had to balance these competing demands with pre-existing family stressors that were evident prior to the cancer diagnosis. Some husbands reported a decrease in social and recreational activities, as they had to direct more of their energies to maintain the day-to-day interworkings of their families.

Some researchers have investigated how family members manage the many demands that breast cancer creates within the family. Stetz, Lewis, and Primomo (1986) studied the coping strategies of families with school-aged children, and they found that the most common strategy was making alterations in household management, including greater coordination of efforts among family members, altering household routines, and providing one another with added assistance. Other commonly used strategies included seeking assistance from people outside the family and mobilizing the family to solve problems that arose. The investigators found that most families were very resourceful and self-reliant; they tried to resolve their own problems within the family and seldom sought help from others.

Lewis and Hammond (1992) found that the functioning of the households of women with breast cancer generally became stable over time. Families that were functioning at a high level initially continued to function well over time. However, families who were initially functioning at a low level continued to function poorly. These families were not able to improve the functioning of their household, even though the demands of the illness decreased over time.

Vess, Moreland, and Schwebel (1985) found that open communication among family members was one of the key factors that helped families to manage the many changes brought on by cancer. They found that the family members' ongoing ability to communicate with one another and to negotiate role changes helped the family to maintain a sense of cohesion and to reduce their conflicts with one another.

Even though breast cancer places additional or different social demands on the family, the research indicates that most families are able to use coping strategies that help them to adapt to these changes. Families that

may need more assistance from nurses and other health professionals are those families that exhibit greater difficulty managing household changes initially or who have restricted communication patterns that inhibit family members from negotiating role changes with one another.

FACTORS THAT HELP FAMILY MEMBERS ADAPT TO THE ILLNESS

There are a number of factors that influence how well spouses and other family members adapt to the stress and strain associated with breast cancer. These factors include the amount of support families perceive, the amount of physical distress patients experience, the health status of family caregivers, the amount of concurrent stress in the family, and the amount of hopelessness experienced by family members. The role of each of these factors is described briefly below.

Social Support

Although social support has been identified as an important factor that helps women adjust to breast cancer, it has only recently been identified as an important factor for spouses and other family members. Northouse (1988) interviewed husbands of breast cancer patients and found that those who perceived more support reported less emotional distress and fewer adjustment problems than those who felt they had less support. When women's and husbands' levels of support were compared, husbands perceived that they had less support than their wives, particularly from health professionals.

Even though spouses and other family members have their own needs for support, they often have difficulty obtaining it (Oberst & James, 1985). Husbands of mastectomy patients said that they were essentially on their own during their wives' diagnosis, surgery, and hospitalization, with little opportunity to discuss their concerns with family members or friends, especially male friends (Sabo, 1990).

Friends and acquaintances focus primarily on the needs of the patient and overlook the spouses' needs for support (Oberst & James, 1985). In some situations, professionals and friends assume that spouses have an intuitive sense of how to help their partners and therefore have little need for additional support or affirmation from others (Northouse & Peters-Golden, 1993).

The research is clear that spouses and other family members have needs for support and that they cope better when they receive it. Family members need the opportunity to verbalize their feelings of distress to an understanding listener. They benefit when others acknowledge their efforts to help the patient.

Symptom Distress

A second factor that influences the adjustment of family members is the amount of symptom distress experienced by the woman with breast cancer. In a recent study, Northouse et al. (1995a) examined which factors were the strongest predictors of husbands' adjustment to their wives' recurrent breast cancer. They found that symptom distress was the strongest predictor of husbands' emotional distress and role problems. The more symptom distress experienced by the wives, the more adjustment difficulties reported by husbands.

Symptom distress is especially difficult for family members to manage. They often lack the knowledge and skills to alleviate symptoms such as pain, nausea, and anorexia. Furthermore, family members feel frustrated and helpless when they cannot decrease the suffering created by these symptoms. The patient's distress also adds to the demands placed on family members; as patients are less able to care for themselves, they require more assistance from spouses and other family members.

Given the added demand that symptom distress can place on family members, health professionals need to develop strategies that teach both patients and their family members to manage symptom distress. Mood (1993) developed an intervention protocol in which pa-

tients viewed a series of videotapes that described radiation therapy and the possible side effects that they might encounter with it. In addition, patients were given a set of cards that listed common side effects as well as a list of ways to handle the side effects if they should occur. Patients who received the information intervention were able to counter the nausea and anorexia associated with treatment and significantly increased their caloric and protein intake. In an upcoming study, Mood and her colleagues will be including family members in the intervention protocol. More interventions such as these are needed to help patients and family members manage symptom distress caused either by the disease or by its treatments.

Caregiver's Health

A third factor that influences adjustment is the health status of the family caregiver. Hilton (1993) studied the challenges faced by families coping with breast cancer and found that spouses often had their own medical problems, such as cardiovascular disease and arthritis, which required medical attention. These medical problems often created physical limitations in spouses and interfered with their ability to provide physical care to their wives following breast surgery.

Northouse et al. (1995a) found that half of the husbands of women with recurrent breast cancer reported some type of current health problem of their own, such as hypertension, diabetes, or heart disease. In addition, they found that husbands' health problems accounted for a significant amount of variance in husbands' adjustment to their wives' breast cancer. Husbands with more health problems reported significantly more role adjustment problems than husbands without current health problems.

It is not surprising that the health of the caregiver has a significant influence on the caregiver's adjustment to the patient's illness. What is surprising is that this factor is seldom taken into consideration when medical decisions are made that require the assistance of a family caregiver. For example, women with breast cancer are often discharged within 24 to 48 hours after surgery, and it is often assumed that a family member is available and able to assist with the woman's recovery. Although in many cases families are able to meet the needs of their ill members, health professionals need to evaluate not only the availability of a family caregiver but also the health and well-being of the family member who will assume the caregiving role.

Concurrent Stress

A fourth factor that influences family members' adjustment to breast cancer is the number of other concurrent stressors that they are dealing with at the same time they are dealing with the impact of breast cancer. Breast cancer never occurs in a vacuum or at a peaceful time. Rather, it often piles on top of other pre-existing family stressors. Hilton (1993) found that family members of breast cancer patients were often in the middle of resolving other major crises or changes (e.g., death of a parent, household renovations or relocations) when breast cancer was diagnosed. Some of the family members in Hilton's study talked about the overload of events that they were experiencing and how these events made it more difficult for them to cope with the breast cancer.

Young families coping with breast cancer appear to be especially vulnerable to the stress of many competing demands. Preliminary results from a study of couples' adjustment to breast cancer indicated that younger women reported more emotional distress following the diagnosis of breast cancer, more role problems especially in the domestic area, and a greater number of other life stresses than older women with breast cancer (Northouse, 1994). Younger husbands also reported more adjustment problems, especially in the domestic area, and a greater number of other stressors than older husbands.

While there is no good time to get breast cancer, health professionals need to keep in mind that certain families are already dealing with a number of other life stressors at the time the breast cancer is diagnosed, and they will be more vulnerable to the stressful effects of the illness. These families may need help dealing with the other stressors in their lives, which are further exacerbated by the patient's cancer, as well as needing help with the illness-related stressors. Goldberg and Wool (1985) conducted a counseling intervention with cancer patients and their spouses, and they found that many of the spouses wanted to use the counseling sessions to work on these other concerns rather than just focus on the problems associated with the illness. Families who are helped to resolve some of these pre-existing problems will have more energy to manage the difficulties created by breast cancer.

Hopelessness

A fifth factor that influences the adjustment of spouses and family members to the patient's illness is the attitude they have about the illness—specifically the amount of hope or hopelessness they have about the future. In two recent studies conducted with women during the diagnostic phase of breast cancer and during the recurrent phase of breast cancer, hopelessness was a key factor related to husbands' levels of adjustment during both phases of illness (Northouse, Jeffs, Cracchiolo-Caraway, Lampman, & Dorris, 1995b; Northouse et al., 1995a). Husbands in both studies who reported more hopelessness had poorer adjustments at the time of their wives' diagnosis and in other cases when their wives' cancer recurred.

Concern about the future and progression of the disease are common worries of families facing breast cancer; it is often difficult for spouses and family members to maintain a positive outlook. Husbands of breast cancer patients discussed their feelings of uncertainty about the future and expressed frustration at their inability to predict what might happen; nearly half of the husbands discussed their fears about losing their wives to the breast cancer (Zahlis & Shands, 1991). Although these worries seem overwhelming at times, husbands of breast cancer patients said that their ability to maintain a positive attitude was a major factor that helped them cope with the uncertainty and the worry associated with the disease (Northouse, 1989). Husbands also reported that their wives' positive attitudes helped them maintain their own positive outlook toward the disease, suggesting that there may be a reciprocal relationship or mutual influence between the degree of hope held by women with breast cancer and that held by their family members. Health professionals need to continue to find ways to foster hope in both patients and their family members, because this positive view of the illness is important to their adjustment.

GUIDELINES FOR CLINICAL PRACTICE

Three general guidelines for clinical practice emerge from the studies reviewed. First, it is important for nurses and other professionals to foster contact with spouses and other family members. Too often family members are left on their own to provide complex physical care and emotional support to the patient, with little help from health professionals. Nurses and other health professionals need to take on more responsibility for seeking out family members, for asking them if they have any questions, and for providing them with information that will facilitate their understanding and adjustment to the illness. It is helpful in clinic settings for family members to be invited to join the patient in the interview room with the physician so that family members can get first-hand information as well as have the opportunity to get their questions answered. Attempts such as these will help family members feel more a part of the recovery process, and it will also facilitate their opportunities to receive information and support from health professionals.

Second, it is important to assess the impact of the illness on the family as well as on the patient. A family-focused assessment does not need to be long or cumbersome. Rather, it can include a few pointed questions to determine how the family is adjusting and whether or not a more in-depth assessment is needed. For example, the nurse could ask the husband of a breast cancer patient the following questions: "How have you been managing since your wife was diagnosed with breast cancer? What aspect of the illness is the most difficult for you? Do you need any extra help at this time?" Questions such as these would give the nurse an initial indication of how the husband is coping with the illness and help the nurse to determine if additional assistance is needed.

Third, it is important to direct information and support to patients as well as their family members. It is helpful when both understand the typical course of physical and emotional recovery from breast cancer. It is also useful when spouses or other family caregivers are included in teaching sessions that discuss the side effects of radiation or chemotherapy. Helping family members learn how to manage symptom distress associated with the treatments will add to their competence as family caregivers. Furthermore, as family members are helped to understand the illness and its treatments, they will be in a better position to assist the patient by reinforcing the information that was discussed or by encouraging adherence to the regimen prescribed (i.e., diet plan, medications).

In summary, breast cancer affects the lives of women as well as their family members. Although breast cancer creates specific emotional, physical, and social demands on family members, nurses and other health professionals can help families to cope by keeping in contact with family members, assessing their needs, and providing them with information and support.

ACKNOWLEDGMENT

Research for this chapter was supported in part by a grant from the National Institute for Nursing Research, NIH (R29 NR02019).

References

Baider, L. A., & Kaplan De-Nour, A. (1988a). Breast cancer—A family affair. In C.L. Cooper (Ed.), *Stress and breast cancer* (pp. 155–169). New York: John Wiley and Sons.

Baider, L. A., & Kaplan De-Nour, A. (1988b). Adjustment to cancer: Who is the patient—The husband or the wife? *Israel Journal of Medical Sciences, 24,* 631–636.

Clipp, E. C., & George, L. K. (1992). Patients with cancer and their spouse caregivers. *Cancer, 69,* 1074–1079.

Given, B., & Given, C. W. (1992). Patient and family caregiver reaction to new and recurrent breast cancer. *Journal of the American Medical Women's Association, 47,* 201–206.

Goldberg, R. J., & Wool, M. S. (1985). Psychotherapy for spouses of lung cancer patients: Assessment of an intervention. *Psychotherapy and Psychosomatics, 43,* 141–150.

Gotay, C. C. (1984). The experience of cancer during early and advanced stages: The view of patients and their mates. *Social Science and Medicine, 18,* 605–613.

Halliburton, P., Larson, P. J., Dibble, S., & Dodd, M. J. (1992). The recurrent experience: Family concerns during cancer chemotherapy. *Journal of Clinical Nursing, 1,* 275–281.

Hilton, B. A. (1993). Issues, problems, and challenges for families coping with breast cancer. *Seminars in Oncology Nursing, 9,* 88–100.

Lewis, F. M., Ellison, E. S., & Woods, N. F. (1985). The impact of breast cancer on the family. *Seminars in Oncology Nursing, 1,* 206–213.

Lewis, F. M., & Hammond, M. A. (1992). Psychosocial adjustment of the family to breast cancer: A longitudinal analysis. *Journal of the American Medical Women's Association, 47,* 194–200.

Mood, D. (1993). Promoting patient self-care during cancer treatment. *Proceedings of the Seventh Annual Meeting of the European Society of Psychosocial Oncology,* Jerusalem, p. A74.

Northouse, L. L. (1988). Social support in patients' and husbands' adjustment to breast cancer. *Nursing Research, 37,* 91–95.

Northouse, L. L. (1989). The impact of breast cancer on patients and husbands. *Cancer Nursing, 12,* 276–284.

Northouse, L. L. (1994). Breast cancer in younger women: Effects on interpersonal and family relations. *Journal of the National Cancer Institute, 16,* 183–190

Northouse, L. L., Dorris, G., & Charron-Moore, C. (1995a). Factors affecting couple's adjustment to recurrent breast cancer. *Social Science and Medicine, 41,* 69–76.

Northouse, L. L., Jeffs, M., Cracchiolo-Caraway, A., Lampman, L., & Dorris, G. (1995b). Diagnosing breast cancer: The emotional distress reported by women and husbands prior to a breast biopsy. *Nursing Research, 44,* 196–201.

Northouse, L. L., & Peters-Golden, H. (1993). Cancer and the family: Strategies to assist spouses. *Seminars in Oncology Nursing, 9,* 74–82.

Northouse, L. L., & Swain, M. A. (1987). Adjustment of patients and husbands to the initial impact of breast cancer. *Nursing Research, 36,* 221–225.

Oberst, M. T., & James, R. (1985). Going home: Patient and spouse adjustment following cancer. *Topics in Clinical Nursing, 7,* 46–57.

Packard, N. J., Haberman, M. R., Woods, N. F., & Yates, B. C. (1991). Demands of illness among chronically ill women. *Western Journal of Nursing Research, 13,* 434–457.

Sabo, D. (1990). Men, death anxiety, and denial: Critical feminist interpretations of adjustment to mastectomy. In C. Clark, J. Fritz, & P. Rieder (Eds.), *Clinical sociological perspectives on illness and loss* (pp. 71–84). Philadelphia: Charles Press.

Stetz, K. M. (1987). Caregiving demands during advanced cancer: The spouse's needs. *Cancer Nursing, 10,* 260–268.

Stetz, K. M., Lewis, F. M., & Primomo, J. (1986). Family coping strategies and chronic illness in the mother. *Family Relations, 35,* 515–522.

Vess, J. D., Moreland, J. R., & Schwebel, A. I. (1985). A follow-up study of role functioning and the psychological environment of families of cancer patients. *Journal of Psychosocial Oncology, 3,* 1–13.

Wilson, S., & Morse, J. M. (1991). Living with a wife undergoing chemotherapy. *Image, 23,* 78–84.

Zahlis, E. H., & Shands, M. E. (1991). Breast cancer: Demands of illness on the patient's partner. *Journal of Psychosocial Oncology, 9,* 75–93.

CHAPTER 15

When a Mother Has Breast Cancer

Parenting Concerns and Psychosocial Adjustment in Young Children and Adolescents

Lizbeth A. Hoke, PhD

Breast cancer is the most common type of cancer experienced by American women and the leading cause of cancer deaths among women ages 15 through 54 (Boring, Squires, Tong, & Montgomery, 1994). As such, it is one of the serious medical illnesses that families with young children encounter most frequently. A report by Cancer Care, Inc., in 1977 called for increased awareness of the impact of parental cancer on children (Buckley, 1977), and researchers continue to comment on the lack of attention to this area (Lewis, Hammond, & Woods, 1993; Northouse, 1984; Wellisch, 1985). Despite its prevalence, few empirical studies have examined the effects of maternal breast cancer, or any other types of parental medical illness, on children's adjustment. Yet, parents report that the impact of their illness on their children is a primary concern (Grandstaff, 1976; Hymovich, 1993; Siegel, Mesagno, & Christ, 1990).

As health care providers treating women, it can be easy to overlook the effects of our patients' illnesses on their children, especially because there are so many issues and concerns about the patient herself that need to be addressed. However, a diagnosis of breast cancer in a mother influences the whole family, and the family's responses to the illness, as well as the mother's child-related concerns, affect her adjustment to her diagnosis and treatment.

This chapter focuses on the effects of breast cancer on parenting and young children and adolescent's adjustment. Findings from both the research and clinical literature on maternal breast cancer, as well as other forms of parental cancer, are presented, along with some clinical observations from our ongoing study of women with breast cancer and their children. This chapter aims to increase health care professionals' awareness of parents' concerns and children's responses when a mother has breast cancer, so that they can better address these issues with their patients and their patients' families.

LITERATURE REVIEW

Mothers' Concerns About Their Children

In talking with mothers with breast cancer, we have found that they present with a variety of concerns about their children. These concerns range from questions about what will happen if she dies (e.g., Will my husband be able to care for our children without me? Who will take care of my children?) to questions about everyday disruptions (e.g., What if I am too sick during chemotherapy to take care of my child? Who will take my child to school when I have to go to the hospital for treatments? Who will cook dinner?). More immediately, there are questions about what and how to tell her child about her diagnosis, and if the illness is terminal, how to address the issue of death.

The mother's concerns about the impact of her diagnosis and treatment on her children, coupled with her need to cope with her own emotions and changing outlook on life, may only increase her guilt and worry, as she feels unable to address her children's needs adequately. She may feel that her own difficulties will cause problems for her children (Siegel, Mesagno, & Christ, 1990), and she is likely to experience substantial distress when they are upset over her (Hymovich, 1993). At the same time, she may be confused or hurt if her children respond with anger toward her or if they seem unaffected by her disease. Help in understanding her children's responses can mitigate some of her anxiety and concern.

Children's Reactions to Mother's Breast Cancer

When a mother is diagnosed, children's sense of safety and security is seriously threatened, and the normalcy and predictability of their daily lives are disrupted. Several research studies (Buckley, 1977; Lichtman, Taylor, Wood, Bluming, Dosik, & Leibowitz, 1984; Siegel, Mesagno, Karus, Christ, Banks, &

Table 15-1   Reactions of Children to Parents' Cancer

Mood and self-esteem changes
   Crying
   Anger
   Fearfulness
   Anxiety

Academic changes
   Poor concentration
   Declining academic performance
   Low self-esteem

Somatic symptoms
   Stomach aches
   Appetite disturbance
   Difficulty sleeping

Social and interpersonal changes
   Acting out
   Denial
   Withdrawal from social relationships
   Loss of interest in extracurricular activities

Moynihan, 1992) suggest that children can experience serious adjustment difficulties or significant distress, even though differences in the methodology of these studies limit the comparability of their findings.

A variety of reactions in children have been reported in the clinical and research literature, including crying; fearfulness; lower self-esteem; declining academic performance; somatic symptoms, such as stomach aches and appetite disturbance; trouble sleeping; increased clinging behavior; increased acting out and anger; denial; and withdrawal from family, friends, and activities (Adams-Greenly & Moynihan, 1983; Buckley, 1977; Lewis, 1990; Lichtman et al., 1984; Wellisch, 1981) (Table 15-1).

Northouse (1984), writing about the impact of cancer on the family, identified three periods during the course of an illness—the initial, adaptation, and terminal phases—which present different challenges for the cancer patient and family members. Differences in the effects on children's adjustment of the phase of the mother's illness have not been systematically assessed, though it appears that children experience more difficulties when a parent is in the terminal phase.

A well-designed study comparing children of parents with terminal cancer (40% of cancer patients were women) with a matched community sample found that children of cancer patients experienced significantly more depression and anxiety and lower self-esteem, in addition to more behavior problems and lower social competence, than the matched sample (Siegel et al., 1992).

Another study of parents with advanced cancer (48% with breast cancer) found that 38% of children experienced increased behavior problems during their parent's illness (Buckley, 1977). Other medical variables suggestive of more severe illness have been associated with worse adjustment in children, including longer duration of illness (Buckley, 1977), poorer prognosis, and mastectomy versus less severe surgery (Lichtman et al., 1984).

Some studies suggest that children of mothers with breast cancer generally are doing well (Lewis, 1990; Lichtman et al., 1984), and positive changes in the mother-child relationship have been reported in response to the mother's diagnosis (Lichtman et al., 1984). One report focused on coping in children and families where a mother was diagnosed within the past 2½ years (Issel, Ersek, & Lewis, 1990). Researchers found that children identified four broad categories of adaptive coping: 1) trying to anticipate what the mother would want or need, for example, helping out around the house or trying to be nicer to family members; 2) trying to maintain a sense of normalcy by avoiding the illness or engaging in normal activities; 3) doing things together as a family or with friends; and 4) talking about feelings with other family members or thinking through feelings with oneself. Even children who do well, however, can be expected to experience distress, which can result in the temporary loss of developmental accomplishments, such as regression to younger

behaviors, transient school problems, or increased conflict at home and with peers.

Emotional Effects on Family

A substantial impact comes from the emotional and behavioral effect of the illness on the family. Precisely at the time when a child may need more support and understanding, the mother with breast cancer is faced with one of the most difficult challenges of her own life, coming face to face with her own mortality, and frequently enduring debilitating cancer treatments. The mother may be physically less available to the child when she is busy with her treatment schedule and experiencing medical side effects. Disruptions also can occur in the family's routine as family members attempt to adjust to the maternal illness and changes in roles (Issel et al., 1990). The well parent may need to take over more child care and household related tasks (Siegel, Raveis, Bettes, Mesagno, Christ, & Weinstein, 1990), while children may be required to assume new responsibilities. Families may experience financial strain due to medical expenses and lost income from interruptions in work.

Parents' emotional reactions to the maternal illness, as well as their ability to manage disruptions caused by the illness, influence the extent to which children may feel frightened, overwhelmed, and guilty, or calm and reassured about their own well-being, as well as that of their parents (Buckley, 1977; Lichtman et al., 1984; Siegel, Mesagno, & Christ, 1990). Though most women diagnosed with breast cancer do not develop long-term psychiatric problems (Royak-Schaler, 1991), elevated levels of depression (Lasry et al., 1987), anxiety, hostility, and somatic symptoms (Bloom & Psychological Aspects of Breast Cancer Study Group, 1987) are common in breast cancer patients. Mood disturbances also have been documented in spouses of breast cancer patients (Northouse & Swain, 1987). Parental depression is a well-established risk factor for adjustment problems in children (Downey & Coyne, 1990), and two studies of children of cancer patients suggest that parents' levels of distress and negative experiences with the illness are related to their children's adjustment. Buckley (1977) found, in her study of parents with advanced cancer, that 70% of the children with behavior problems had parents who were depressed. In another study, worse maternal adjustment was related to greater deterioration in the mother-child relationship (Lichtman et al., 1984). The mothers' ratings of unpleasantness of treatments, rather than the presence of radiation or chemotherapy, were significantly related to their reports of these negative changes.

When a woman has breast cancer, her partner must deal with his or her own emotional reactions to the illness, the emotional reactions of the ill spouse, and the changes and disruptions in their daily lives due to the treatment and its side effects. As Taylor and Aspinwall (1990) observed in their review of social supports, partners may be unable to provide adequate support for women with breast cancer because they themselves are experiencing a loss of support. Spouses also may have difficulty helping their children. A study of families where a parent had terminal cancer found that the majority of spouses viewed themselves as less responsive to their children's emotional needs and less able to provide consistent discipline (Siegel et al., 1990). Another study of families with a mother who was recently diagnosed with breast cancer found that fathers who reported more frequent interactions with their children reported significantly better child functioning (Lewis et al., 1993). This finding suggests that a positive and close relationship with the well parent may help protect the child from negative consequences of the mother's illness.

Factors Influencing Children's Adjustment

The strengths and vulnerabilities that a child brings to the crisis of breast cancer influence his or her responses to it. The research and

Table 15-2 Factors Influencing Children's Adjustment to Maternal Breast Cancer

Individual strengths and vulnerabilities
Cognitive capacities
Developmental level
Age
Gender
Previous behavioral or emotional problems
Financial resources/reserve
Marital discord
Family functioning/communication
Individual relationships with each parent

clinical literature have identified several child characteristics that affect how a child understands and adjusts to a parental illness. These include the child's cognitive capacities, developmental level or age, and gender (Table 15-2). Other risk factors not specific to parental illness that can leave children more vulnerable to life stressors also have been identified. These include a history of previous behavior or emotional problems, having a family with few financial resources, and marital discord between the parents (Coie et al., 1993). It is important to consider these factors as they shape the child's experiences, needs, and responses to the maternal illness. For instance, a clinician must be aware that certain reactions that signal a maladaptive response for some children, may be appropriate and expected for children at another developmental level.

Cognitive Capacity. What the child comes to believe about what caused the maternal illness or how it happened, whether it is contagious, how it affects the body, and what happens when someone dies is related to his or her ability to organize and integrate information and to anticipate the future. Children's concepts of illness and death follow a continuum that reflects their capacity for causal reasoning and the degree to which they differentiate themselves from their parents and the outside world (Bibace & Walsh, 1980). In a study of children's explanations of death, Koocher

(1974) identified a continuum of understanding that ranged from concrete thinking to abstract reasoning. While children moved toward abstract reasoning as they got older, he observed variability among same-aged children and advised that it is important to assess a child's understanding independent of age.

Developmental Age. The developmental tasks being negotiated at the time of the mother's illness also color the child's responses to the maternal illness. In their study of children's coping, Issel, Ersek, and Lewis (1990) found that younger children, who developmentally are very dependent on their parents, were more vulnerable to issues about the safety of their family. Adams-Greenly and Moynihan (1983) observed that when a parent dies, preschool children usually believe that death is reversible, and may wonder why their parent is not returning. Children at this age may fear for their own safety and may feel that their thoughts and feelings are somehow responsible for the death (Adams-Greenly & Moynihan, 1983).

School-age children frequently want information about the illness, are concerned about the future, and may wonder if what they are told about the illness is accurate (Lewis, 1990). However, they can be easily overwhelmed by their feelings, making it hard for them to use their cognitive abilities to understand and integrate information (Adams-Greenly & Moynihan, 1983). In one study of children of terminally ill parents, Rosenheim and Reicher (1985) found that children ages 10 to 12 experienced more anxiety than younger and older children. They hypothesized that, unlike younger children, these children could fully understand the finality of death and its implications; at the same time, they lacked the ego-strength of children who were older.

Adolescents fully understand the meaning of death and loss, and developmentally are moving toward increased self-sufficiency and the establishment of separate identities from their parents. In their study of children's cop-

ing with maternal breast cancer, Issel, Ersek, and Lewis (1990) observed that older children could recognize the illness as separate from themselves, but they experienced conflicts around gaining independence from their parents. Others also have suggested that adolescents may feel guilt and anger because they want to be with friends and participate in outside activities, yet feel pulled toward the needs at home (Adams-Greenly, Beldoch, & Moynihan, 1986; Buckley, 1977; Lichtman et al., 1984; Wellisch, 1979). These internal struggles may be expressed through increased conflict with parents, poor school performance, and problem behaviors outside the home.

Gender. There is some suggestion within the clinical and research literature that female children, particularly adolescent daughters, have more difficulties in response to a mother's breast cancer. In a recent report on adolescent stress and coping, Compas, Orosan, and Grant (1993) stated that their research team found higher levels of depression and anxiety in adolescent girls whose mothers had cancer when compared with younger children, boys, or children whose fathers had cancer. A variety of reasons for gender differences in children's responses have been suggested, but have not been tested empirically. For example, breast cancer, more so than other types of cancer, may present daughters with particular challenges. Wellisch (1981, 1985), writing from his clinical experience, suggested that daughters may act out sexually in response to discomfort and heightened competition in the mother-child relationship when the mother's breast is removed or disfigured from surgery. He theorized that daughters unconsciously help their mothers experience a "vicarious sense of sexual freedom" (Wellisch, 1985, p. 198) that is lost when the mother loses her breast. Lichtman et al. (1984) observed that problems in daughters were more severe and that mothers were more distressed by their daughters' problems than their sons' problems. They suggested that mothers with breast cancer rely more heavily on their daughters for support, often in ways that are difficult for their daughters to manage. They also observed that daughters may be more fearful of inheriting breast cancer. Daughters may identify with mothers and feel more vulnerable about their sexuality and body integrity; they may worry about getting breast cancer themselves, and their mothers may expect more help and nurturance from them during their illness.

Responses of boys are less frequently described in the literature, though a range of reactions has been reported, including increased and ongoing somatic symptoms (Grandstaff, 1976), concerns about body integrity, discomfort over the loss of the mother's breast, fearfulness about the mother's well-being, denial of the illness, and aloofness (Lichtman et al., 1984).

INTERVENTIONS

Parental Communication

The importance of parents communicating clearly and openly with their children about the illness is emphasized repeatedly in the literature (Adams-Greenly & Moynihan, 1983; Buckley, 1977; Siegel, Mesagno, & Christ, 1990; Wellisch, 1981). One study of families containing a parent with terminal cancer (Rosenheim & Reicher, 1985) found that children who were not informed by their parents about the cancer diagnosis reported significantly more anxiety than children whose parents informed them. Additionally, in a study of families with newly diagnosed breast cancer patients (Lewis et al., 1993), parents who reported more introspective coping and who talked with each other more frequently about how they dealt with illness reported better functioning in their children and better relationships between the child and the well parent.

Sharing of information and feelings about the parental illness can benefit children in several ways (Adams-Greenly & Moynihan, 1983; Rosenheim & Reicher, 1985; Siegel, Mesagno, & Christ, 1990). Talking with children enables them to express and begin to work through their own painful feelings. Often children harbor incorrect beliefs and fears about what is happening, or, in the absence of information, may develop their own explanations, which can be more upsetting than the truth. For example, a child may feel somehow responsible when the mother is tired and irritable in response to chemotherapy; talking with the child can help identify and correct these feelings and beliefs. Through discussion of events related to the illness, children can be helped to prepare for changes that may take place as a result of the mother's illness, treatment, and in some cases, death.

Despite this widespread support for open family communication, parents frequently are concerned that talking about the parental illness will increase their children's distress and even overwhelm them. Especially when experiencing emotional pain themselves, parents' desires to protect their children from suffering may be heightened (Hymovich, 1993); however, when the topic of the parental illness is avoided, it can have the opposite effect intended by the parents (Siegel et al., 1990).

In talking with children of recently diagnosed breast cancer patients, we have observed that children often are very aware of their parents' distress, even when it is not discussed openly. They follow their parents' cues and may feel that they cannot express their feelings directly when parents do not talk about the illness. We have found that children usually are reassured by their parents' openness, even when they see their parents as being distressed. They can more readily trust that their parents are being truthful, which, in turn, reduces their anxiety that they will be surprised by unexpected events. The parents' confidence in the child's ability to handle the information also contributes to the child's feeling that he or she is not making the problem worse and that the child can do something to help. The opportunity to help out in age-appropriate ways enables children to feel included and gives them a positive role in the family.

Most of what is written about talking with children when a parent has cancer deals with the situation of the terminally ill parent (Adams-Greenly & Moynihan, 1983; Koocher, 1974). When a parent is dying, one of the main tasks of communication is helping the children to anticipate and prepare for the loss and to grieve the loss once it occurs. It is important for the surviving parent to be truthful with children, in order to foster their trust (Siegel et al., 1990). When the mother is newly diagnosed with a good or uncertain prognosis, parents frequently have questions about how much to tell their children about risks for the mother and for their daughters. In this case, it is also important to answer the children's questions honestly and to anticipate and discuss issues that they are likely to hear about from sources outside the family, such as friends, school, and the media. Children are exposed to many sources of information, and hearing about aspects of the mother's illness from persons other than the parents can be more upsetting than hearing it from the parents. There also is an increased risk that information the child obtains will be incorrect or not applicable to the mother's particular situation.

The level of distress experienced by the parents and the types of coping used to deal with the illness will influence their ability to communicate openly and honestly with their children. Buckley (1977) observed that parents who were able to confront the illness and talk frankly between themselves were better able to help their children cope with the illness. When parents are unaccustomed to sharing information and unable to acknowledge their own feelings, forced openness on the part of the parents can leave the children without the emotional support they need to understand and integrate information about the parental illness (Rosenheim & Richter, 1985).

Early Intervention

When a family is faced with a serious parental illness, helping the patient and her partner feel like they are being effective parents can enable them to feel better about themselves and to support their children more effectively. The importance of early intervention to help with parenting has been emphasized by several researchers (Buckley, 1977). Siegel, Mesagno, and Christ (1990) have developed a prevention program for bereaved children that aims to help children grieve the loss of their parent more adaptively. In this intervention, which begins prior to the ill parent's death, the clinician works primarily with the well parent to support the parent's grief, to provide information and foster understanding about the children's needs and reactions, and to facilitate communication between parents and children.

Other promising interventions include support groups for children of cancer patients (Call, 1990), some of which also feature concurrent groups for parents (Greening, 1992; Taylor-Brown, Acheson, & Farber, 1993). When children can talk with other children in similar situations, they learn that they are not alone. These programs have in common an emphasis on providing accurate information about the parent's illness and opportunities for open communication.

It is not necessary, however, to be a child or family therapist to help these children and their parents. Health care providers treating women with breast cancer can support their patients and their patients' children more effectively through greater awareness and understanding of issues and concerns that confront families with maternal breast cancer. Even women who are very satisfied with the quality of their medical care frequently report that it would be helpful to acknowledge and discuss with their treatment providers issues related to their own adjustment and the impact of their illness on their families. These women and their partners can benefit from recognition of their concerns for their children. Acknowledgement that, at times, their own needs may conflict with the needs of their children can help parents feel less guilty and inadequate in their roles as parents. Information about how to talk with their children about the illness can help parents communicate with their children and respond more supportively to their questions. Knowledge about normal reactions and signs of more serious adjustment problems can help parents better understand their children's responses and identify children who may need professional services. Health care providers can facilitate parents' use of resources by being aware of services in the community and making available informational pamphlets, such as those about parental cancer and children published by the American Cancer Society and the National Cancer Institute. When health care providers can take an active role in supporting mothers with breast cancer, they also are helping these mothers to better support their children.

ACKNOWLEDGMENTS

This work was supported by the Trustees Under the Will of Herman Dana and the American Cancer Society, Mass. Division, Inc.

References

Adams-Greenly, M., Beldoch, N., & Moynihan, R. (1986). Helping adolescents whose parents have cancer. *Seminars in Oncology, 2*, 113–118.

Adams-Greenly, M., & Moynihan, R. (1983). Helping the children of fatally ill parents. *American Journal of Orthopsychiatry, 53*, 219–229.

Bibace, R., & Walsh, M. E. (1980). Development of children's concepts of illness. *Pediatrics, 66*, 912–917.

Bloom, J. R., & Psychological Aspects of Breast Cancer Study Group (1987). Psychological response to mastectomy: A prospective comparison study. *Cancer, 59*, 189–196.

Boring, C. C., Squires, T. S., Tong T., & Montgomery, S. (1994). Cancer statistics, 1994. *CA—A Cancer Journal for Clinicians, 44*, 7–26.

Buckley, I. G. (1977). *Listen to the children: A study of the impact on the mental health of children of a parent's catastrophic illness.* New York: Cancer Care, Inc.

Call, D. (1990). School-based groups: A valuable support for children of cancer patients. *Journal of Psychosocial Oncology, 8*, 97–118.

Coie, J. D., Watt, N. F., West, S. G., Harkins, J. D., Asarnow, J. R., Markman, H. J., Ramey, S. L., Shure, M. B., & Long, B. (1993). The science of prevention: A conceptual framework and some directions for a national research program. *American Psychologist, 48*, 1013–1022.

Compas, B. E., Orosan, P. G., & Grant, K. E. (1993). Adolescent stress and coping: Implications for psychopathology during adolescence. *Journal of Adolescence, 16*, 331–349.

Downey, G., & Coyne, J. C. (1990). Children of depressed parents: An integrative review. *Psychological Bulletin, 108*, 50–76.

Grandstaff, N. W. (1976). The impact of breast cancer on the family. *Frontiers of Radiation Therapy and Oncology, 11*, 146–156.

Greening, K. (1992). The 'bear essentials' program: Helping young children and their families cope when a parent has cancer. *Journal of Psychosocial Oncology, 10*, 47–61.

Hymovich, D. P. (1993). Child-rearing concerns of parents with cancer. *Oncology Nursing Forum, 20*, 1355–1360.

Issel, L. M., Ersek, M., & Lewis, F. M. (1990). How children cope with mother's breast cancer. *Oncology Nursing Forum, 17* (Suppl.), 5–13.

Koocher, G. P. (1974). Talking with children about death. *American Journal of Orthopsychiatry, 44*, 404–411.

Lasry, J. C., Margolese, R., Poisson, R., Shibata, H., Fleischer, D., Lafleur, D., Lagault, S., & Taillefer, S. (1987). Depression and body image following mastectomy and lumpectomy. *Journal of Chronic Disease, 40*, 529–534.

Lewis, F. M. (1990). Strengthening family supports. Cancer and the family. *Cancer, 65*, 752–759.

Lewis, F. M., Hammond, M. A., & Wood, N. F. (1993). The family's functioning with newly diagnosed breast cancer in the mother: The development of an explanatory model. *Journal of Behavioral Medicine, 16*, 351–370.

Lichtman, R. R., Taylor, S. E., Wood, J. V., Bluming, A. Z., Dosik, G. M., & Leibowitz, R. L. (1984). Relationships with children after breast cancer: The mother-daughter relationship at risk. *Journal of Psychosocial Oncology, 2*, 1–19.

Northouse, L. (1984). The impact of cancer on the family: An overview. *International Journal of Psychiatry in Medicine, 14*, 215–242.

Northouse, L. L., & Swain, M. A. (1987). Adjustment of patients and husbands to the initial impact of breast cancer. *Nursing Research, 36*, 221–225.

Rosenheim, E., & Reicher, R. (1985). Informing children about a parent's terminal illness. *Journal of Child Psychology and Psychiatry, 26*, 995–998.

Royak-Schaler, R. (1991). Psychological processes in breast cancer: A review of selected literature. *Journal of Psychosocial Oncology, 9*, 71–89.

Siegel, K., Mesagno, F. P., & Christ, G. (1990). A prevention program for bereaved children. *American Journal of Orthopsychiatry, 60*, 168–175.

Siegel, K., Raveis, V. H., Bettes, B., Mesagno, F. P., Christ, G., & Weinstein, L. (1990). Perceptions of parental competence while facing the death of a spouse. *American Journal of Orthopsychiatry, 60*, 567–576.

Siegel, K., Mesagno, F. P., Karus, D., Christ, G., Banks, K., & Moynihan, R. (1992). Psychosocial adjustment of children with a terminally ill parent. *Journal of the*

American Academy of Child and Adolescent Psychiatry, 31, 327–333.

Taylor, S. E., & Aspinwall, L. G. (1990). Psychosocial aspects of chronic illness. In P. T. Costa & G. R. Vanden Bos (Eds.), *Psychological aspects of serious illness: Chronic conditions, fatal diseases, and clinical care* (pp. 3–60). Washington, DC: American Psychological Association.

Taylor-Brown, J., Acheson, A., & Farber J. M. (1993). Kids can cope: A group intervention for children whose parents have cancer. *Journal of Psychosocial Oncology, 11,* 41–53.

Wellisch, D. K. (1979). Adolescent acting out when a parent has cancer. *International Journal of Family Therapy, 1,* 230–241.

Wellisch, D. K. (1981). Family relationships of the mastectomy patient: Interactions with the spouse and children. *Israel Journal of Medical Science, 17,* 993–996.

Wellisch, D. K. (1985). The psychologic impact of breast cancer on relationships. *Seminars in Oncology Nursing, 1,* 195–199.

PART 6 | Innovative Community Models or Interventions

CHAPTER 16

Breast Cancer Early Detection and Control
Strategies for Community Outreach

Sandra Millon Underwood, PhD, RN

Despite the unprecedented explosion in scientific knowledge and the phenomenal capacity of medicine to diagnose and control breast cancer, many women are not benefitting fully from the advances being made in science (Figures 16-1 and 16-2). Current national data indicate that breast cancer is the most common form of cancer observed in American women (American Cancer Society [ACS], 1995; Boring, 1992; Byrd & Clayton, 1993; Clayton & Byrd, 1993; U.S. Department of Health and Human Services [USDHHS], 1993, 1994; U.S. Public Health Service, 1990) (Figure 16-3). Yet, despite the strides that have been made in the area of early detection and diagnosis, and the fact that breast cancer can be successfully treated with surgery, radiation therapy, and chemotherapy, it continues to be among the leading causes of cancer death (Figure 16-4).

Reports from the National Cancer Institute indicate that between 1989 and 1992 the national death rate from breast cancer fell almost 5% (the largest short-term decline in four decades) (USDHHS, 1994; USDHHS, 1993). However, on close examination of the data, it appears that the rate for white women fell 5.5%, the rate for African American women actually rose 2.6% and the rate for women of other minority groups was unreported (Figure 16-5) (ACS, 1995; USDHHS, 1994; USDHHS, 1993).

Several explanations for the variations noted in breast cancer mortality have been postulated. While recent studies suggest that a more deadly form of breast cancer occurs among select ethnic groups, most experts agree that the major reasons are related to trends in health promotion and breast cancer detection, timeliness in which medical care is sought once a breast lump is found, the stage of disease at time of diagnosis and first treatment, the availability of state-of-the-art facilities and resources for early detection, screening, and early care (ACS, 1995; Joslyn, Eley, & Hill, 1995; Eley, 1994; Freeman, 1994; National Cancer Advisory Board [NCAB], 1994; Roberson, 1994; Long, 1993).

Fig 16-1   Breast Cancer Incidence Rates Per 100,000 Population by Race/Ethnic Group, 1977–83

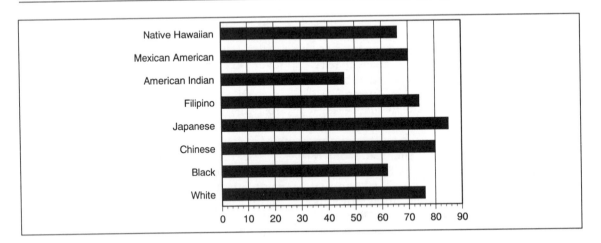

Note. Data from *1991 ACS Cancer Facts and Figures for Minority Americans* by the American Cancer Society, 1991, Atlanta: American Cancer Society. Copright 1991 by the American Cancer Society. Reprinted by permission.

Fig 16-2   Five-Year Breast Cancer Survival Rates (%) by Racial/Ethnic Group, 1975–84

Note. Data from *1991 ACS Cancer Facts and Figures for Minority Americans* by the American Cancer Society, 1991, Atlanta: American Cancer Society. Copright 1991 by the American Cancer Society. Reprinted by permission.

Statistics demonstrate with sharp clarity that many American women do not receive adequate early, routine, and preventive health care. Studies have demonstrated that programs emphasizing screening mammography and clinical breast examinations are effective in increasing compliance with recommended screening schedules, and thereby reducing breast cancer mortality (Ansell, 1994; Brown & Williams, 1994; Greenberg, 1994; King, 1994; NCAB, 1994). However, while breast self-examination and mammography are becoming more frequently used than was true in the early 1980s, significant under-use by many

Fig. 16-3   Cancer Cases by Site

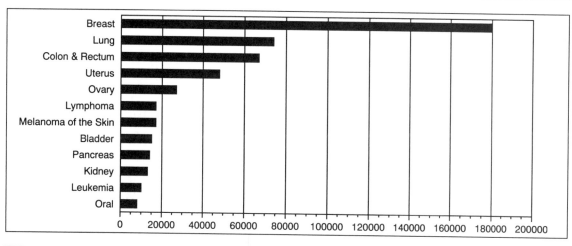

Note. Data from *1995 ACS Cancer Facts and Figures,* by the American Cancer Society, 1995, Atlanta: American Cancer Society. Copyright 1995 by the American Cancer Society. Reprinted by permission.

Fig 16-4   Cancer Deaths by Site

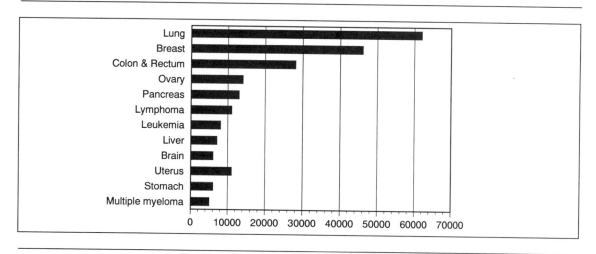

Note. Data from *1995 ACS Cancer Facts and Figures,* by the American Cancer Society, 1995, Atlanta: American Cancer Society. Copyright 1995 by the American Cancer Society. Reprinted by permission.

women is still noted (ACS, 1995; Ansell, 1994; USDHHS, 1994; USDHHS, 1993; Long, 1993).

The extensive under-use of breast self-examination, screening mammography, and clinical breast examination is considered to be largely due to the lack of breast health and breast cancer programs and resources targeted to high-risk groups. Multiple reports have been cited, indicating that many women who are at high risk of breast cancer (1) fail to receive directives from their health care providers regarding the importance of monthly breast self-examination, regular clinical breast examinations, and regular mammography; (2)

Fig 16-5   Female Breast Cancer Mortality Rates (United States, 1973–1992)

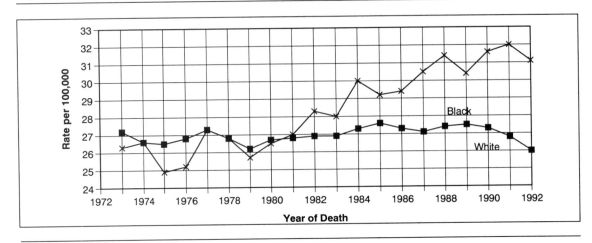

Note. From *Breast Cancer Mortality Rates, 1973–1992*, by the National Cancer Institute, 1995. SEER program data.

fail to receive information from their health care providers regarding the advances that have been made in the areas of the early detection, diagnosis, and treatment of breast cancer; and (3) fail to receive information from their providers that would allow them to take advantage of available early detection, screening, and treatment options/programs (ACS, 1995; NCAB, 1994; Underwood, 1994; Underwood and Hoskins, 1994; Underwood, Hoskins, Morris, & Williams, 1994; USDHHS, 1994; USDHHS, 1993).

COMMUNITY-BASED HEALTH CARE: A STRATEGY FOR EFFECTING CHANGE

In spite of the devastating disparities in cancer incidence and mortality, it has been asserted that given what is currently known about cancer control through health promotion, risk reduction, early detection, and treatment, the health status of our nation's women could be significantly enhanced (NCAB, 1994; Public Health Service [PHS], 1990). Many existing national health care efforts have been implemented in an attempt to lessen the cancer burden among American women. However, an increasing body of research has described the use of community-based health care models as being among the most effective method for promoting women's health and wellness (NCAB, 1994; PHS, 1990; USDHHS, 1993).

While drawing on as many aspects of community life as possible, community-based health care models have proven to be successful in their attempts to assist clients to overcome many of the barriers and bridge many of the gaps that currently exist within the health care system. Research has demonstrated that by carefully designing programs that emphasize health promotion, risk reduction, early detection, and early treatment of disease in a supportive community environment, these programs can positively influence health, health behaviors, and health outcomes.

DESIGNING A COMMUNITY BREAST HEALTH INTERVENTION: BUILDING SUCCESS

The literature contains numerous reports completed by nurses and professionals from other disciplines, which describe models of care that have been developed to address many of the breast health care needs of our nation's women. Most notable among these reports are models that attempted to reduce the health disparities through the implementation of interventions focused specifically on health promotion through education, early detection, and the coordination of health care services and resources (Eng, 1993; Holland, Foster, & Louria, 1993; Lacey, 1993; Suarez, Nichols, & Brady, 1993).

Many of these models engaged health-oriented institutions peripheral to the community in the development of community based breast health care systems (Kang & Bloom, 1993; Rudolph, Kahan, & Bordeau, 1993). Other community-based breast health care models have used community settings that are more engaged in the social structure of the community, such as religious institutions, housing units, community centers, and civic centers, as the point of access to this population (Eng, 1993; Holland et al., 1993; Lacey, 1993; Rubin & Black, 1992; Thomas, Quin, Billingsley, & Caldwell, 1994).

Reports highlighting the impact of these models demonstrate that involving institutions that are perceived as being outside the community often fails to achieve optimal involvement. However, they suggest that there is a far greater benefit to working closely within settings that are frequented by large numbers of people and those that also play a strong role in the life of the people within the community.

Also highlighted in the literature are other community-based breast health care models that addressed the breast health needs of the community through the incorporation of natural helpers, peer role models, lay health educators, informants, and other persons indigenous to the community into the structure of the health care team (Dingman, 1990; Eng, 1993; Rubin & Black, 1992; Suarez et al., 1993). It has been suggested that their increased familiarity with the lifestyles, values, and beliefs of the target community makes them uniquely qualified to serve in this capacity.

The literature suggests that the involvement of persons indigenous to the community in the process of community outreach, health promotion, and health education facilitates the organization, motivation, and mobilization of populations often difficult to access. Their use of techniques and strategies that "model" behaviors that are familiar to persons within the community has been shown to be consoling to those who are struggling with serious problems of life (Dingman, 1990; Eng, 1993; Rubin & Black, 1992; Suarez et al., 1993).

THE NURSING CHALLENGE

Recognizing that multiple factors affect health, health behavior, health care, and health care outcomes, public health officials have challenged nurses to further design interventions to address the health disparities known to occur among our nation's women. Yet, while the literature is replete with reports that define the health status and the health care dilemma faced by women, and reports that describe models of care that have been successful in addressing many of the health care needs of the population, the disparities in health and barriers to access to health care continue to persist.

Current data suggest that modifications in certain health care practices would significantly decrease breast cancer mortality and increase breast cancer survival (ACS, 1995; Eley, 1994; Freeman, 1994; Greenberg, 1994; Long, 1993; NCAB, 1994; PHS, 1990; USDHHS, 1994; USDHHS, 1993). Modifications advocated include increased participation in breast cancer screening (and follow-up) programs and increased enrollment in breast cancer trials that focus on early detection, early diagnosis, and state-of-the-art treatment. It is believed that excess breast cancer mortality could be significantly reduced if the current knowledge were effectively communicated to and used by women with breast cancer and women who are at risk of breast cancer (ACS, 1995; Long, 1993; NCAB, 1994; PHS, 1990; USDHHS, 1994; USDHHS, 1993).

In 1990, the U.S. Department of Health and Human Services released "Healthy People 2000," which outlines general health objectives for the nation and specific health objectives for high-risk groups (PHS, 1990). The year-2000 cancer goals have major implications for health care professionals. There has been a call for an increase in the number of primary care providers, including practicing nurses, who routinely counsel patients and educate consumers (within the health care system and within the community) about the availability of early detection of cancer, as well as diagnostic and treatment options. Efforts by nurse educators, nurse scientists, nurses representing private and public industry, and nurses representing community advocacy groups have similarly been recommended (NCAB, 1994; PHS, 1990; Thomas, Pinto, Roach, & Vaughn, 1994; Underwood, 1995; USDHHS, 1994; USDHHS, 1993).

Nurses are in key positions to play a significant role in achieving these goals. Nurses have been observed to have a critical influence on the lives of both sick and well people. People look to nurses for education and counseling about their health. Their ongoing interaction with patients, families, and community groups in a wide array of settings provides an excellent opportunity for nurses to serve as cancer control advocates (Cassidy & MacFarlane, 1991; Eng, 1993; Lacey, 1989; Lacey, 1993; Long, 1993; Phillips, 1991; Roberson, 1994; Willis, 1989).

Nurses, more often than any other health care professional, are "positioned" to provide health education, identify patients who exhibit multiple high-risk behaviors and patients who are otherwise at high risk, and initiate a patient referral. The nurse is often the first health care professional the patient encounters on arrival at a health care facility, and the last encountered prior to departure. In this position, the nurse may be the critical link in identifying patients with significant breast cancer risk, symptoms suggestive of neoplastic breast disease, and high-risk behaviors.

A nurse's awareness of the current screening and procedures for breast cancer can facilitate planning the inclusion of screening diagnostics in the treatment plan. A nurse's

awareness of the current early detection, screening, and treatment programs and trials may also aid the physician, the nurse practitioner, and the clinical scientist in determining if a patient is eligible to serve as a participant in a breast cancer early detection and control program or trial. And, in this position, the nurse may be the best vehicle through which to ensure that women with breast cancer and women who are at risk of breast cancer (1) receive directives regarding the importance of monthly breast self-examination, regular clinical breast examinations, and regular mammography; (2) receive information regarding the advances that have been made in the areas of early detection, diagnosis, and treatment of breast cancer; and (3) receive information from their health care providers that would increase the likelihood that they would take advantage of available early detection, screening, and treatment options/programs.

References

American Cancer Society. (1995). Cancer facts and figures—1995. Atlanta: American Cancer Society.

Ansell, D. (1994). A nurse-delivered intervention to reduce barriers to breast and cervical cancer screening in Chicago inner city clinics. *Public Health Reports, 109* (1), 104–111.

Boring, C. (1992). Cancer statistics, 1992. *CA—A Journal for Clinicians, 42* (1), 19–38.

Brown, L., & Williams, R. (1994). Culturally sensitive breast cancer screening programs for older Black women. *Nurse Practitioner, 19* (3), 21–27.

Byrd, W., & Clayton, L. (1993). The African American cancer crisis: A prescription. *Journal of Health Care for the Poor and Underserved, 4* (2), 102–116.

Cassidy, J., & Macfarlane, D. (1991). The role of the nurse in clinical cancer research. *Cancer Nursing, 14* (3), 124–131.

Clayton, L., & Byrd, W. (1993). The African American cancer crisis: The problem. *Journal of Health Care for the Poor and Underserved, 4* (2), 83–101.

Dingman, M. (1990). The role of focus groups in health education for cervical cancer among minority women. *Journal of Community Health, 15* (6), 369–375.

Eley, W. (1994). Racial differences in survival from breast cancer: Results of the National Cancer Institute Black/White cancer survival study. *Journal of the American Medical Association, 272,* 947–955.

Eng, E. (1993). The Save Our Sisters Project: A social network strategy for reaching rural black women. *Cancer, 72* (3), 1071–1077.

Freeman, B. (1994). Fighting a taboo that can lead to a deadly tragedy. *Emerge, 5,* 64.

Greenberg, D. (1994). Rethinking the cancer programs. *Lancet, 344,* 1075.

Holland, B. K., Foster, J. D., & Louria, D. B. (1993). Cervical cancer and health care resources in Newark, New Jersey, 1970 to 1988. *American Journal of Public Health, 83* (1), 45–48.

Joslyn, S., Eley, W., & Hill H. (1995). Racial differences in survival from breast cancer. *Journal of the American Medical Association, 273,* 1000.

Kang, S. H., & Bloom, J. R. (1993). Social support and cancer screening among older black Americans. *Journal of the National Cancer Institute, 85* (9), 737–742.

King, E. (1994). Promoting mammography use through progressive interventions: Is it effective? *American Journal of Public Health, 84* (1), 104–106.

Lacey, L. (1993). Cancer prevention and early detection strategies for reaching underserved urban, low-income black women: Barriers and objectives. *Cancer, 72* (3 Suppl.), 1078–1083.

Long, E. (1993). Breast cancer in African-American women: Review of the literature. *Cancer Nursing, 16* (1), 1–24.

National Cancer Advisory Board. (1994). Cancer at a crossroads: A report to Congress. Bethesda, MD: National Cancer Advisory Board.

Phillips, J. (1991). Cancer control by the year 2000: Implications for action. *Journal of the National Black Nurses' Association, 5,* 42–48.

Public Health Service. (1990). Summary of healthy people 2000: National health promotion and disease prevention objectives. Washington, DC: American Public Health Association.

Roberson, N. (1994). Breast cancer screening in older Black women. *Cancer, 74,* 2034-2042.

Rubin, F. H., & Black, J. S. (1992). Health care and consumer control: Pittsburgh's town meeting for seniors. *Gerontologist, 32* (6), 853–855.

Rudolph, A., Kahan, V., & Bordeu, M. (1993). Cervical cancer prevention project for inner city black and Latina women. *Public Health Report, 108* (2), 156–160.

Suarez, L., Nichols, D. C., & Brady, C. A. (1993). Use of peer role models to increase Pap smear and mammogram screening in Mexican-American and black women. *American Journal of Preventive Medicine. 9* (5), 290–296.

Thomas, C., Pinto, H., Roach, M., & Vaughn, C. (1994). Participation in clinical trials: Is it state-of-the-art treatment for African Americans and other people of color? *Journal of the National Medical Association, 86* (3), 177–182.

Thomas, S. B., Quinn, S. C., Billingsley, A., & Caldwell, C. (1994). The characteristics of northern black churches with community health outreach programs. *American Journal of Public Health, 84* (4), 575–579.

Underwood, S. (1994). Access to health care in America: The dilemma faced by the poor in seeking cancer care. *Seminars in Oncology Nursing, 10* (2), 89–95.

Underwood, S. (1995). Enhancing the delivery of cancer care to the disadvantaged. *Cancer Practice, 3* (1), 31–36.

Underwood, S. & Hoskins, D. (1994). Cancer and the poor: Focusing the challenge. Atlanta: American Cancer Society.

Underwood, S., Hoskins, D., Morris, K., & Williams, A. (1994). Obstacles to cancer care: Focus on the economically disadvantaged. *Oncology Nursing Forum, 21* (1) 47–52.

U.S. Department of Health and Human Services. (1993). The national strategic plan for the early detection and control of breast and cervical cancers. Bethesda, MD: U.S. Department of Health and Human Services.

U.S. Department of Health and Human Services. (1994). SEER cancer statistics review, 1973–1991. Bethesda, MD: U.S. Department of Health and Human Services.

Willis, M. (1989). Interagency collaboration: Teaching breast self-examination to Black women. *Oncology Nursing Forum, 16* (2), 171–177.

CHAPTER 17 | **Rural Care Cost Issues**

Nancy J. White, RN, MS, OCN
Barbara A. Given, PhD, RN, FAAN

The diagnosis of breast cancer, requiring treatment with the possibility of side effects, thrusts upon patients and their families a variety of challenges and may result in tremendous disruption. As new role demands arise for patients and those who care for them, they must develop strategies to help each other cope.

In the last several years, the role of the family in coping with breast cancer has been examined and the costs of breast cancer have been documented. The costs of breast cancer include not only formal medical costs, but also additional expenses incurred by patients and families. These additional expenses include time lost from work, out-of-pocket medical care expenses, and costs associated with family labor when care is needed but not covered through skilled home care.

Nowhere are these burdens and costs more evident than in rural families dealing with the diagnosis of breast cancer. In addition to financial burdens, rural breast cancer pa-

tients face significant barriers to needed care and support services. Providing cancer care to rural breast cancer patients requires multiple strategies and creative problem solving to support families and reduce the costs of cancer care. In this chapter, data from a research project, the "Rural Partnership Linkage for Cancer Care" (grant No. 5 R01 CA56338, funded by the National Cancer Institute), which uses a nursing intervention model to deliver supportive and continuing care to breast cancer patients, is used to explore several issues. In addition, this chapter defines roles for rural oncology nurses caring for patients with breast cancer.

BACKGROUND

It is estimated that in 1990, 6.5 billion dollars was spent on breast cancer treatment in the United States. This figure does not include the cost of screening and diagnosis (Brown &

Fintor, 1994). These formal costs of breast cancer treatment are only a portion of the financial picture.

Studies show that financial strain is also a critical personal issue for the family facing cancer and its treatment. In a study of 12 breast cancer patients and their families, Hilton (1993) interviewed the women at five intervals, beginning at the time of diagnosis to 1 year following diagnosis. Though their stage of diagnosis varied slightly, 9 of the 12 had undergone conservative treatment including radiation therapy and partial mastectomy. None of the study participants was reported to be in a terminal phase of cancer. Over the course of the five interview periods, 7 of the 12 families cited financial concerns as a major issue.

Other studies have also indicated financial issues as a problem. In a study that included 182 breast cancer patients, Mor, Guadagnoli, and Wool (1988) reported 14.9% of the women receiving adjuvant treatment (n = 84) needed assistance with finances. Another 8.4% of women undergoing palliative treatment (n = 98) either sought financial advice or had the need unmet.

The costs of cancer on psychosocial adjustment are another consideration. Costs include traditional medical care, but also such things as transportation expenses, child care, medical supplies, and nutritional supplements. Costs create significant strain for most patients and may even cause disruption in the patient's treatment (Berkman & Sampson, 1993).

Cost-related issues are magnified in the rural community. It is reported that 25% of the population of the United States resides in rural areas. One third of the elderly population lives in rural areas and one out of six lives in poverty (Office of Technology, 1990).

This underserved population is at a greater risk of delaying the diagnosis and treatment of cancer for a variety of reasons, including lack of finances or insurance coverage. Initial evidence indicates that the less educated, poorer, and older rural population has less access to screening and detection programs (Monroe, Ricketts, & Savitz, 1992). This delay in diagnosis results in cancer being detected at more advanced stages, thereby increasing health care costs.

Additional barriers exist for the rural population. Often, rural cancer patients must travel great distances to access health care and to continue treatment. In many rural areas, public transportation is limited or nonexistent. Volunteer organizations have difficulty recruiting drivers to travel to major cancer treatment centers. The cost of traveling long distances for treatment has been identified as a major obstacle for poor and middle class patients, regardless of whether or not their actual cancer treatment is covered by insurance (Murphy et al., 1993).

Rural patients may also be asked to accept fragmented medical care due to the lack of oncology services in the rural community. A consultant model, as described by Curtiss (1993), provides intermittent visits by specialized physicians and nurses. The success of this design is based on the need for knowledgeable local team support. A strong local network of formal caregivers with cancer expertise, including persons such as clergy, educators, nurses, and home health care or hospice staff, is necessary or the fragmentation will continue (Watson, 1993).

INFORMAL COSTS OF CARE

Researchers have documented and quantified cancer costs beyond formal third-party insurance payments and medical bills. Stommel, Given, and Given (1992) conceptualized the informal costs of care to include direct out-of-pocket expenditures that are not reimbursed by insurance or other sources, loss of employment earnings for both the patient and caregivers, and the indirect cost of family labor in caring for the patient.

Categories of informal costs are defined as follows. Direct out-of-pocket expenditures include nine specific categories: hospital and physician services, nursing homes, medications, visiting nurses, home health aides, and the purchase of special equipment, supplies, food, and supplements. Labor costs of the caregiver providing services is a dollar figure assigned to the actual time spent providing "tangible care." Last, wages in dollars lost as a result of the cancer diagnosis were measured for both the patient and caregiver.

Stommel, Given, and Given (1992) found there were significant expenses in all three areas across the cancer trajectory for a group of 192 patients with cancer and their primary caregivers. Stommel linked cost to dependency in activities of daily living (ADL) and found that ADL dependency was a significant predictor of increasing costs. Patients' stage of disease was another significant predictor. As patients neared death, informal costs rose an additional 9%. Unlike past research that directly links formal costs to undergoing treatment, informal costs are directly related to a patient's physical functioning and nearness to death.

The data on 62 breast cancer patients and their families, who were involved in the larger cost study, were analyzed independently (Given, Given, & Stommel, 1994; White, Stover, Given, & Stommel, 1994). Based on the cancer trajectory, the women were divided into two groups: survivors (women who remained alive 6 months after the initial interview) and decedents (those who died prior to the 6-month interview).

Both groups were evaluated by studying informal costs of care in relationship to disease status and ADL dependencies. Given, Given, and Stommel (1994) reported the following characteristics within the surviving group (n = 49).

1. Mean family income was $34,000, with a range of $12,500 to $60,000.
2. The mean age of the caregivers was 55; the mean age of the patients was 56.
3. Mean time since diagnosis was 45 months.
4. A high level of independence was documented in the area of ADL.
5. Fifty-nine percent of caregivers were employed full time or part time outside the home.

Table 17-1 Out-of-Pocket/Labor Expenses for Survivors/Nonsurvivors with Breast Cancer (3-Month Period)

Expenses	Survivors (n=49)	Nonsurvivors (n=13)
Out-of-pocket	$ 548 (92%)	$1,125 (100%)
Labor	$1,586 (52%)	$3,444 (70%)
	(18 hrs/wk)	(46.3 hrs/wk)

% = Percent of total patients/caregivers reporting expenses in this category.

Comparing this group with the decedents or nonsurvivors, one sees the following:

1. The household incomes were similar, with a mean of $36,667.
2. The mean ages were similar, with a mean age of 51 for the caregivers and 55 for the patients.
3. The functional status of the nonsurvivors was, as expected, less optimal, with a mean of 3.85 ADL dependencies. Sixty-one percent of those who died reported needing assistance. Nine of the 13 (70%) needed assistance with specific medical treatments or procedures.
4. Most caregivers were spouses residing with the patient; 62% of the caregivers were employed full time.

Table 17-1 documents the informal expenses of the groups over a 3-month period.

Out-of-pocket expenses included hospital and physician services, nursing homes, medication, visiting nurses, home health aides, special equipment, supplies, food, and supplements. Patients were asked if, during any month, they had paid out of pocket for any of these services. In both groups, significant cost was incurred in buying services, supplies, and equipment. In a 3-month period, the survivors saw a mean expense of $548, with 92% of the group having expenses. The nonsurvivors had a mean expense of $1,125, with all 13 (100%) having incurred expenses.

Second, the survivors' caregivers' labor expenses were roughly 18 hours of labor per week (mean cost was $1,586; 52% incurred expenses). The nonsurvivors' caregivers' hours of labor more than doubled to 46.3 hours per week, with mean labor costs calculated at $3,444 (70% incurred expenses). These hours are reported by caregivers after being defined as hours spent providing tangible and direct care ("keeping company" was not included).

Finally, Given, Given, and Stommel (1994) documented the cost and hours other family members spent rendering care. In the larger group of survivors, extended family spent only 8 hours per week assisting with the patient's care. Far more significant is that during the terminal phase of the disease, extended family estimated that they spent 29 hours per week supporting the patient and the primary caregiver.

Earnings lost by patients and caregivers are not included in these data. In this particular group of women with breast cancer, minimal lost earnings were reported. In a 3-month period, patients reported an average loss of $1,258, with a range of $0 to $9,375. Family members reported an average loss of $214, with a range of $0 to $5,418.

These data further illustrate the financial constraints breast cancer patients face and the enormous number of hours caregivers spend supporting patients and managing the medical treatments, especially during the terminal phase of care.

The next section briefly describes the findings from our current work with a small number of rural women who are participating in a nurse-directed intervention designed to reduce costs, manage symptoms, and improve patient and family access to supportive care in the community.

"RURAL PARTNERSHIP LINKAGE FOR CANCER CARE" BREAST CANCER DATA

The challenges of caring for the rural woman with breast cancer were documented in the

Table 17-2 Age, Marital Status, and Insurance Status of Women with Breast Cancer from the Rural Cancer Care Project

Patient No.	Age	Insurance	Marital Status
1	37	Private	Married
2	53	Private	Married
3	59	None	Married
4	74	Medicare/private	Married
5	67	Medicare/private	Married
6	42	Medicaid	Married

first year of implementation of the Michigan State University's "Rural Partnership Linkage for Cancer Care" (Rural Cancer Care Project). The goal of the project is to improve rural cancer care by designing, implementing, and measuring an advanced practice nursing model of direct care in rural communities of Southwest Michigan.

In the first few months, seven women with breast cancer enrolled in the study. Their stories help clarify the oncology nurse's role in meeting their needs in a rural setting. It is important to look at their breast cancer experiences to answer the question of what actual expenses remain after the formal costs are paid by third-party insurance. Telephone interviews also illustrate the true concerns and symptoms experienced as compared with what is actually documented by the health care professionals. Their experience also helps confirm the complexity of the health care system and how few resources are provided to support them during the treatment process. Data from six of the seven women were reviewed for this chapter. Both medical records and initial telephone interviews were used for analysis. Several significant issues should be noted. The women ranged in age from 37 to 74 years, with an average age of 55. All were Caucasian and married. Two of the women had private insurance coverage, two were insured through both Medicare and secondary private insurance, one had Medicaid, and one had no medical insurance. Table 17-2 summarizes these data.

Table 17-3 Diagnostic, Treatment, Symptom, Functional, Comorbid, and Teaching Status of Women

Patient No.	Stage at Diagnosis	Treatment	No. of ADL Dependencies	No. of Comorbid Conditions	Symptoms Recorded on Chart	Symptoms Recorded on Phone	Teaching Encountered
1	IV	Radiation therapy, bone marrow transplant, chemotherapy	3	0	6	4	7
2	I	Chemotherapy	4	4	5	19	3
3	II	Chemotherapy	0	1	3	10	1
4	II	Hormone and radiation therapy	1	4	2	8	0
5	I	Chemotherapy, hormone therapy	4	2	2	3	4
6	I	Chemotherapy, hormone therapy	5	4	2	17	0

On further examination of their breast cancer experience, additional similarities can be identified. Only one subject was diagnosed at an advanced stage (patient no. 1). This patient was a young woman whose cancer remains aggressive. Patient no. 4's cancer, though diagnosed at an early stage, quickly metastasized despite treatment. Since diagnosis, four of the six women have experienced significant ADL dependencies in instrumental activities of daily living, such as household management, and they have identified numerous role changes within their family structure.

Another common issue among these breast cancer patients was the number of symptoms or complications documented in their medical records. While undergoing adjuvant treatment, the number of symptoms and complications experienced by the women ranged from as few as two to as many as six. At the time of the initial telephone interview, each woman reported many more problems to the interviewer (a range from 3 to 19). Some symptoms, such as fatigue, weakness, and shortness of breath, were individually reported during the interview and, if caused by low hemoglobin, may be translated into anemia. However, there was little documentation in patients' medical records of problems such as pain or fatigue, which may be a result of the anemia's being addressed. In at least one situation, the problem identified in the telephone interview was the most disruptive to the patient and her husband. However, concerns about sexuality and associated physical changes were not documented in her medical record.

Comorbid conditions are also a recurring theme in all of the cases. Breast cancer is one of several chronic medical conditions to which these women have needed to adjust over time. Common conditions for these women included diabetes, cardiac disease, arthritis, and hypertension.

Despite numerous cancer-related problems identified and various chronic diseases complicating the cancer experience, few community resources were used. When the Rural Cancer Care Project Clinical Nurse Specialist (CNS) served as a case manager and identified needs, resources such as indigent drug programs and support group programs were accessed. Home care nursing was not used by any of the patients. The young woman with stage IV disease underwent a bone marrow transplant at an out-of-state cancer center and returned home with no community service referrals to assist her.

The records further reflected a minimal amount of patient and family teaching in physicians' offices or in outpatient chemotherapy clinics. Teaching was done by either the Rural Cancer Care Project CNS or the chemotherapy nurse at one of the rural hospitals. During telephone contacts, little teaching was documented in an outpatient setting. Table 17-3 summarizes these data.

In examining the financial issues surrounding care, key points are discussed. Table

Table 19-4 Income, Employment, Disease-Related Expenses, and Service Characteristics of Women in the Rural Cancer Care Project

Patient No.	Income	Employment Status	Disease-Related Expenses	Sites of Service	No. of Doctors
1	$60,000–69,999	Full time	Work; used 10 vacation days; $50/mo. meds; $1,200 for Texas apartment/gas; still owes 20% of $175,000 bone marrow transplant	5	6
2	$30,000–34,999	Full time	$2,600 lost work; $220 meds./dressings	2	3
3	$10,000–14,000	Unemployed due to cancer	$12,000 hospital/physician bills; $900 meds.; $500 office visits	4	3
4	$20,000–24,999	Retired	$100 labs; $600 meds	5	4
5	$15,000–19,999	Homemaker	Approx. $50	3	3
6	$5,000–9,999	Homemaker	$50 meds; $30/month gas	2	2

17-4 lists each family's reported household income.

All but one of the families were considered middle- or low-income. Two women continue to work full time, even though both reported lost wages due to treatment and health problems. One woman was unemployed as a direct result of the breast cancer diagnosis. She had no health insurance.

The amount of direct out-of-pocket expenses or lost wages incurred as a result of the cancer experience was remarkable. The range of reported direct expenses in a 3-month interval ranged from $50 to $13,400. These expenses were for various needs, but three patients discussed the cost of gasoline needed to drive to physician visits, laboratory tests, and chemotherapy or radiation treatments. Table 17-4 also lists the number of different sites of medical care and physicians seen. The number of medical delivery sites and distance traveled directly influenced out-of-pocket expenses as well as lost wages from work. This illustrates the struggles of rural patients, both in facing cancer financially and coordinating the often fragmented care. Some remaining expenses are staggering. Though patient no. 1 had a high family income, the family's remaining expenses are conservatively estimated at over $40,000. Patient no. 3 lost her service worker job due to her disease, yet still faces over $13,000 in medical expenses. She has little prospect of obtaining insurance.

THE RURAL ONCOLOGY NURSE: A MODEL TO ASSIST THE BREAST CANCER PATIENT

The Nursing Role

The barriers faced by the rural breast cancer patients and their families, the financial expense of cancer treatment, and the challenges of providing patient care in the rural community create an opportunity for the rural oncology nurse. The advanced-practice model tested in the "Rural Partnership Linkage for Cancer Care" provides a basis for role development for all health care practitioners wishing to link specialty services with supportive care for chronic illnesses in rural communities.

The patient care intervention is based on a comprehensive nursing approach to supportive cancer care and includes the following components: knowledge, information, symptom management, psychological counseling, support, monitoring disease and treatment, implementing the medical plan of care, mobilizing and coordinating community services, maximizing patient and family resources, and integrating cancer care services into the plan.

The intervention model, designed for advanced practice, was based on the Oncology Nursing Society standards for continuing and supportive care. The intervention model ensures a comprehensive approach that includes the family and considers the environment in which the individual lives.

This model of care affects the health status of the patient through prevention and early detection of complication, symptom management, and improved overall mobility and functional status. The goal of the model is to increase the appropriate use of health care service and prevent unnecessary and excessive cost of both formal and informal care. The model allows us to describe the nursing pattern of care and provides a method to track and quantify patient problems and problem resolution, knowing both the strategies used and outcomes achieved. The program was designed to be as long as 16 weeks in length, including in-person visits and phone contacts.

Rural Case Management

It has been stated that the most comprehensive and practical method of caring for the rural cancer patient is to offer care (case) management services to coordinate care (Given, Given, & Harlan, 1994). The Rural Cancer Care Project has implemented this concept throughout several counties. Similar programs have been piloted in other communities (Bryant, 1993; Watson, 1993). The focus continues to be coordination of multiple resources, assistance with symptom management, triage for medical care, ongoing monitoring of patient care, and retention of rural patients in specialized care despite the barriers to care and regardless of the community selected.

Case management in a rural area holds many distinctive challenges as a result of the same barriers cancer patients face: long travel distances; limited community, personal, and social resources; financial constraints; and staffing issues (Parker et al., 1992).

Despite the complexity and inherent limitations, advanced-practice oncology nurses serving as case managers and care team directors can have a major impact on rural breast cancer patients. Several key areas are worth further examination.

Assessment

All too often, oncology nurses define their role to a narrow focus and do not look at the cancer patient and family from a multidimensional perspective. Nurses neglect to understand the community or system surrounding patients. Oncology nurses must broaden their initial assessment of breast cancer patients and their family to include many additional areas not usually considered central to their care. These areas include the following:

- Financial and employment status of the patient, caregiver, and extended family;
- Support services available in the rural area;
- Family's readiness to use support services or community resources;
- Social and community networks;
- Comorbid conditions of the patient;
- Caregiver's health history;
- Resources available, such as wigs, wheelchairs, and the like.

Oncology nurses who are serving as the primary care provider need a clear understanding of variables influencing the patient and not limit their scope of care. People residing in rural areas (Eggebeen & Lichter, 1993) report poorer health. Their perception will direct our care and certainly influence their tolerance to cancer treatment offered. An assessment of the family care for cancer patients is listed in Table 17-5 and provides a framework for examining the family system (Given & Given, 1991).

One of the mandates of providing comprehensive care in a rural setting is to have adequate knowledge and skills to deal with the other chronic diseases the breast cancer patient faces. By assisting with such other problems as hypertension or diabetes, we can

Table 17-5 Assessment for Family Care

Type and quality of prior relationships:
1. What was the quality of the relationship between the patient and family prior to cancer diagnosis?
2. What is the usual decision-making and communication pattern within the family?
3. How has the relationship with the patient been altered by cancer and cancer treatment?
4. How has the relationship among other family members been altered by cancer and cancer treatment?
5. How has the family used outside support and resources in the past?

Initiation and maintenance of the role of family care:
1. When was the original diagnosis made? What has been the course of the illness?
2. What is the duration of the "care" relationship?
3. What changes in the family situation might influence the decision to continue care?
4. What changes in the patient might lead the family member to consider institutionalization or discontinue care?

Patient characteristics:
1. What are the signs and symptoms that require assistance?
   a) Behavioral and emotional reactions and mental health status
   b) Side effects of disease or treatment
   c) Functional disability level (ADLs and IADLs)
2. How long have the signs and symptoms and disability been present?
3. Which symptoms or functional deficits are most problematic to the patient?
4. What seems to cause the patient the most difficulty?
5. What is the subjective well-being of the patient?
6. What are the needs for care (functional levels)?
   a) ADL and IADL
   b) Treatments and other health care activities
   c) Symptom management and control
   d) Outlook and quality of life

Caregiver characteristics:
1. What is the relationship to the patient of those assisting with care?
2. What other family, work, or social roles exist for those helping with care?
3. What roles have been given up by the family to maintain the care relationship (work, family, social)?
4. What conflicts exist that interfere with the other role obligations of the family?
5. Does the family feel they have adequate knowledge/skills needed to provide care (ADL, IADL, treatments, symptom management, emotional support)?
6. Is the family aware (informed) of the patient's health status/condition?
   a) Expectations of course of treatment?
   b) Expectations around patient's health improving/declining?
7. Is the family aware of changes to expect in patients' condition?
8. What psychological resources—optimism, hardiness, self-esteem—do family members demonstrate?

Care requirements:
1. Which symptoms or behaviors are most problematic to the family?
2. What are the care requirements?
   a) ADL and IADL
   b) Treatments and other health care activities
   c) Symptom management
   d) Emotional problems
3. How long has the family provided care?
4. What are the hours of care per week?
5. What is the intensity of care?

Table 17-5   *Continued*

Support and resources for care:
  1. What other family members are available to assist with care?
  2. What family support is utilized to help with care?
  3. Is there adequate support available? Is it satisfactory?
  4. What formal agency support is used? Is it needed?
  5. What social support is used from friends or informal groups?
  6. What respite services or supports are used and available?
  7. Are more in-home, chore, and respite services needed?
  8. Are needed services affordable?
  9. What resources exist with friends and family?
 10. Do prior financial commitments interfere/enhance situation?
 11. What are the living arrangements?
 12. What insurance benefits and other financial resources are available?

Family member responses:
  1. What negative responses to care are evident?
  2. What is the perceived impact of care on the family member's physical and mental health?
  3. How does the caregiver perceive that caregiving affects daily activities and other role responsibilities?
  4. Does the family caregiver feel supported by other family members? By the patient?
  5. Does the caregiver perceive a caregiving role responsibility?
  6. What have been the benefits derived from being in the care situation?
  7. Has there been a change in financial/legal situations?
  8. Has there been a change in living arrangements?
  9. What is the perceived quality of family life?
 10. Has there been a change in the work situation?

eliminate unnecessary visits to various medical sites and reduce the fragmentation of care.

The cases of the breast cancer patients previously discussed also illustrate that even in the early stages of breast cancer, multiple needs exist and ADL dependencies are present. The Rural Cancer Care Project's breast cancer patients, though primarily early-stage, did have ADL dependencies and multiple symptoms due to treatment effects with which nursing can assist. It is, therefore, important to address all physical and psychosocial issues with each patient and caregiver, and it is equally critical to review these issues periodically as needs and priorities change in every situation.

It has been documented as well that the symptoms associated with cancer and cancer treatment continue for an extended period after treatment has ended. The nurse's role continues, therefore, long after the technical function of administering chemotherapy or radiation treatment ends.

Symptom Management and Teaching

The role of the rural oncology nurse in symptom management and patient and family teaching is clearly evident in the care of the six breast cancer patients previously discussed. The teaching that has already been carried out is helping patients and their spouses cope with the side effects of chemotherapy or radiation therapy and the fatigue commonly experienced by breast cancer patients. The stress that spouses and families experience while assisting their loved ones is well documented (Northouse & Peters-Golden, 1993). This research helps identify specific nursing interventions that can improve coping and reduce the disruption of side effects. In the following sections, we explain some of the aspects of patient care and treatment roles that have emerged as central to nursing intervention.

Individualized Treatment

The Rural Cancer Care Project CNS must serve as a patient advocate in designing a cancer treatment plan that is not only medically appropriate, but feasible for the rural family. When designing a treatment plan, ask the following: Have we limited the need to travel long distances by ordering the appropriate amount of laboratory tests? Have we looked to local resources to assist in performing tests or administering treatment, assuming the nurse is certified? Have we accessed home care services, community services, equipment, or supplies to supplement services; or used volunteer organizations, church networks, or natural helpers such as extended family or friends to assist with transportation? Often, the husband of the breast cancer patient must leave work to accompany her for treatment or diagnostic tests. This creates additional strain for the family and increases the financial crisis.

The treatment centers have historically designed their hours of service based on employee desires or the traditional 9-to-5 outpatient clinic. These hours are not in the best interest of the breast cancer patient who attempts to maintain her own job or depends on extended family for such support as child care or transportation. A creative solution might be extended treatment hours or developing a volunteer program to staff a playroom at the cancer center for patients' children.

Discharge Planning

The rural cancer patient faces more difficulty when returning home after discharge from a tertiary or urban hospital, if the discharge planning has been inadequate. In a descriptive survey of rural case managers, Parker et al. (1992) documented that urban discharge planners are not often knowledgeable about rural resources nor are they aware of what informal resources may be available.

The inpatient oncology nurse often is responsible for teaching the family how to care for the patient upon discharge. All too often we do not begin by identifying all family members and friends involved in the care at home when we target who should receive instructions or learn a task. The primary caregiver is asked to learn several tasks, coordinate appointments, contact resources, and obtain supplies. The health care team divides these jobs among an RN, aide, social worker, and others; perhaps we need to do the same for each family—building a stronger, better "team" in the home.

The Rural Cancer Care Project CNS has demonstrated the success of "bridging the gap" from hospital to home by helping families access resources, following through on referrals, and coordinating the team, which can include, as in one situation, the nurse, a case worker from the Department of Social Services, the inpatient hospital social worker, the outpatient chemotherapy nurse, a juvenile court representative, and the local visiting nurse service.

Families have also expressed a sense of abandonment by the medical team. This may occur when the patient's disease status enters a terminal phase (Buehler & Lee, 1992). It also occurs when adjuvant treatment is concluded. The case management of the rural oncology nurse helps counterbalance that sense of abandonment and can identify earlier the need for hospice, thereby introducing an additional support service for the final phase of the disease process. The rural cancer nurse as case manager can then remain involved, providing knowledge and understanding in dealing with disease progression and complications.

Community Education and Service Development

An additional role of the Rural Cancer Care Project CNS has been one of community educator, with a goal of achieving cancer program development. The rural community is in need of community information that will assist in early detection and successful screening programs. The rural oncology nurse must enter the next decade as a leader in supporting the proven methods of early detection and prevention (Swanson, 1992). This message must be carried into the rural community in creative places such as county fairs, women's church meetings, service clubs, Cooperative Extension services, and Farm Bureau meetings. Hometown health fairs are an example of what is being done in New York. In cooperation with the local American Cancer Society, the Healthy Heart Program modeled a community outreach program after a "country fair" and had a wonderful response (Michela & Kozubek, 1992).

The rural oncology nurse must also overcome the psychological barriers that limit breast cancer patients' use of services. Interviews with senior citizens in rural communities indicate that services are perceived to cost too much and create a sense of dependence that is undesirable (Roberto, Richter, Bottenberg, & MacCormack, 1992). This same research confirmed this feeling by documenting that professionals feel rural seniors are more physically and emotionally independent compared with urban seniors. The need to develop a trusting long-term relationship that allows for rural women's use of complementary resources is a critical goal of the rural oncology nurse.

One of the most promising opportunities of rural outreach through the nurse-directed supportive care program for rural areas has been to work with the medical, service, hospital, and other institutions to develop new resources to reduce costs and improve patient care services within the community. Examples to date include:

- A "chronic disease" support group developed by a collaborative effort of the local hospital, hospice, community leaders, and the local American Cancer Society;
- A community task force to design and implement a high school-based smoking cessation program;
- High-risk-targeted prostate screening program;

- Facilitating one county's first "I Can Cope" program in several years;
- A county-based cancer resource guide for professional and lay use.

Several of these activities have directly assisted the breast cancer patients enrolled in the study, and in one county the caregiver husband has led the formation of the support group.

CONCLUSION

It is important to consider the comprehensive needs of rural patients with breast cancer. The nature of the disease and the lack of health care and financial and psychosocial resources make care to rural women quite challenging. A combination of creativity by the health care professional and enhanced community-based services and linkages is needed to improve the care of women with breast cancer living in rural areas. This need is particularly important as debate at the national level continues on how to reform health care for all U.S. citizens. As managed care programs begin to extend beyond urban areas, the role of the rural cancer nurse becomes an essential part of a collaboration between urban-based specialty care and local supportive care. By providing high-quality care within the community, costs to the system and patients can be reduced, services can be coordinated, and patients and their families will experience outcomes similar to those of persons with cancer who reside in urban areas. As the health care community assumes a broader view of care for cancer patients and as the charges for that care are assigned to a single system, there will be far greater motivation to extend needed care to rural areas and to ensure that the rural cancer patients and their families are satisfied with the services they are receiving.

ACKNOWLEDGMENT

This research was supported by grant #5 R01 CA56338, "Rural Partnership Linkage for Cancer Care," funded by the National Cancer Institute, Charles W. Given, PhD, Principal Investigator.

References

Berkman, B. J., & Sampson, S. E. (1993). Psychosocial effects of cancer economics on patients and their families. *Cancer, 72,* 2846–2849.

Brown, M., & Fintor J. (1994). Economic burden of cancer care. In P. Greenwald, B. Kramer, and D. Weed (Eds.), *Cancer prevention and control* (pp. 69–81). New York: Marcel-Dekker.

Bryant, B. (1993). Strategies increase access to care in rural areas. *Oncology Nursing Forum, 20,* 1436.

Buehler, J. A., & Lee, H. J. (1992). Exploration of home care resources for rural families with cancer. *Cancer Nursing, 15*(4), 299–308.

Curtiss, C. P. (1993). Trends and issues for cancer care in rural communities. *Nursing Clinics of North America, 28*(1), 241–251.

Eggebeen, D. J., & Lichter, D. T. (1993). Health and well-being among rural Americans: Variations across the life course. *The Journal of Rural Health, 9*(2), 86–98.

Given, B. A., & Given, C. W. (1991). Family caregivers of cancer patients. In S.M. Hubbard, P. E. Greene, M. T. Knobf (Eds.), *Current issues in cancer nursing practice* (pp. 1–9). Philiedelphia: J. B. Lippincott.

Given, B. A, Given, C. W., & Harlan, A. N. (1994). Strategies to meet the needs of the rural poor. *Seminars in Oncology Nursing, 10*(2), 114–122.

Given, B. A., Given, C. W., & Stommel, M. (1994). Family and out-of-pocket costs for women with breast cancer. *Cancer Practice, 2*(3), 187–193.

Hilton, B. A. (1993). Issues, problems, and challenges for families coping with breast cancer. *Seminars in Oncology Nursing, 9,* 88–100.

Michela, N. J., & Kozubek, M. (1992). Hometown health fairs. *Oncology Nursing Forum, 19,* 93.

Monroe, A. C., Ricketts, T. C., & Savitz, L. A. (1992). Cancer in rural versus urban populations: A review. *Journal of Public Health, 8*(3), 212–220.

Mor, V., Guadagnoli, E., & Wool, M. (1988). The role of concrete services in cancer care. *Advanced Psychsomatic Medicine, 18,* 102–118.

Murphy, G. P., Prestifilipp, J., Antman, K., Berkman, B. J., Huber, S. L., Kaufman, D., Knox, W. A., Lawrence, W., Levine, R. J., & Young, F. E. (1993). The economic impact of therapy on cancer patients. *Cancer, 72*(Suppl. 9), 2862–2864.

Northouse, L. L., & Peters-Golden, H. (1993). Strategies to assist spouses. *Seminars in Oncology Nursing, 9*(2), 74–82.

Office of Technology. (1990). *Office of technology assessment: Health care in rural America* (OTA Publication No. OTA-H-435). Washington, DC: U.S. Government Printing Office.

Parker, M., Quinn, J., Viehl, M., McKinley, A. H., Polich, C. L., Hartwell, S., Van Hook, R., & Detzner, D.F. (1992). Issues in rural case management. *Community Health, 14*(4), 40–60.

Roberto, K. A., Richter, J., Bottenberg, D. J., & MacCormack, R. A. (1992). Provider/client views: Health care needs of the rural elderly. *Journal of Gerontological Nursing, 18*(5), 31–37.

Stommel, M., Given, B. A., & Given, C. W. (1992). The cost of cancer home care to families. *Cancer, 71,* 1867–1874.

Swanson, G. M. (1992). Breast cancer in the 1990s. *Journal of the American Medical Women's Association, 47*(5), 140–148.

Watson, A. C. (1993). The role of the psychosocial oncology CNS in a rural outreach program. *Clinical Nurse Specialist, 7,* 259–265.

White, N. J., Stover, D., Given, B. A., & Stommel, M. (1994, January). *The cost of continuing care for women with breast cancer.* Paper presented at the American Cancer Society National Conference on Cancer Nursing Research, Newport Beach, CA.

CHAPTER 18

The Mastectomy Nurse Prosthetist
An Innovative Community-Based Rehabilitation Program

Johanna Lombardo Ehmann, RN, AAS, OCN

BREAST CANCER REHABILITATION

Breast cancer rehabilitation is the dynamic process of assisting women who are recovering from breast cancer (Ehmann, 1994b). It is comprehensive, ongoing, and most effective when begun at diagnosis. Rehabilitation is best conducted by a team including all persons caring for the patient. The nurse specializing in the care of women with breast cancer has a vitally important role as a member of the rehabilitation team, shaping the patient's and family's experience during all aspects of the rehabilitation process (Staiger & Harkings, 1993)

A useful definition of body image is "the self-perception of one's body structure and function as dynamic and different from all others (one component of self-concept)" (Clark & McGee, 1992). Body image can be affected by the diagnosis and treatment of breast cancer, thus a program of body image restoration may be needed during breast cancer rehabilitation.

This chapter describes an innovative breast cancer rehabilitation program that fo-cuses on body image restoration after mastectomy. The role of the mastectomy nurse practitioner in a community-based setting is described. Innovative interventions for body image restoration are also discussed.

DEVELOPMENT OF THE MASTECTOMY AND LUMPECTOMY OPTIONS PROGRAM

Several factors led to the development of the mastectomy and lumpectomy options (MALO) body image restoration program. These include clinical experience (through case studies), patient needs assessment, and a nurse questionnaire. The following case example is representative of the concerns many women have about body image after mastectomy.

Case Example

"I was administering chemotherapy to a 50-year-old white female who was 2 weeks postmastectomy. She informed me that she rejected her husband's invitation to spend Valentine's Day in a hotel because she couldn't find a mastectomy swimsuit for the jacuzzi. Her concern was that she would look different if she wore a tee-shirt over her regular swimsuit to hide the loss of her breast. A colleague contacted the American Cancer Society (ACS) Reach to Recovery volunteers, who provided a list of mastectomy suppliers in the area. However, a swimsuit was not available in the winter months. Unable to obtain a swimsuit, the patient chose not to accompany her husband."

Patient Needs Survey

In 1989, a survey of 28 postmastectomy women was conducted to determine a need for improved postmastectomy image restoration. Twenty-two women responded to the survey. Twenty had undergone a modified radical mastectomy, and two had undergone a simple mastectomy. Ages ranged from 20 to 89 years. Eighty-eight percent of the women expressed dissatisfaction with the temporary cotton puff supplied by the Reach to Recovery Program of the ACS. They delayed returning to the workplace, citing insecurity with obtaining a symmetrical appearance with the stuffed cotton filler. Eighty-two percent were unaware of product options such as presized, unweighted breast forms. Women reportedly used BB pellets, fish sinkers, bird seed, and drapery weights to weigh down the temporary products. Forty-one percent wanted premastectomy education and counseling about image restoration, and 23% would have preferred the education immediately postoperatively (Ehmann, Sheehan, & Lombardo, 1992).

Nurse Questionnaire

A questionnaire was then sent to two local institutions and five surgical practices to determine how much nurses knew about the image restoration options available after mastectomy. Of the 14 nurses responding to the questionnaire, 38% thought that women were satisfied with the

prosthesis provided by the program. Fewer than 20% were familiar with product options such as sleep forms, nipples, and temporary breast forms. The costs of prostheses were unknown by 86%, and 57% did not know when a woman could begin wearing a permanent prosthesis (Ehmann et al., 1992).

THE MALOCARE CONSULTATION

The surveys of women and nursing staff led to the development of the MALOcare Consultation, which is a specialized program designed for women undergoing mastectomy. Pre- and postmastectomy consultations are available with mastectomy nurse prosthetists who are oncology nurses certified in breast prosthetics (Ehmann, 1994b). The goal of the program is to provide preventive, restorative, supportive, and palliative nursing interventions. The role of the mastectomy nurse prosthetist is similar to other oncology nursing roles in the provision of nursing assessment, image restoration, education, counseling, and referral for women diagnosed with breast cancer. Several programs, offered by the mastectomy nurse prosthetist, can be incorporated into oncology nurses' practice. *Nursing assessment* includes information of the patient and family knowledge needs, progressive body image and goal needs, response to diagnosis and breast surgery, and support needs and resources.*Image restoration* includes assistance with the selection and fitting of prostheses, bras, and clothing options; and the selection and fitting of temporary product options to be worn 1 to 4 weeks following breast surgery. The following should also be provided: *Education and counseling* about surgical procedures (mastectomy and breast conserving surgery); progressive mastectomy and lumpectomy prosthetics; product and clothing options; clothing and dressing hints for swimming, exercising, and intimacy; arm and hand care; range-of-motion exercises; breast self-examination; and information on insurance reimbursement. *Referral* to local community and national support organizations is made as needed.

Figure 18-1   Image Counseling: The Presurgical Patient Interview

What type of surgery has been recommended?

Will your underarm lymph nodes be removed?

Where will the surgical incisions be placed?

Did you know that you could wear your favorite brassiere to the doctor to ask if the surgical incision could be placed within the bra lines?

Are you aware of image restoration product options?

Would you like to see an external breast prosthesis?

Are you aware of your option of reconstructive surgery?

Do you know that you can consult with a reconstructive surgeon before your breast surgery?

Would you like more information on breast reconstruction?

Did you know that you will be unable to wear your own bra upon hospital discharge?

Would you like assistance with the selection of a postsurgical brassiere?

Would you like assistance with the selection of an unweighted breast form to be worn in the postsurgical brassiere?

Are you aware that you will be taught exercises to regain range of motion of the affected arm?

Would you like to learn these exercises today?

Did you know that the nurse in the hospital will help you to look at the surgical incisions before hospital discharge?

Note. Copyright 1993 by Johanna Lombardo Ehmann, RN. Reprinted with permission.

PRESURGICAL IMAGE COUNSELING

A presurgical image counseling session helps a woman prepare for changes in her body image as a result of surgery and helps to preplan interventions. This session includes an assessment of the woman's knowledge and level of communication with her physician, provision of several educational resources, fitting for temporary prosthesis postsurgical bra, and referral as needed to national support organizations.

Nursing Assessment.   The presurgical patient interview (Figure 18-1) aids the mastectomy nurse prosthetist in counseling a woman who

anticipates an alteration in body image. The assessment guides the nurse in the preparation of individualized patient teaching packets. The nurse also encourages the patient to communicate with her physician.

Educational Resources.   Books and videos are provided as educational resources during a presurgical consultation to reinforce teaching and to empower women facing breast cancer surgery. The provision of individual patient teaching packets with a limited but select group of materials will help a woman make informed choices without overwhelming her during the decision-making process.

Table 18-1   Progressive Image/Comfort Needs and Care of Postmastectomy Women

Time Frame	Week 1	Week 2-4	After Week 4
What to Expect:	swelling chest/arm	reduced swelling chest/arm	reduced swelling chest/arm
	restricted motion in affected arm	improved motion in affected arm	improved motion in affected arm
	adjustment to change in body image	adjustment to change in body image	adjustment to change in body image
What to Do:	exercise per doctor	exercise per doctor	exercise per doctor
	meet with certified prosthetist to select image product options	meet with certified prosthetist to select image product options	meet with certified prosthetist to select image product options
What to Wear:			
Lingerie:	unrestrictive front opening postsurgical bra, tee	unrestrictive front opening postsurgical bra, tee	bra, tee, camisole
Breast Form:	temporary unweighted breast form[a]	temporary unweighted breast form	permanent weighted breast form
Clothing:	loose, comfortable clothing, oversized sweaters, tees, shoulder pads, scarf dressing	loose, comfortable clothing, oversized sweaters, tees, shoulder pads, scarf dressing	silks, knits, fitted clothing
Swimwear:		mastectomy/regular	mastectomy/regular

(Approximate times vary with individual progress.)

[a] Temporary unweighted breast forms may be purchased presized and should be kept in place by using a strip of elastic attached to the postsurgical bra and underwear or worn in a specially designed postsurgical brassiere with a wide camisole strap.

Note. Developed by Johanna Lombardo Ehmann, RN, OCN, Johanna's of Albany Ltd., Cancer Rehabilitation Nurse Consultants. Reprinted by permission.

Maintaining a Positive Image with Breast Cancer Surgery, developed by the author (1990), addresses the physical, emotional, and sexual concerns expressed by women with body image concerns. The booklet, written in a question-and-answer format, contains a progressive image and clothing options chart that provides a time frame to guide women in understanding their progressive image and comfort needs during and after their surgical recovery.

The Progressive Image and Comfort Needs and Care of Postmastectomy Women (Table 18-1) is a teaching tool that indicates what prosthetic, lingerie, and clothing options are suggested after mastectomy. This tool guides women in un-

derstanding what arm limitations to expect, what to do to help themselves, and what to wear to accommodate image and comfort needs. Figure 18-2 can also be used by nurses for a quick reference.

A video, *Maintaining a Positive Image with Breast Cancer Surgery, with Johanna Ehmann* (Ehmann, 1994a) is another patient education tool. The video contains demonstrations of various prosthetic, lingerie, clothing, and swimwear options and their appropriate use after mastectomy. It can be viewed by the patient in the privacy of her home, in the hospital and/or surgeon's office, or in a support group setting. The video can also be used as a training tool for Reach to Recovery volunteers, oncology nurses, and nursing students.

Fitting.   Fitting for temporary product options, unweighted breast forms and surgical brassieres, helps a woman adjust to her change in body image. Clothing and dressing hints are provided to help the patient disguise asymmetry of the chest while wearing an unweighted breast form. A demonstration of image product options to familiarize the woman with permanent postmastectomy products to be worn after healing is also provided.

Referrals.   Referrals to local and national support organizations, such as the National Breast Cancer Coalition (NBCC) and the Y-Me organization for breast cancer, provide up-to-date information on breast cancer treatment and rehabilitation for women seeking additional information and support. Local chapters of the ACS provide pre- and postsurgical Reach to Recovery volunteer services. The following case example illustrates the success of a presurgical image counseling session.

Case Example

A 42-year-old, married school teacher and mother of two girls, ages 11 and 6, was diagnosed with inflammatory breast cancer. Her treatment plan included high-dose chemotherapy, followed by a modified radical mastectomy, bone marrow transplant, and possible radiation therapy.

When I met her she was postchemotherapy and 2 weeks premastectomy. Her oncology nurse referred her for presurgical image counseling. At consultation, she presented with alopecia and was wearing a baseball cap. She began to cry when I extended my hand to greet her. I reviewed the patient intake form that provided me with information regarding her age, occupation, diagnosis, treatment plan, physicians, and insurance carrier. She had written, "inflammatory breast cancer" on the form, which indicated that she was knowledgeable about her disease.

A few minutes into the interview, she stated, "Even though this sounds crazy, I need to know what I will wear in the hospital, at home, and for swimming. The doctors don't care about that!" I reassured her that I could help by providing her with information and product options that would allow her to maintain confidence and dignity in her appearance during the recovery process. I asked her whether she had discussed reconstruction with her doctor. She stated that she "got the impression" that she was not a candidate for immediate reconstructive surgery because of her aggressive cell type and risk of recurrence. She had concerns about implants. I informed her that she could think about reconstructive surgery at a later date and offered her an article (Leigh & Webb, 1994) describing how the authors took the time to seek information and used the decision-making process about the feasibility of reconstruction.

With the understanding that immediate reconstruction was not an option, we discussed her impending surgery. She was told that she was having a total mastectomy in which her breast would be removed but her muscles would remain intact. It was recommended that she have a level-one lymph node removal. However, she had not made her decision to accept this procedure because she feared developing lymphedema and she felt that she already had "big arms." I asked if she knew why lymph nodes would be removed. She stated that if the lymph nodes were determined to be positive, she would have to have radiation therapy. She was opposed to radiation unless it was absolutely necessary, because of her concern over skin changes and swelling. After verbalizing her concerns, she was more comfortable with the decision to have lymph node dissection in the hopes of avoiding radiation therapy.

She asked what she could wear in the hospital and at home during recovery, and how soon she could wear a bathing suit to be "normal" with her children. She indicated that her brother and sister-in-law would be visiting 2 days after her surgery, and she didn't want to look like a "freak" to them. We discussed product options, and she was fitted for a postsurgical, cotton cropped camisole and unweighted presized breast form, to be worn upon hospital discharge and at home during recovery.

She said that she hoped to wear her own bras after healing had taken place and that she wore front-hook bras with very little fabric. I suggested that she wear her favorite bra to the doctor's office to ask if the incision could be placed inside the bra lines. Next, I asked her if she had ever seen a weighted breast prosthesis. She said that she hadn't, but that she would like to see one. I showed her a self-supported silicone breast form that could be worn directly on the body or in the pocket of a bra after healing had taken place.

Another concern she had was how to address her 11-year-old daughter, who wondered what the mastectomy incision would look like. The daughter wanted to be prepared as well. I let her watch a video, which showed a mastectomy incision and placement of a self-supporting breast form, and loaned her the video to share with her spouse and her daughter at the appropriate time. She was glad to learn what an incision would look like and to be better equipped to share this information with her daughter.

Finally, I told her that she could expect temporary limited range of motion of the affected arm following removal of underarm lymph nodes. We discussed the need for exercise to regain full range of motion. She was scheduled for surgery at a hospital that did not use the Reach to Recovery Program. I provided her with their booklet on postmastectomy exercise (American Cancer Society, 1982a), reviewed a few of the exercises, and emphasized the importance of asking her surgeon how soon she could begin to practice the exercises illustrated in the booklet.

I informed her that she could expect to have a chest drain in place for a couple of days after surgery to prevent fluid accumulation in the chest wall, and that she would experience some swelling and discomfort of the surgical side immediately postoperatively. To help her adapt to her change in body image, I suggested that she select a nurse with whom she was comfortable to help her view the incision when the bandages were removed for the first time.

On leaving the office, she said that she felt 100% better, and that our visit enabled her to face her mastectomy.

PROGRESSIVE IMAGE AND COMFORT NEEDS AFTER SURGERY

A woman's progressive image and comfort needs and care following mastectomy, lumpectomy, and breast reconstruction are different for each individual. However, general expectations can guide women in their recovery.

Postmastectomy Comfort Needs

Week 1.   Because the lymph nodes under the arm are removed during surgery, it is often difficult for women to raise their arms over their head for about 1 to 2 weeks after surgery. Initially, women feel most comfortable in a loose-fitting nightgown or pajamas that open in the front to allow for ease in dressing. The bandage over the incision may be bulky, and a chest drain may be in place. An open-front cotton tank, loose-fitting camisole, or specially designed bra may be useful at this time to be worn under sleepwear.

Week 2.   Women are encouraged to choose comfortable, loose-fitting clothing that opens in the front. Shoulder pads and/or dolman sleeves may help keep shirt material away from the incision. Women may want to wear the cotton puff and bra or a presized unweighted breast form and specially designed pocketed, cropped camisole. The unweighted breast form will stay in place by wearing it on adjustable straps under a front-opening cotton tank or without the straps in a specially designed pocketed, cropped camisole. If the cotton puff is worn in a regular bra, it must be kept in place by securing a strip of elastic tacked to the bra and pinned to the underwear.

Weeks 3 to 6.   Following surgery, it is important for a woman to replace her natural breast weight in order to keep her body balanced. Back, shoulder, and neck discomforts are common problems when the body is not properly balanced. The two choices for replacing the natural body weight are wearing a breast prosthesis or having reconstructive surgery. Image product options include weighted breast forms made of cloth or silicone. Weighted fabric breast forms allow for a soft cotton material against the chest wall. They are useful for women who desire a modestly priced breast form, who want a second form for everyday or casual wear, or who perform strenuous activities such as gardening, bicycling, and exercising.

Silicone breast forms are very soft and are made of naturally shaped silicone gel. They are available in a variety of shapes, shades, and sizes. The silicone "tawny" designed for the African American woman is a form closer to her skin tone, and is available in silicone or cotton. The newest development in breast forms is the self-supporting prosthesis that adheres directly to the body with skin-friendly adhesive, relieving weight from the shoulders. It may be worn with or without a bra, and comes with a silicone nipple prosthesis. A bra-supported breast form is worn in the pocket of a bra. Other types of breast forms include sleep forms and swim forms. Permaform bras with a built-in prosthesis are useful for women with limited dexterity, for the physically or mentally disabled, or for women who do not want to deal with placing the breast form in the bra or on the chest wall. Another image product option is called "Extrinsic Breast Reconstruction." This custom-designed breast prosthesis adheres to the chest wall with or without a bra and is individually designed and sculpted.

PRIMARY SURGERY AND RADIATION THERAPY

If axillary lymph nodes are removed during surgery, many women find it difficult to raise their arm over their head for about 1 to 2 weeks following surgery. Initially, most women prefer to wear open-front nightgowns and robes to allow for ease in dressing. The bandage over the incision may be bulky and women may experience some expected swelling under the arm as well as discoloration and tenderness in the breast. In such instances, a supportive cotton bra with a wide camisole strap is useful to support the surgical and nonsurgical breast.

Following lumpectomy, women are scheduled for radiation therapy for 6 weeks. The radiated area of the breast is usually marked with gentian violet to map out the treatment area. A cotton tank or soft stretch bra with wide camisole straps may help protect clothing. Side effects of radiation therapy to the breast may include redness, itching, and skin sensitivity. Thus, the soft cotton tank or a cotton stretch bra will also protect the sensitive breast. Depending on the extent of local surgery, a partial breast form may be needed to fill the bra cup completely.

BREAST RECONSTRUCTION

Prosthesis, lingerie, and clothing options after breast reconstruction are dependent on the type of reconstructive surgery. It is recommended that a woman select lingerie and clothing that will accommodate any bulky bandaging immediately following breast reconstruction. The surgeon may recommend that a supportive stretch bra be worn following surgery once the compressive bandage is removed. However, reconstructive surgeons differ in their opinion as to whether or not a brassiere is needed. A partial breast form (enhancer) may be needed to fill the cup of the bra on the reconstructed breast or contralateral breast to obtain symmetry. However, in these cases, the surgeon will usually suggest surgery of the contralateral breast. Surgery may include a breast reduction for women with large, pendulous breasts or a tuck/lift for women with small, sagging breasts. For women who do not want additional surgery on the opposite breast, a supportive underwire bra is recommended to lift the healthy breast and obtain a symmetrical appearance with the reconstructed side. For women who are undergoing the tissue expander method, the expander must first be overexpanded before an implant may be inserted. An enhancer may be needed to fill the cup of the bra of the healthy breast before the implant is inserted and the reconstructive process is completed. A silicone nipple prosthesis may be placed directly on the skin instead of nipple reconstruction if desired.

POSTMASTECTOMY/LUMPECTOMY IMAGE COUNSELING

Similar to the presurgical image counseling session, the postmastectomy/image counseling session incorporates patient assessment and education. The MALOcare patient teaching flow sheet assists the nurse in conducting a nursing assessment of patient needs, providing patient teaching, and suggesting interventions (Figure 18-2).

Patient education addresses the individual needs of the postmastectomy/lumpectomy woman. Information about image restoration product options, dressing hints for swimming and intimacy, range-of-motion exercises, self-examination instruction, insurance reimbursement procedure, and financial assistance programs are provided.

The following patient booklets and videos, developed by the author, the American Cancer Society, and Foresight Communications, Inc., are useful in improving or maintaining a positive image after surgery:

1. "Intimate Interludes," in *Maintaining a Positive Image with Breast Cancer Surgery*, 1990, provides helpful hints offered by mastectomy patients to help women select lingerie for intimacy.
2. *Maintaining a Positive Image with Hair Loss and Cancer Therapy* (Ehmann, 1989) assists women who are anticipating hair loss due to chemotherapy.
3. *Maintaining a Positive Image with Cancer Therapy* (Ehmann, 1991c) is a wellness workbook and personal journal for those scheduled to receive chemotherapy and/or radiation therapy. This book of esteem cards provides basic information on exercise, nutrition, relaxation, and inti-

macy to help women participate actively in their recovery.
4. Range-of-motion exercise is reinforced using the Reach to Recovery booklets, *Exercises After Mastectomy Patient Guide* (American Cancer Society, 1982a) or *Exercises After Lumpectomy Patient Guide* (American Cancer Society, 1982c).
5. Video resources include *In Touch for Life: A Wellness Program for Mastectomy Patients* (1991a) and *In Touch for Life: A Wellness Program for Lumpectomy Patients* (1991b). Patients are encouraged to view the videos in the office so that they have a better understanding of how to perform the exercises at home. Women are encouraged to listen to their favorite music when practicing range-of-motion exercises.
6. The Reach to Recovery booklet, *An Ounce of Prevention: Suggestion for Hand and Arm Care* (American Cancer Society, 1982b), is provided to teach women how to protect themselves from lymphedema. Patients may also be referred to the National Lymphedema Network (NLN).

Follow-up Care

Women need to be taught that an important step in their continued recovery is to follow the ACS guidelines for cancer prevention and detection, available through pamphlets distributed by their local ACS office, their physician, or nurse, and through cancer screening and wellness programs. Regular breast self-examination (BSE) including the surgical side, keeping scheduled visits to their physician, and follow-up mammography are essential components of continued health care. BSE and self-examination of the surgical side are taught to familiarize women with their change in body image. A mammography may be performed on the surgical side following lumpectomy and mastectomy. It may also be performed on the reconstructed breast.

Figure 18-2   MALOcare Patient Teaching Flow Sheet

MALOcare Consultation
(Mastectomy and Lumpectomy Options)

Date: _____   Physician: _____

Patient: _____   Therapy: _____

DOB: _____   Date of surgery: _____

Nursing Assessment   **Comments**

Mastectomy/lumpectomy risk/status   _____

Mastectomy/lumpectomy anatomy knowledge   _____

Emotional response to breast cancer   _____

Arm/hand/wound care knowledge   _____

ROM exercise knowledge/practice   _____

Self-exam knowledge/practice   _____

Progressive image needs/goals   _____

Support needs/resources   _____

Patient Education	**A**	**B**	**C**	**D**
Image restoration product options	☐	☐	☐	☐
Dressing hints for swimming and intimacy	☐	☐	☐	☐
ROM exercises	☐	☐	☐	☐
Self-examination instruction	☐	☐	☐	☐
Insurance reimbursement procedure	☐	☐	☐	☐
Financial assistance programs	☐	☐	☐	☐

Nursing Interventions   **Comments**

Prosthesis selection/fitting   _____

Clothing selection: swimwear/lingerie   _____

Emotional support/counseling   _____

Referrals to financial/support resources   _____

Instructional booklet, "Maintaining A Positive
   Image With Breast Cancer Surgery"   _____

A = Verbal instruction given to patient/family; B = Patient/family given written instruction and
encouraged to review literature; C = Patient/family verbalizes understanding of instruction; D =
Return demonstration given by patient family

Signature: _____

Women should be told to ask their physician how often they should have a mammogram on the surgical and nonsurgical sides following these surgeries.

Women are also encouraged to share the information of prevention and early detection with their mothers, grandmothers, aunts, sisters, friends, and daughters. An innovative communication strategy is a music video geared toward teens and developed to create a positive message regarding BSE. "BSE RAP: It's Your Body, Check Yourself Out!"(Ehmann, 1991a) is a 5-minute video that features students singing and dancing to rap music, practicing BSE on a silicone model, and learning hand positioning for BSE on a doll. It teaches BSE in an upbeat, nonthreatening manner and provides a woman the opportunity to discuss the need for prevention and early detection practices with her daughter.

The Breast Health Diary (Ehmann, 1991b) is a workbook written to help women monitor their own breast health and communicate their breast history to their doctor. It is another form of breast health material offered to the patient and other adult family members and friends. Information regarding low-cost mammography programs is also provided.

RECOMMENDATIONS FOR INCORPORATING BREAST CANCER REHABILITATION SERVICES INTO PRACTICE

The following suggestions are offered for nurses interested in incorporating breast cancer rehabilitation services into their practice.

Collaboration with Community Organizations. Networking with community organizations is an effective way to use the expertise of various health professionals and businesses involved in the care of women with breast cancer. The Service and Rehabilitation Committee of the ACS is an excellent resource for identifying, coordinating, and incorporating rehabilitation services into existing programs.

Rural Outreach Programs. These programs are vital to provide rehabilitation services in hard-to-reach areas. Our mobile office, or "Esteemobile," is used to bring services to the rural Northeast region. Mastectomy nurse prosthetists staff the 26-foot van and provide teaching through videotapes, audiotapes, and distribution of pamphlets, books, and articles that have been previously described in this chapter. These materials may be part of a lending library, to be left with nurses at the facility that is visited for a specific period of time.

Development of an Image Product Display. An image product display may be established at a hospital or an outpatient facility to help familiarize women with prosthetic product options.

Support Through the Oncology Nursing Society. A National Oncology Nursing Chapters Special Projects grant funded through the Oncology Nursing Foundation provided the opportunity to invite nurses and their patients to a special program focusing on image restoration and cancer rehabilitation (Ehmann & Decker, 1991). The success of this program has spurred other similar programs in two other communities. One rural area of upstate New York provided a program that specifically addressed the rehabilitation needs of breast cancer survivors.

Nurses are in a crucial position to assist women who have an alteration in body image resulting from breast cancer surgery, because they have the unique opportunity to counsel women before, during, and after breast surgery. By incorporating image restoration as an integral component of comprehensive breast cancer rehabilitation, nurses will assist in the adaptation of women following a diagnosis of breast cancer.

References

American Cancer Society. (1982a). *Reach to recovery exercises after mastectomy patient guide.* New York.

American Cancer Society. (1982b). *An ounce of prevention: Suggestions for hand and arm care.* New York.

American Cancer Society. (1982c). *Exercises after lumpectomy patient guide*. New York.

Clark, J., & McGee, R. (1992). *Core curriculum for oncology nursing*. Philadelphia: W. B. Saunders.

Ehmann, J. (1989). *Maintaining a positive image with hair loss and cancer therapy*. Schenectady, NY: Genium Publishing.

Ehmann, J. (1990). *Maintaining a positive image with breast cancer surgery*. Albany, NY: Johanna's On Call to Mend Esteem, Inc.

Ehmann, J. (1991a) *BSE RAP: It's your body, check yourself out!* Atlanta: ISIP and Johanna's On Call to Mend Esteem, Inc.

Ehmann, J. (1991b) *The breast health diary*. New Orleans: Spectra Communications.

Ehmann, J. (1991c) *Maintaining a positive image with cancer therapy*. Albany, NY: Kermani Press..

Ehmann, J. (1994a) *Maintaining a positive image with breast cancer surgery, with Johanna Ehmann*. Albany, Johanna Lombardo Ehmann Production.

Ehmann, J. (1994b). Breast cancer rehabilitation: Exploring the role of the mastectomy nurse prosthetist. *Innovations in Oncology Nursing 10* (1), 14–17.

Ehmann, J., & Decker, G. (1991). *Nurses and patients together: Maintaining a positive image with cancer therapy*. Oncology Nursing Society Special Projects Funding.

Ehmann, J. Sheehan, A., & Lombardo, A. (1992). *Restoring image after mastectomy: The need for proactive nursing*. The American Cancer Society Second National Conference on Cancer Nursing Research, Baltimore, Jan. 30–Feb. 1992.

Foresight Communication, Inc. (1991a). In touch for life: A wellness program for mastectomy patients.

Foresight Communication, Inc. (1991b). In touch for life: A wellness program for lumpectomy patients.

Leigh, S., & Webb, N. (1994). To reconstruct or not to reconstruct: That is the question! *Innovations in Oncology Nursing 10* (1), 1–25.

Staiger, M., & Harkings, (1993). Advances in the diagnosis of breast disease. *Innovations in Oncology Nursing 1*, 2–12.

PART 7 | Ethnicity and Culture in Breast Cancer

CHAPTER 19

Breast Cancer and African American Women

Janice Mitchell Phillips, PhD, RN

Breast cancer is the second leading cause of cancer death for women in the United States; however, it is the leading cause of cancer death for African American women. Existing data indicate that African American women have experienced a poorer survival rate from breast cancer when compared with their white counterparts. The potential for reducing this disparity lies in earlier detection and subsequent treatment.

The purpose of this chapter is to synthesize some of what is known about breast cancer and African American women. This chapter begins with a discussion of the incidence, mortality, and survival related to breast cancer, with an emphasis on black and white differences. This is followed by a discussion on the breast cancer screening practices of African American women. The chapter concludes with implications for promoting breast cancer control among African American women through practice and research.

BREAST CANCER INCIDENCE

Epidemiologists estimate that in 1995, 182,000 new invasive cases of breast cancer will be diagnosed in the United States (American Cancer Society, 1995). Although only 25% of breast cancers can be linked to any identifiable risk factor, the risk of developing breast cancer varies according to age, race, and sex (Seldman, Stellman, & Mushinski, 1982).

Incidence rates in white women are approximately 20% higher than in African American women (Hankey, Brinton, Kessler, & Abrams, 1993). Although the overall incidence of breast cancer is higher in white women when compared with African American women, the reverse is true for African American women under the age of 45 years (Miller et al., 1993). An analysis of incidence trends by race revealed that since 1973, there has been an average increase of 1.8% per year for white women and an average increase of 2.0% for

African American women (Spratt, Donegan, & Sigdestad, 1995). Part of the increase in cancer incidence is partly due to the detection of asymptomatic cancers in both African American and white women.

Of interest is the influence of socioeconomic status (SES) on breast cancer incidence for both African American and white women. Several studies have shown that African American and white women of similar SES have comparable breast cancer rates (Devesa & Diamond, 1980; McWhorter, Schatzkin, Horm, & Brown, 1989). Devesa and Diamond (1980) were among the first to examine the association of breast cancer incidence based on income and education among both African American and white women. They found that highest level of education completed had the most significant influence on breast cancer incidence for African American women. Age at first pregnancy, a variable sometimes associated with level of education, also influenced breast cancer incidence among African American women. Women with higher education levels tended to delay age at first pregnancy compared with women with lower education levels. Thus, the investigators concluded that SES, education, and age at first pregnancy were associated. African American women with higher levels of education and delayed age at first pregnancy had an increased risk of developing breast cancer comparable with that of their white counterparts (Devesa & Diamond, 1980).

Similarly, McWhorter et al. (1989) examined the contribution of SES to racial differences in cancer incidence among twelve cancer sites, including the breast. The investigators also found that differences in breast cancer incidence among black and white women were largely attributed to SES rather than race.

While further investigations assessing the link between SES and breast cancer incidence are needed, the aforementioned studies as well as others suggest directions for examining the etiology of breast cancer. More importantly, these studies begin to provide direction for developing interventions for high-risk populations.

BREAST CANCER MORTALITY

Projections indicate that there will be 46,240 deaths attributed to breast cancer in 1995 (46,000 women, 240 men) (American Cancer Society, 1995). As previously mentioned, while breast cancer is the second leading cause of cancer death in white women, it is the leading cause of cancer death for African American women (American Cancer Society, 1991). In 1990, the breast cancer mortality for white women was 27.4 per 100,000 compared with 31.7 per 100,000 for African American women (Miller et al., 1993). According to Surveillance, Epidemiology, and End Results (SEER) data, during the years from 1973 to 1990, the breast cancer mortality rate for women under the age of 50 decreased nearly 11% due to the decreasing mortality trend in white women. However, breast cancer mortality increased by 2.5% in African American women (Miller et al., 1993). Figure 19-1 depicts age-adjusted breast cancer incidence and mortality rates for African American and white women.

BREAST CANCER SURVIVAL

Perhaps more striking is the difference in breast cancer survival between African American and white women. For example, the 5-year relative survival rate in African American women is 63% compared with 78% for white women (American Cancer Society, 1994). This difference is partly attributed to the late stage at diagnosis for African American women.

When compared with their white counterparts, African American women were less likely to present with breast cancers at an early stage when potentials for cure were greatest (Bang,1994; Eley et al., 1994; Long, 1993).

According to SEER data during 1988 – 1990, more white women presented with breast cancers classified as stage I, whereas the

Figure 19-1   Breast Cancer Incidence and Mortality: White Females vs. Black Females

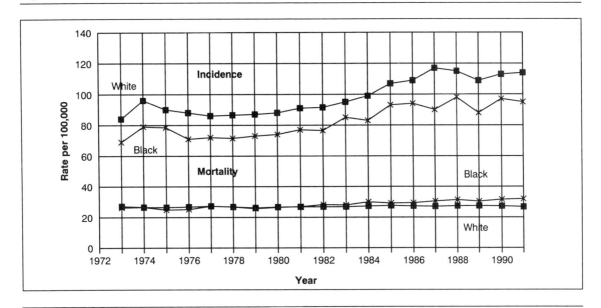

Note. From "SEER Cancer Statistics Review, 1973–1991: Tables and Graphs, National Cancer Institute. NIH Pub No 94-2789," by L. A. G. Reis, B. A. Miller, B. F. Hankey, C. L. Kosary, A. Harras, and B. K. Edwards, p. 134.

proportion of breast cancers classified as stage IV was higher in African American women. However, both racial groups presented with a similar proportion of in situ cancers (Miller et al., 1993). Figure 19-2 presents breast cancer stage distribution according to race.

In a review of the literature, Long (1993) found that SES, particularly low SES, was the most significant factor contributing to lower survival rates from breast cancer among African American women. Other factors contributing to lower survival rates among African American women included late stage at diagnosis, diagnostic and treatment delays, treatment differences, and biological and constitutional factors.

In a study on stage at diagnosis in breast cancer, race, and socioeconomic factors, Wells and Horm (1992) reported that although there were black and white differences related to breast cancer mortality and survival, both African American and white women of lower median education and incomes have breast

cancers diagnosed at a later stage. In contrast, African American women of higher education and income levels presented with breast cancers at an earlier stage at diagnosis similar to white women.

Further, to date, the largest study to examine black and white differences related to breast cancer survival, The National Cancer Institute's Black and White Cancer Survival Study, included 612 African American and 518 white women ranging in age from 20 to 79 years (Eley et al., 1994). Researchers pointed out that approximately 40% of the difference in African American survival from breast cancer was attributed to the more advanced disease stage at diagnosis among African American women. African American women scored lower on measures of disease stage, tumor size, number of cancerous lymph nodes, and receptor status. Eley et al. (1994) concluded that 15% of the African American/white survival was explained by histological differences of tumor

Figure 19-2   Breast Cancer Stage Distribution: 1991

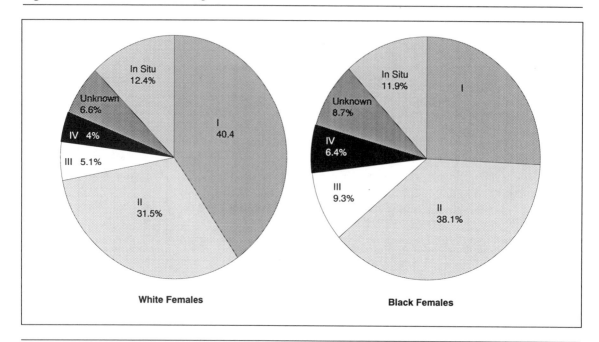

Note. From "SEER Cancer Statistics Review, 1973–1991: Tables and Graphs, National Cancer Institute. NIH Pub No 94-2789, " by L. A. G. Reis, B. A. Miller, B. F. Hankey, C. L. Kosary, A. Harras, and B. K. Edwards, p. 128.

grade. Furthermore, when compared with white women, African American women were more likely to be classified as being overweight and more likely to die of breast cancer.

Finally, in a review of the literature, Pace and Johnson (1994) identified additional factors influencing survival among African American women, including early age of breast cancer development, significantly higher incidence of positive lymph node involvement, and less favorable negative hormone receptor status. Although somewhat controversial, differences in tumor histology were also implicated. Some investigators posited that African American women present with more aggressive tumor types that are less responsive to treatment. The literature also indicated that African American women may receive different treatment compared with other groups. For example, African American women may receive less aggressive

therapy or may lack access to state of the art cancer treatment.

BREAST CANCER SCREENING PRACTICES AMONG AFRICAN AMERICAN WOMEN

To date, there is no known method to prevent breast cancer; rather, the greatest hope for reducing mortality is within the area of early detection through secondary prevention: monthly breast self-examination (BSE), regular mammography, and annual professional breast examination. In support of the need to reduce breast cancer mortality among African American women, the 1991 landmark document *Healthy People 2000: National Health Promotion and Disease Prevention Objectives* identified specific goals to target low-income and African American women. Table 19-1 depicts 1987 baseline data and year-2000 target goals for breast cancer screening.

In order to increase the percentage of African American women being screened for breast cancer, an examination of the breast cancer screening practices and related factors of this population is warranted. In recent years more research has focused on assessing breast cancer among women in general and among African American more specifically. Several national studies compared the breast cancer screening practices of both African American and white women (Dawson & Thompson, 1989; Horton, Romans, & Cruess, 1992; Piani & Schoenborn, 1993; Romans, Marchant, Pearse, Gravenstine, & Sutton, 1991). Findings from the 1987 National Health Interview Survey, a national household survey examining selected health practices of a nonprobability sample of the U.S. population, revealed that 18% of African American women reported not knowing how to perform BSE compared with 9% of white women. However, among BSE performers, African American women reported more frequent performance than white women. Similarly, a higher percentage of African American women (22%) reported having received a professional breast examination compared with white women (14%). Finally, the 1987 findings showed that a higher percentage of white women (39%) reported having received a mammogram compared with African American women (30%) (Dawson & Thompson, 1989).

When the National Health Interview Survey was repeated in 1990, data showed that African American women who knew how to do BSE were more likely than white women to actually do so (51% and 42%, respectively). Both African American and white women reported mammography screening at a similar rate; thus, proportional differences in mammography use according to race and ethnic group were not statistically significant. Finally, African American women aged 18 to 29 years were more likely than white women of comparable age to have had a professional breast examination in the past year. However, both African American and white women

Table 19-1   Special Population Targets

Clinical Breast Exam and Mammogram Received	1987 Baseline	2000 Targets
Received at some previous time Low income women age 40 and older (annual family income < $10,000)	20%	80%
Black women age 40 and older	28%	80%
Received within preceding 2 years Low-income women age 50 and older (annual family income < $10,000)	15%	60%
Black women age 50 and older	19%	60%

Note. From *Healthy People 2000: National Health Promotion and Disease Prevention Objectives* (1991), p. 428. (DHHS Publication No. PHS 91-50212). Washington, DC: U.S. Government Printing Office.

ranging in age from 30 to 65 years and older reported having received a professional breast examination in the past at a similar rate (Piani & Schoenborn, 1993).

In examining mammography use among women age 40 and older, results from two additional studies—The Mammography Attitudes and Usage Study (MAUS) conducted in 1990 and 1992—showed that mammography use was higher among white women than among African American women, 65% and 58%, respectively, in 1990 and 76% and 56%, respectively in 1992 (Horton et al., 1992; Romans et al., 1991). Between 1990 and 1992, researchers noted an increase in mammography use among two groups of white women—better educated women and women with higher incomes. The finding that mammography use did not increase among African American women during this time is disturbing and underscores the ongoing need for education, encouragement, referral, access to screening, and further delineation of barriers related to screening for this population.

Several researchers studied factors related to breast cancer screening using African American women exclusively (Bloom, Grazier, Hodge, & Hayes, 1991; Jacob, Penn, &

Brown, 1989; Nemcek, 1990; Phillips & Wilbur, 1995; Price, Desmond, Slenker, Smith, & Stewart, 1992). Jacob, Penn, and Brown (1989) found that African American women who performed BSE were more likely to be older, had higher incomes, and were more likely to believe that BSE was beneficial. Further, African American women who had been taught how to perform BSE were more likely to perform BSE than those who had not received instruction. Finally, African American women who perceived social approval for performing BSE were more likely to continue doing so than African American women who did not perceive social approval for performing BSE.

In a sample of 95 African American women, Nemcek (1990) examined their health beliefs and BSE practices. Findings revealed that African American women reporting fewest barriers were more likely to practice BSE on a monthly basis compared with women reporting more barriers. Further, BSE frequency was associated with health motivation. African American women who were concerned about their health were more likely to examine their breasts than were women who were not as concerned about their health (Nemcek, 1990). The researcher concluded that in order to enhance BSE frequency among this population, providers must identify barriers related to BSE performance and consider health motivation when teaching and encouraging BSE.

Phillips and Wilbur (1995) examined factors related to breast cancer screening (BSE, mammography, professional breast examination) among 154 low- and middle-income African American women. Results showed that when compared with BSE nonperformers, African American women who performed monthly BSE were married women, had private insurance, had been taught BSE, perceived fewer barriers to BSE, had received high scores on the knowledge measure on BSE, and intended to continue BSE in the future.

Using only samples of African American women, researchers also identified factors related to mammography use among this population (Bloom, Grazier, Hodge, & Hayes, 1991;

Phillips & Wilbur, 1995; Price et al., 1992). Using a sample of 418 African American women age 35 and older, Bloom et al. (1991) found that both older African American women and African American women who examined their breasts were more likely to have received a mammogram. Interestingly, having insurance and having received an annual professional breast examination were not significantly related to mammography use.

Using a total of 186 low-income African American women, Price et al. (1992) studied differences in perceptions of breast cancer and mammography use between African American women who wanted a mammogram and African American women who did not want a mammogram. Discriminant analysis revealed that African American women who wanted a mammogram had a greater perceived risk about breast cancer and identified more benefits with mammography in comparison with African American women who did not want a mammogram. Researchers concluded that educational interventions need to consider perceptions of risk and benefits of mammography screening when encouraging African American women to seek mammography.

Phillips and Wilbur (1995) found that African American women age 48 to 55 were least likely to have received an age-related mammogram when compared with African American women age 40 to 47 and 56 to 65—a disturbing finding because the incidence of breast cancer increases with age. Further, African American women with private insurance and those who had received information on mammography were more likely to have an age-related mammogram when compared with African American women who did not have private insurance or had not received mammography information. Of note, the number one reason for lack of mammography screening was lack of provider recommendation, a finding consistent with previous research. Researchers point out the need to target all African American women for mammography screening. However, special efforts are needed for African American women in the 48 to 55 years age group and particularly for

African American women lacking insurance or access to care. (Phillips & Wilbur, 1995).

Germane to any discussion on the breast cancer screening practices of African American women is the discussion of the current debate on the importance of mammography screening for women under age 50. The current debate on the efficacy of mammography screening in women under age 50 poses unique concern and confusion for African American women, particularly because African American women under age 45 experience an increased incidence from breast cancer. To briefly summarize, in the fall of 1993, the National Cancer Institute (NCI) announced a revision of their mammography guidelines; they were no longer recommending mammography screening for women age 40 to 49. After critical analysis of previous clinical trials, the NCI concluded that clinical trials were statistically inconclusive in showing a clear benefit for mammography screening for women age 40 to 49. Rather, the NCI advised women in this age group to consult with their health care provider regarding their breast cancer screening needs (National Cancer Institute, 1993).

In a recent commentary by Patterson (1994), the author identified the limitations of using data from previous clinical trials as a basis for determining mammography screening guidelines for African American women. Patterson (1994) asserted that previous clinical trials did not include adequate and representative samples of African American women. An exception to this was the Breast Cancer Detection Demonstration Project (BCDDP), initiated in 1970; this trial included approximately 5% African American women. However, because of its nonrandomization, this study should not be considered as a basis for determining mammography screening guidelines. Patterson (1994) concluded that because of the increased breast cancer incidence noted among African American women under age 45, the recommendation to screen women age 40 to 49 should continue.

Although further research in this area is needed, it is imperative that health care provid-

ers assist African American women in understanding the current controversies surrounding mammography screening guidelines. Health care providers are particularly challenged to assist African American women in making informed decisions regarding their breast health needs, including BSE, professional breast examination, and mammography. Of utmost importance is the need for accessible and available breast health services that promote breast health and breast cancer awareness, early detection, and treatment for African American women regardless of age.

IMPLICATIONS FOR PRACTICE AND RESEARCH

Practice

The information presented in this chapter provides some direction for nursing practice and research. The goal to promote breast cancer control among African American women may not be realized without comprehensive efforts and programs that provide breast cancer education, early detection, and treatment. Nurses working with African American women both on an individual and/or community basis are ideally positioned to inform African American women about breast cancer. Nurses working with this population must seize the opportunity to initiate discussion, provide education, and make referrals for screening and/or treatment in both practice and nonpractice settings.

Any educational effort must include an appraisal of attitudes, myths, and misconceptions held by this population regarding cancer, and specifically breast cancer. For example, in a review by Clarke-Tasker (1993) and Underwood (1995), African Americans, regardless of gender, tended to underestimate cancer incidence, held a pessimistic and fatalistic view about cancer, and were hesitant to seek care when confronted with symptoms. Moreover, the author has encountered African American women who mistakenly believe that breast cancer is a white woman's disease. Part of this misconception may be due to the limited number of African American role models depicted in media messages focusing on breast cancer screening and early detection. Thus, nurses must be mindful to assess and address these and other attitudes, beliefs, and practices that may interfere with the early detection and/or treatment of breast cancer. Misconceptions must be replaced with factual information in a culturally appropriate and sensitive manner.

When educating African American women on breast health and breast cancer screening, particular attention should be paid to addressing any fears or pessimisms related to either cancer in general or breast cancer. As previously mentioned, African American women frequently present with breast cancer symptoms in a more advanced stage than their white counterparts. Although, every effort should be made to explore reasons why African American women may delay seeking care for breast symptoms, educational messages should stress that early detection makes an enormous difference in terms of mortality and survival. Again, messages should be culturally specific and acceptable to the target population, making sure that African American women representative of diverse SES and walks of life are depicted. Nurses involved with promoting breast cancer awareness among this population may find it essential to elicit the support of African American women when developing messages and/or interventions to promote breast cancer screening, early detections, and treatment.

Akin to need for education is the need for empowerment. African American women may need assistance and encouragement in making informed decisions about their breast health needs. More importantly, they need to know that it is their right to communicate with their provider about such needs. Assisting African American women in identifying resources for screening and treatment, along with obtaining information on how to navigate the health care system to get the desired care, is of utmost priority. This is especially true for low-income individuals who may find it difficult to interact with health care professionals. In concert with other organizations, health care providers, and policy makers, nurses must work to identify and support existing programs and strategies that promote early detection and breast cancer control within the African American community.

Research

Although the body of research addressing breast cancer and African American women is growing, opportunities for research in this area remain plentiful. First, nurses seeking to conduct research with this population must be mindful of the meaning of research as viewed by the African American community. Many African Americans today remain skeptical of research and thus may be reluctant to participate in research in general and clinical trials specifically. Briefly, this skepticism dates back to before the infamous Tuskegee Syphilis Study that began in 1932 and ended in 1970. Approximately 400 African American males were enrolled in the Syphilis Study primarily to undergo diagnostic testing and be observed for the effects of untreated syphilis. African American males remained untreated despite the discovery of penicillin as a treatment (Jones, 1981). Inequities in research along with difficulties encountered when interfacing with the health care delivery system only begin to partially explain why African Americans may be reluctant to participate in research.

As generators of research, there is a critical need to establish partnerships that will maximize collaboration and cooperation with the African American community. Individuals wishing to conduct research with African American women are particularly challenged to seek the assistance of African American women prior to initiating research to gain insight into problems related to breast cancer control. When conducting research with African American women, every effort should be made to ensure that the target population benefits in some way. Compensation for participation can include, but need not be limited to, money, breast health education, and resources and referral for screening and treatment.

Second, because of the limited body of knowledge on biologic differences and etiologic factors noted among African American women, nurses are particularly needed to advocate for the conduct and expansion of breast cancer research and clinical trials that will include representative samples of African American women. Nurses conducting their own research must be mindful to include diverse samples of African American women in order to better understand the diversity that exists within and among African American women.

Third, in order to achieve breast cancer control among this population, potential research questions should include the following.

1. What factors influence the successful recruitment and retention of African American women into clinical trials?
2. What teaching strategies best promote long-term adherence to breast cancer screening guidelines among African American women?
3. How have recent legislative initiatives influenced the breast cancer screening practices of low-income African American women?

CONCLUSIONS

This brief overview on breast cancer and African American women only begins to identify some of the issues and implications related to breast cancer control in this population. While further delineation of barriers and facilitators related to early detection and treatment for this population is needed, nurses and health care providers must seize every opportunity to establish partnerships with the African American community that will help to enhance participation in breast cancer control activities. As we move toward achieving the objectives outlined in *Healthy People 2000*, nurses in concert with other health care providers and policy makers must continue to advocate to ensure that all women have access to state-of-the art screening and treatment. Education and encouragement of African American women and their health care providers are essential if we are to realize early detection and improved breast cancer outcomes for this population.

References

American Cancer Society. (1991). *Cancer facts and figures for minority Americans.* Atlanta: American Cancer Society.

American Cancer Society. (1994). *Cancer facts and figures.* Atlanta: American Cancer Society.

American Cancer Society. (1995). *Cancer facts and figures.* Atlanta: Author.

Bang, K. M. (1994). Cancer and black Americans. In I. Livingston (Ed.), *Handbook of black American health: The mosaic of conditions issues, policies, and prospects* (pp 77–93). Westport: Greenwood Press.

Bloom, J. R., Grazier, K., Hodge, F., & Hayes, W. (1991). Factors affecting the use of screening mammography among African American women. *Cancer Epidemiology, Biomarkers, and Prevention, 1,* 75–82.

Clarke-Tasker, V. A. (1993). Cancer prevention and early detection in African Americans. In M. Frank-Stromborg & S. J. Olsen (Eds.), *Cancer prevention in minority populations* (pp 142–197). St. Louis : Mosby.

Dawson, D. A. & Thompson, G. B. (1989). Breast cancer risk factors and screening: United States, 1987. *National Center for Health Statistics, Vital and Health Statistics, 10* (172).

DeVesa, S. S., & Diamond, E. L. (1980). Association of breast cancer and cervical cancer incidence with income and education among whites and blacks. *Journal of the National Cancer Institute 65* (3), 515–528.

Eley, J. W., Hill, H. A., Chen, V. A., Austin, D. F., Wesley, M. N., Muss, H. B., Greenberg, R. S., Coates, R. J., Correa, P., Redmond, C. K., Hunter, C. P., Herman, A. A., Kurman, R., Blackow, R., Shapiro, S., & Edwards, B. K. (1994). Racial differences in survival from breast cancer: Results of the National Cancer Institute Black/White Survival Study. *Journal of the American Medical Association, 272* (12), 947–954.

Hankey, B. F., Brinton, L. A., Kessler, L. G., & Abrams, J. (1993). Breast. In B. A. Miller, L. A. G. Ries, B. F. Hankey, C. L. Kosary, A. Harras., S. S. Devesa, & B. K. Edwards (Eds.), SEER Cancer Statistics Review: 1973–1990, National Cancer Institute. NIH Pub. No. 93–2789, 1993 (p. iv.1).

Horton, J. A., Romans, M. C., & Cruess, D. F. (1992). Mammography attitudes and usage study, 1992. *Women's Health Issues, 2,* 180–188.

Jacob, T. C., Penn, N. E., & Brown, M. (1989). Breast self-examination: Knowledge, attitudes, and performance among black women. *Journal of the National Medical Association, 81* (7), 769–776.

Jones, J. (1981). *Bad blood: The Tuskegee syphilis experiment. A tragedy of race and medicine.* New York: The Free Press.

Long, E. (1993). Breast cancer in African American women: Review of the literature. *Cancer Nursing, 16*(1), 1-24.

McWhorter, W. P., Schatzkin, A. G., Horm, J. W., & Brown, C. C. (1989). Contribution of socioeconomic status to black/white differences in cancer incidence. *Cancer, 63* (5), 982–987.

Miller, B. A., Reis, L. A. G., Hankey, B. F., Kosary, C.L., Harras, A., Devesa, S. S., & Edward, B. K. (Eds.). (1993). SEER Cancer Statistics Review: 1973–1990. National Cancer Institute. NIH Pub. No. 93–2789

National Cancer Institute. (1993). Updating the guidelines for breast cancer screening. Bethesda: National Cancer Institute.

Nemcek, M. A. (1990). Health beliefs and breast self-examination among black women. *Health Values, 14* (5), 41–52.

Pace, B. W., & Johnson, H. (1994). Racial differences in breast cancer: Fact or fiction? In L. Wise & H. Johnson (Eds.), *Breast cancer: Controversies in management* (pp 507–516). New York: Futura.

Patterson, E. A. (1994). Screening guidelines for African American women: Looking at the facts and sorting out the confusion. *Journal of the National Medical Association, 86* (6), 415–416.

Phillips, J., & Wilbur, J. (1995). Adherence to breast cancer screening guidelines among African American women of differing employment status. *Cancer Nursing : An International Journal for Cancer Care, 18* (4), 258–269.

Piani, A., & Schoenborn, C. (1993). Health promotion and disease prevention: United States, 1990. *National Center for Health Statistics, Vital and Health Statistics, 10* (185), 6–30.

Price, J. H., Desmond, S. M., Slenker, S., Smith, D., & Stewart, P. W. (1992). Urban black women's perceptions of breast cancer and mammography. *Journal of Community Health, 17* (4), 191–204.

Romans, M. C., Marchant, D. J., Pearse, W. H., Gravenstine, J. F., & Sutton, S. M. (1991). Utilization of screening mammography, 1990. *Women's Health Issues 1* (2), 68–73.

Seldman, H., Stellman, S. D., & Mushinski, M. H. (1982). A different perspective on breast cancer risk factors: Some implications of the nonattributable risk. *CA—A Cancer Journal for Clinicians, 32,* 301–303.

Spratt, J. S., Donegan, W. L., & Sigdestad, C. P. (1995). Epidemiology and etiology. In W. L. Donegan & J. S. Spratt (Eds.), *Cancer of the breast* (pp 116–142). Philadelphia: Mosby.

Underwood, S. M. (1995). Cancer among black Americans. In R. W. Johnson (Ed.), *African American voices : African American health educators speak out* (pp 31–51). New York: National League for Nursing Press.

United States Department of Health and Human Services. (1991). *Healthy People 2000: National Health Promotion and Disease Prevention Objectives* (DHHS Publication No. PHS 91–50212). Washington, DC: U.S. Government Printing Office.

Wells, B. L., & Horm, J. W. (1992). Stage in diagnosis in breast cancer: Race and socioeconomic factors. *American Journal of Public Health, 82* (10), 1383–1385.

CHAPTER 20 | Issues Affecting Asian American and Pacific American Women

Marjorie Kagawa-Singer, PhD, RN, MN

Asian Pacific Americans (APAs) constitute the fastest growing population in the United States. The population is now about 3% of the total U.S. population. By the year 2050, this percentage will increase to 10.7%. (Lin-Fu, 1993). APAs labor under the myth that they are a healthy population without unique, ethnically related needs and problems. Statistics indicate that overall, the APA group has about one half to three fourths the rate of cancer incidence as white Americans (U.S. General Accounting Office [GAO], 1990). However, as discussed in the next section, these aggregate statistics are deceiving. For example, Native Hawaiian women have a rate of cancer of 111 in 100,000 compared with the white rate of 86 in 100,000. Lung cancer is 18% higher; liver cancer in Chinese and Southeast Asians is twelve times the rate of white Americans (Lin-Fu, 1994).

Cultural practices such as not asking for assistance, the demeanor of stoicism, and underutilization of mental health services by

APA women (compared with their percentage in the population) also result in the invisibility of potential and actual physical and emotional distress. These practices further support the myth that the health of APAs is not problematic. The seminal work by Sue and Morishima (1982) began to dispel this myth. Their work indicated that Japanese Americans and Chinese Americans underutilized mental health services despite indications that the incidence of mental disorders and distress were similar to that of the white population. Subsequent work in ethnic mental health has supported this initial finding and documented enormous unmet needs in sixty or more groups that compose the APA population. As yet, however, research on the physical health of APAs lags about 15 years behind mental health research in general (Zane, Takeuchi, & Young, 1994). Almost no work specifically in cancer care exists, except in epidemiology (Jenkins & Kagawa-Singer, 1994; Jones, 1989.) The emotional needs of Asian Pacific American women

229

with breast cancer are essentially unknown. There is only one published work to date on Chinese women and breast health (Mo, 1992), and none on APA women with breast cancer.

The following section provides a brief overview of the demographic characteristics of the APA population. Most notable is the bimodal pattern of overrepresentation within this group at both ends of the spectrum for income, education, and social status. This disparity is usually not apparent in most data bases because the APA groups are aggregated together and the resulting figures are confounded as a statistical mean.

SOCIODEMOGRAPHIC FACTS

Asian Pacific Americans are the fastest growing ethnic group in the United States. The 1990 census indicates that APAs now compose 2.9% of the total U.S. population, a growth of 107.8% since the 1980 census (U.S. Bureau of Census, 1990). Women constitute 51% (3,715,624) of the population and men 49% (3,558,038). This rapid growth will continue, and estimates now predict that the APA population will approach 10.7% of the U.S. population by the year 2050 (Lin-Fu, 1993). The 1990 census designates 71 different ethnic, cultural, national, and regional groups as Asian Pacific Americans (Table 20-1). The five largest groups of APAs are Chinese (1,645,472), Filipino (1,406,770), Japanese (847,562), Asian Indians (815,447), Korean (798,849), and Vietnamese (614,547).

Fifty-six percent of APAs live in the three western states, California, New York, and Hawaii, and 40% live in California (U.S. Bureau of Census, 1990). Of those living in California, 45% live in Los Angeles and Orange Counties (U.S. Bureau of Census, 1990). Because the APA population is relatively sparse and widely distributed in the rest of the United States, many of the statistics presented in this chapter were obtained from California and the National Cancer Institute Surveillance, Epidemiology and End Results (SEER) data bases. The latter also includes Hawaii.

Table 20-1 U.S. Demographics

Ethnicity	Year	
	1990 (%)	2050 (%)
APA	3	10.7
African American	11.5	16.2
Hispanic	9	18
White	75	52.7

Note. Data from "Asian and Pacific Islander Americans: An Overview of Demographic Characteristics and Health Care Issues" by J. S. Lin-Fu, 1994, *Asian American and Pacific Islander Journal of Health*, 1(1), pp. 20–36.

The percentage of foreign-born APAs is varied but significant, and directly affects their patterns of health service use, because of their recent arrival. Approximately 30% of Japanese Americans are foreign-born. Since 1965, with the great influx of many of the other Asian populations, 62% of the Chinese, 92% of the Vietnamese, and 67% of the Filipinos are now foreign-born (Zane et al., 1994). Much of the data on health status and health care use by "Asians" is based on Japanese American and Chinese American populations. Part of the reason for this is their longer length of time in the United States and their sociocultural history when compared with other Asian groups. In addition, Japanese and Chinese Americans tend to be the most acculturated of the Asians, the most educated, have the greatest English fluency, and are more familiar with the purpose of research studies.

Poverty within the APA population is 13%. Contrary to popular belief, this level is greater than the national average of 11%. This fact, as well as others covered throughout this chapter, is often obscured by the myth of the model minority syndrome, which bases much of its information on the Japanese American and Chinese American populations. These two groups have been in the United States for 140 to 225 years, or for more than seven generations. Very often in studies, these groups are aggregated in the total sample, because it is felt they have assimilated into standard Caucasian American society. Yet, studies have demonstrated that even highly acculturated

Table 20-2 Poverty Levels (1990 Census)

Ethnic Group	Percentage of Group
U.S. total population	12.5
Filipino	7
Japanese	7
Asian Indian	10
Chinese	14
Korean	15
Other Asian	17
Pacific Islander	20
Vietnamese	25
Southeast Asian	46
Laotians	65.9

Note. Data from "The State of Asian Pacific America: Economic Diversity, Issues, and Policies" by P. Ong (Ed.), 1994, LEAP Asian Pacific American Public Policy Institute and UCLA Asian American Studies Center.

Table 20-3 Educational Levels of APAs

Level (>25 yoa)	% APAs	% Total Population
0-4 Years Elementary School	5.3	2.4
Women	6.2	2.1
High School	81.8	78.4
Laotian	26.5	
Cambodian	37.5	
College	39.1	21.5

Yoa, years of age.

Note. Data from "Asian and Pacific Islander Americans: An Overview of Demographic Characteristics and Health Care Issues" by J. S. Lin-Fu, 1994, Asian American and Pacific Islander Journal of Health, 1 (1), pp. 20–36.

Asian Americans still retain identifiable Asian cultural beliefs and practices (Fugita & O'Brien, 1991), and these beliefs and practices appear to influence the experience of breast cancer for APA women (Kagawa-Singer, Wellisch, & Durvasula, 1995).

Only 6.6% of Japanese Americans live below the poverty level; the highest median household income is $36,784. But almost 66% of Cambodians live below the poverty level compared with 6.6% of Caucasians. Whites have an average household income of $31,435; Latinos, $24,156; Native Americans, $24,156; and African Americans, $19,758 (Hubler, 1992). However, for the APAs, the figures noted could be much lower, because the data collection method obscures differential living patterns. Many Asian households have several wage earners (and sometimes several whole families) who pool their incomes to support the group, which inflates the figure per household. Consequently, this reduces the amount of money available for each individual. The per capita income for APA household income exceeded the white household income by about $450, but per capita, APAs made only 71 cents for every dollar a white American made (Hubler, 1992; Ito, Chung, & Kagawa-Singer, 1995) (Table 20-2).

EDUCATION

Education levels are also confounded by aggregated data, which conceal the overrepresentation at both the highest and lowest levels (Table 20-3). Seventy-eight percent of the total U.S. population over the age of 25 has a high school education, and 21.5% have college educations compared with 81.8% and 39.1% of APAs overall for high school and college, respectively. However, only 26.5% of Laotians and 37.5% of Cambodians have high school educations. At the lowest educational levels only 2.1% of American women have 0 to 4 years of elementary school education compared with 6.2% of APA women who fall into this category. Women have been shown to be the major health care decision makers in APA families. This low-education population constitutes a high-risk group for health care use.

The four major demographic variables covered in this section outline the wide variations in the APA population in ethnicity, income, education, and acculturation. To this list must also be added language differences, English fluency, generation, and social class as major modifying variables for health care beliefs, preventive practices, cancer knowledge, and use of health services (Harwood, 1981; Kagawa-Singer, 1995).

APAs are very heterogeneous, both between ethnic groups as well as within each of the groups, according to the variables just mentioned. The impact of breast cancer will likewise vary according to cultural and individual differences. The next section reviews the epidemiological data on the incidence and mortality of breast cancer in APA women.

INTRAGROUP DIVERSITY

Within the APA groups there are further distinctions of ethnicity, religious affiliation, class, different sociocultural histories in their native lands, as well as differing experiences here in the United States (DeVos & Romanucci-Ross, 1982). There are also significantly different levels of acculturation achieved by generation as well as individually. Each group, due to lifestyle habits and social and economic resources, has different health care issues and needs. Moreover, each group also has culturally appropriate ways of dealing with illness and vastly different patterns of disease incidence and mortality, including cancer (Jenkins & Kagawa-Singer, 1994). When these differences are added to the complexities of gender and immigration histories, generalizations about this group as a whole are most inaccurate. Ethnic-specific information and understanding are required to develop effective and efficient screening programs, treatment and care plans, or policy formation.

BREAST CANCER INCIDENCE AND DISTRIBUTION IN THE APA COMMUNITY

In 1984, the National Cancer Institute SEER published the first article documenting cancer incidence in three Asian American groups: Japanese, Chinese, and Filipino (Young, Reis, & Pollack, 1984). Until that time, cancer data categorized APAs in "Other" (see Figure 20-1). It was not until 1988 that the California Tumor Registry listed six separate APA groups. Incidence and mortality *rates,* however, could not be calculated until 1992 when the results of the 1990 census became available. Therefore, the

Figure 20-1

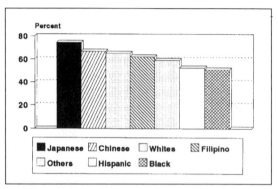

Note. From the California Tumor Registry, 1994, unpublished report.

available data on APA women are extremely limited. The ability to determine any trends and changes as a result of program interventions is also extremely limited (Jenkins & Kagawa-Singer, 1994).

The 1995 Cancer Facts and Figures (American Cancer Society, 1995) notes that breast cancer is the leading type of cancer in all six APA groups. However, the rate of breast cancer varies considerably. Per 100,000, the rate for Chinese American women is about 59.8, 55 for Japanese American women, 41.3 for Filipino women, and 111 for Native Hawaiian women (SEER, 1985).

When stage at diagnosis is noted, APAs in the four SEER groups appear to also present at earlier stages of disease than do Caucasian women. It is true that Japanese American and Chinese American women have a higher percentage of early (stage I and localized) disease at diagnosis than Caucasian women (about 70% compared with 65%). However, fewer Filipino and Native Hawaiian women present with early disease (60% and 48%) (American Cancer Society, 1994) (Figure 20-2).

When these early-stage figures are aggregated, as is most often done when presenting APA rates (as well as other minorities such as "Hispanic" and "black"), the overall incidence appears very similar to the Caucasion population (64% APA, 65% white) and higher than the other ethnic minorities (54% African American and 53% Hispanic) (American Cancer Society, 1994). These figures serve to sustain the myth that the APA population requires fewer early detection and education efforts than other ethnic groups or Caucasian Americans, and that development of culturally competent care is not needed.

However, studies reveal that APA women have the *lowest* rates for participation in early detection and screening programs for breast and cervical cancer (Chen, 1993; Jenkins & Kagawa-Singer, 1994).

Lovejoy et al. (1989) compared screening data for San Francisco's Chinatown women with data of other women in the United States. Eighty-nine percent never had a mammogram, compared with 60% to 85% of U.S. women; 47% had no regular doctor, compared with 8% of U.S. women; and 21% never had a clinical breast exam, compared with 8% of other U.S. women.

Analyses of APAs in clinical trial data are usually nonexistent. The sample size of APA women is usually so small that researchers often drop the APA sample from the analyses (S. Fox, 1992, personal communication). However, some preliminary unpublished data (Kagawa-Singer, 1995) indicate that Asian American women may vary in obtaining "optimal" treatment. According to the California Tumor Registry data, APA women have the lowest rate of breast-conserving therapy among all the ethnic groups (Gillis, Perkins, Snipes, Wright, & Young, 1994). Kagawa-Singer and Wellisch (1994) also found that Japanese American and Chinese American women rarely choose breast-conserving therapy, and use adjuvant therapy at a statistically lower rate than white women (89% compared with 100%). This latter finding would be contrary to the data that Chinese and Japanese American women with breast cancer have better survival rates than any other ethnic group (SEER, 1989). More definitive investigation into this finding is presently ongoing. No other clinical studies exist in the cancer literature on APA women and breast cancer.

THE BREAST CANCER EXPERIENCE AND ITS EFFECT ON APA WOMEN

Empirical evidence regarding the prevalence of cancer or the social or psychological effects of this disease on APA women is virtually nonexistent. Although some studies have been conducted among APAs on health care practices related to cancer (Centers for Disease Control, 1992a, 1992b; Han et al., 1989; Jenkins, McPhee, Bird, & Boknilla, 1990), almost nothing is known about the psychosocial impact of cancer in the APA population. Yet, culture profoundly affects the illness experience through beliefs about the meaning of cancer, use of screening and early detection programs, emotional and physical responses to the treatments, side effects of the treatments, patterns of decision making, and the family dynamics that infuse each step along the continuum of care.

Cultural Beliefs

Cultural differences make a major difference in the response of individuals to the cancer experience. The pathophysiologic *disease* of cancer may be the same objectively measured entity, but the *illness* and the *meaning* of the disease to one's self-concept and social network is culturally framed (Eisenberg, 1979; Kleinman, Eisenberg, & Good, 1982). One's culture frames (1) the meaning of the disease (e.g., Why does it happen now? What caused it to happen?); (2) the problems created by the disease and the illness (e.g., symptom expression and effects on daily responsibilities); and (3) the coping styles used to adapt to the disease and illness by the woman, her family, and friends (e.g., who constitutes the social support network and what is considered appropriate modes of social support) (Kagawa-Singer, 1988).

Table 20-4 indicates the findings from an earlier study by Kagawa-Singer (1988), comparing the impact of cancer on Japanese American and Anglo American patients. The impact of the cancer experience and the modes

Figure 20-2

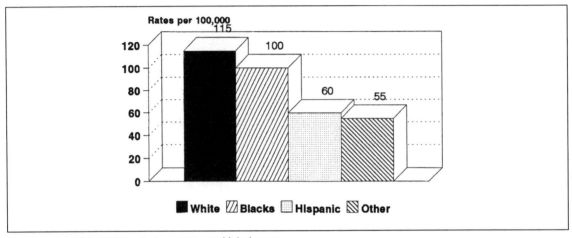

Note. From the California Tumor Registry, 1994, unpublished report.

of coping are different between the two groups. Both groups felt they were coping well. It was apparent that the style of coping was culturally consistent. Moreover, it would be ineffective and probably detrimental for members of one group to use the coping mechanisms of the other. However, cultural modes of coping among Asian women may not be adaptive in a multicultural society where the social network cannot provide culturally appropriate responses. This may be due to employment of daughters and mothers and dispersal of the extended family. The health care system is not responsive to the traditional Asian modes of coping and is as yet unaware of the differences.

Cultural Beliefs About Health and Illness

Part of the difficulty in presenting information about APA women harkens to the diversity between and within the groups. For example, Ito reported differences in concepts of health for APA women between different groups. She found that Chinese American women felt that health was a precarious position, and that ill-

ness may befall one despite precautions taken in dietary and demeanor practices and regular allopathic medical care.

Japanese American women saw health as a matter of will. Focusing upon oneself or even using preventive monitoring was considered self-indulgent and reprehensible: a woman's focus should be on the "others" in one's responsibility (family and friends) rather than on oneself. Sickness can be overcome by focusing outward on one's duties and by ignoring symptoms.

Filipino women, in contrast, saw illness as a moral statement. Catholicism probably has had a strong influence on the cultural beliefs of this population in contrast to Confucianism and Buddhism for the Chinese American and Japanese American women, respectively, in which individual conduct for the welfare of one's primary group is most significant (Ito, 1982).

Each culture defines the meaning of a disease (the illness) when they decide which and what symptoms require outside intervention, what the cause of the disease might be, and what remedial steps should be taken. This cultural perspective depends on the world view of the group, which defines who the indi-

Table 20-4. Associative Differences of the Impact of Breast Cancer Between Japanese American and Anglo American Cancer Patients

	Japanese-Americans	Anglo Americans
Emotional Patterns		
Concept of self	Ego-less	Autonomous
	Part of group identity	Independent
Acceptance	Endure	Fight
	Accommodate	Be assertive
Emotional style of response	Deflect attention	Focus attention
	Suppress dysphoria	Express dysphoria
Cause of cancer	Personal lifestyle choices	Outside forces
Physical Impact		
% Disruption by side effects[a]	0	64
% Decrease in ADL[b]	35	30
Social Support		
Communication	Nonverbal, indirect	Verbal, direct
Relationships	Harmony	Intimacy
	Inner Self	Sharing of feelings
Social needs	Self-sufficiency, 61%	More assistance, 37%
Support source	Inner self	Family/friends

[a] The incidence of side effects from treatment were comparable, but the perceptions and impact on life differed.

[b]Activities of daily living.

Note. From "Bamboo and Oak: Differences in Adaptation to Cancer by Japanese-American and Anglo-American Patients" by M. Kagawa-Singer, 1988, unpublished dissertation, UCLA School of Anthropology.

vidual is, her place in the cosmos, and her role responsibilities within a social network. Therefore, these three APA groups (Chinese, Japanese, and Filipino) have significantly different concepts of illness, its etiology, and how one should respond physically to the medical disease (Ito, 1982).

One's cultural background also prescribes the appropriate interpersonal responses within one's social network. Only very broad generalities can be presented here. It is the responsibility of practitioners to learn about the specific groups that constitute the patient population in their particular geographic area. Frank-Stromborg and Olsen's book, *Cancer Prevention in Minority Populations* (1993), is an excellent beginning to learn about various ethnic groups. Geissler's *Pocket Guide to Cultural Assessment* (1994) describes for oncology practi-

tioners common beliefs and practices of any of the 150 cultures described, such as major religions of each country, predominant sick care practices, dominance patterns, death rites, and food practices and intolerances. However, assuming that the generalities are valid for all members of each of the groups is inaccurate. Interventions based on such superficial knowledge would be, at best, of little use to the patient and her family, and at worst, have effects counter to our intent. Such actions would also indicate a lack of knowledge, caring, and competence on our part as practitioners and would severely undermine our effectiveness and credibility. Such general information serves only as guidelines or hypotheses of beliefs and practices. Quality care requires testing these assumptions for their validity with each individual patient and her family.

Table 20-5   Common Philosophical Heritage of Asian Pacific Americans

- Appropriate behavior and conduct
- Group harmony
- Collectivity
- Hierarchical familial/social relationships
- Reciprocity

CULTURAL BELIEFS ABOUT CANCER

Common Philosophical Values

Table 20-5 lists the common philosophical heritage of the APA cultures. These values reflect the strong Chinese and Indian cultural influence of Confucianism, Buddhism, and Taoism, which stress acceptance, endurance, filial piety, and group welfare over individual needs (Kagawa-Singer, 1988). The concept of appropriate behavior is very much reflected in the value of "face" (Doi, 1985). Face is extremely significant in Asian cultures, for face is a fundamental aspect of maintaining both social respectability and self-respect. Asian cultures are exquisitely aware of their public persona compared with their private self (Doi, 1985). Individuals are seen as both representatives and reflections of their families and primary social groups. Asians with stigmatized illnesses such as cancer may lose face in the community for themselves and for their families, resulting in serious social consequences (e.g., loss of marriageability) (Cheung, 1982; Long & Long, 1982).

In APA cultures, group harmony is valued over individuality and intimacy. Thus, dysphoric feelings are kept to oneself if they might disrupt the well-being of the group, and especially if the situation cannot be changed, as would be the case with a cancer diagnosis. Emotional problems are kept to oneself or, at most, within the family. Sharing such private information with outsiders (anyone not of the immediate family) is considered unacceptable and a sign of inner weakness and family disrespect.

Hierarchical relationships mean that persons in positions of authority and/or those who have education are to be given proper respect. In the clinical setting, asking questions is considered disrespectful, for it implies that the persons questioned did not do their jobs adequately. For practitioners, this valued mode of interaction runs counter to Western training, in which patients/family members are expected to ask questions when they do not understand. These dissonant modes of interaction can potentially result in misunderstandings on the part of both practitioner and patient in issues ranging from pain control to treatment decisions.

Reciprocity is a fundamental dynamic in APA cultures. One incurs debts or obligations that must be reciprocated when any favors or kindnesses are extended to oneself or one's family. An individual must reciprocate in kind or suffer loss of face. The repercussions of this social expectation are critical when social support is offered or required during the cancer experience. Patients and families may actually choose to endure an uncomfortable situation alone rather than request help, because the burden of obligation may exhaust the emotional and/or physical energy the patient and family possesses during this time.

Impact of Breast Cancer on APA Women

The breast cancer literature most often addresses three concerns: (1) body image and sexuality, (2) impact on close interpersonal relationships; and (3) social support.

Body Image.   Body image is affected by breast cancer and its emerging treatment (Schain, Jacobs, & Wellisch, 1984; Wellisch, et al., 1989). Body image research is based on Western concepts of beauty and body image. For APA women, different concepts of both beauty and body image exist. The APA culture places a greater value and emphasis on role fulfillment as a criterion for femininity than on physical attributes. In addition, the significance of body parts and concepts of their beauty also differ. For example, in Japanese culture the nape of the neck and lightness of the skin are central foci of beauty. In Chinese culture, concepts such as deportment are essential to concepts of beauty. One proverb extols the virtues of rounded shoulders versus squared shoulders, indicating submissiveness versus defiance and masculinity. In Korean culture, the shape of the heel of the foot indicates beauty. Physical modesty for APA women in their native countries often focuses below the waist. The significance of the breasts per se in sexuality and body image has significantly less sexual meaning in APA cultures and more functional meaning (breast feeding) than in American and European cultures (Rosaldo & Lamphere, 1974; Chipp & Green, 1980). These variations in concepts about the breast may be reflected by the rarity of psychosocial breast cancer studies in Chinese and Japanese American women (Gillis et al., 1994).

The normative Western therapeutic mode of *interpersonal interaction* is used to discuss and share aspects of the experience of breast cancer (Taylor, Falke, Shoptaw, & Lichtman, 1986; Peters-Golden, 1982). Cross-cultural research shows this may not be the normative style of communication used in close interpersonal APA relationships (Izard, 1980; Ho, 1989). In APA groups, verbalization of intimate subjects with those outside the immediate family is frowned upon (Kagawa-Singer & Chung, 1994). Close interpersonal interactions in APA relationships often are communicated by "doing for" the person in need rather than "talking about" the situation (Kagawa-Singer, 1988).

The literature also indicates that APA women obtain their greatest *social support* from their husbands (Taylor, et al., 1986; Wellisch, Jamison, & Pasnau, 1978). The marital relationship for traditional APA women is not egalitarian, but complementary. These women may not expect emotional support from their spouse, but rather from their related female network. Friends are rarely called upon, because self-sufficiency is highly valued. Friends and family may provide support in the form of material aspects such as cooking, cleaning, shopping, transportation, etc., which can be provided without asking. Emotional support is less often verbalized, but rather demonstrated in the form of caring behaviors.

APA cultures are often stereotyped as somaticizers of psychological distress (Lock, 1983). APAs clearly differentiate psychological from physical distress. Their modes of coping and symptom presentation differ significantly from standard Western culture. Practitioners must become more familiar with assessing these variations so that the proper diagnosis can be made and the appropriate interventions implemented (Kagawa-Singer, 1988; Kagawa-Singer et al., 1995; Kagawa-Singer & Chung, 1994).

CHARACTERISTICS OF SUCCESSFUL CANCER PROGRAMS THAT TARGET THE APA COMMUNITY

Lovejoy and colleagues (1989) have the only published report of a successful program to specifically screen one group of APA women: Chinese. No programs presently exist to address the needs of APA women *with* breast cancer. However, too little is yet known about APA women with breast cancer to design effective programs for the many different cultural groups.

Part of the difficulty in developing programs for this population is the diversity. Each group requires specific cultural sensitivity and competence, but the demographic distribution of this group creates another barrier. Usually the populations in any one community are too small to warrant additional attention or too small to develop cost-effective programs.

RESEARCH RECOMMENDATIONS

As indicated throughout this chapter, very little work has been done regarding the needs of APA women with breast cancer. Studies should be carried out to identify the impact of the experience on APA women along the entire continuum of care, from screening and early detection to treatment choices and side effects, and to rehabilitation or terminal care. Most studies need to be at the descriptive level at this time, and researchers must clearly identify the women's ethnicities, their ages, and their levels of acculturation, class, and education.

A review of the transcultural oncology nursing literature in 1990 uncovered only 14 papers that addressed the emotional needs of ethnic minority populations (Kagawa-Singer, 1990). Since that time, there has been an increase in the number of studies of Hispanics and African Americans, but not of APA women with breast cancer. In the 1994 Oncology Nursing Society announcement of grants, one researcher was given funds to study the attitudes and beliefs of Asian Indians toward breast self-examination. Obviously, more studies are necessary for this population.

Information for the study of breast health and breast cancer in APA women is beginning to appear in several data bases. The SEER data base is the oldest for the largest and highest risk APA groups: Chinese, Japanese, Filipino, and Native Hawaiian. The state Behavioral Risk Factor Surveys are also a source of national data (California State Dept. of Health, 1993). Two national health research centers on APAs are conducting research and developing researchers who will study the health needs of this group: The National Research Center on Asian American Mental Health, based at the University of California Los Angeles (UCLA) headed by Stanley Sue, Ph.D.; and the UCLA/ MEDTEP Medical Outcomes Research Center on Asian and Pacifics, based at the West Los Angeles Veterans Administration Hospital, headed by Takashi Makinoden, PhD. The Asian and Pacific Health Forum based in San Francisco is a national advocacy group for APA health issues and has as one of its missions the dissemination of information about this population. Several community health clinics and consortia of clinics across the United States also provide mental and physical health services to APA women and have developed outreach programs in cancer education, screening, and early detection. These facilities offer a potential source for the study of APA women. One joint project between the

San Francisco unit of the American Cancer Society, the University of California San Francisco, and the Asian Pacific Women's Business Association has developed educational (written and video) materials for the Chinese population (Kagawa-Singer, 1995).

IMPLICATIONS FOR PRACTICE

APA women face two categories of problems that must be simultaneously resolved. The first is structural. This includes such generic problems as accessible, affordable, and logistically convenient health services. However, these problems pose significant barriers to APA women of low acculturation. Specific structural factors that would facilitate use of services for APA women of limited acculturation are (1) the availability of providers of the same ethnicity, (2) bicultural and bilingual staff, (3) respectful communication styles demonstrated by staff,(4) health education materials in the appropriate language and at the correct literacy level, (5) affordability of services, and (6) multiservice centers to reduce the need for multiple appointments in different geographic locations or requiring multiple, uncoordinated visits (Ho, 1991).

The second category of important factors is conceptual issues such as correct knowledge about cancer, and attitudes, beliefs, and values of a particular ethnic group toward cancer in general and specifically toward preventive health care practices, use of screening modalities, and treatment options (Ho, 1989). Many programs on breast health and breast cancer are not appropriate or acceptable to APA women. These programs focus on the individual self and autonomous decision-making styles; they promote modes of communication that are antithetical to the APA rules of interpersonal interactions. They also emphasize concepts of femininity and beauty that may also be inappropriate for APA women. Many of the available interventions encourage women to express and work through their negative emotional responses to the cancer experience. This too might create more discomfort than support for APA women, and it might alienate them from their own social support system. Understanding the knowledge level of the patient and family, the cultural meaning of the disease, and the appropriate communication style will assist the practitioner in eliciting and evaluating valid information.

Screening efforts often use a model that emphasizes individuality and autonomy in the women, which tends to be unsuccessful in ethnic minority communities. The relationship in this paradigm is between the individual and an institution as a resource. In contrast, community programs that appear to be most successful in providing education and early detection and screening frame the programs congruent with cultural values. Generally, a health promotion approach with an educational focus is used. The delivery also emphasizes the value and support of women's roles in the family. Outreach efforts personalize the relationship and foster trust between the provider and the woman. These outreach workers are often respected women from the community who also represent the health agencies.

The effect of culture on specific APA cancer patient care issues is confined to anecdotal information and speculation at this point because there are no empirical data. However, a short guideline can serve to direct practice and begin to build a data base.

In a cross-cultural therapeutic encounter, the practitioner must demonstrate sincere respect, caring, trustworthiness, and competence in order to develop rapport with the patient and family. This rapport building requires that the practitioner be *culturally sensitive* to the beliefs, values, and norms of behavior of the particular ethnic group to which the patient and family belong. When this knowledge and sensitivity is applied to the interview process, the practitioner will more likely elicit accurate information and be able to recommend a plan of action *relevant* to the patient and family. This process requires negotiation on the part of all participants. When a mutually acceptable plan is formu-

lated, adherence to the recommendations will be more likely, the encounter will be mutually satisfactory, and *culturally based and competent* care will be provided.

The four steps of this process compose the acronym KOPF, or "head" in German. *Knowledge* of the specific values, beliefs, and behavioral practices of the particular ethnic groups in one's practice is the first step. This information can be obtained from the literature in transcultural health, and by talking with informed members of the groups themselves, such as community members or religious officials. From these representatives the staff can also learn about the rules and expectations of the communication process; that is, the proper social etiquette, both verbal and nonverbal, as well as the symbolic meanings of body parts.

When language is a barrier, translators are essential, but it is critical that they be well trained. Otherwise, common mistakes such as omissions, editing, and interpretation without the knowledge of the patient or provider can occur.

Observation and openness are required after general knowledge about the particular groups is obtained. This step may offer the key to unlocking perplexing or conflicting information with individual patients and families. Eliciting individualized information requires informed, culturally based *observations* and a *prepared openness* to differentiate between cultural generalities, culturally specific similarities, and individual variances.

Patience is required to develop rapport with individuals who are not of our same ethnic group and who may also be unfamiliar with our health care system. Most people will usually answer our inquiries. However, before divulging or sharing their private beliefs, patients and families may test the practitioner's credibility, trustworthiness, and sensitivity.

Facilitation is the last step. The clinician must use the information obtained in the prior three steps to facilitate the process so that patients and families can best meet their own objectives. New alternatives may be necessary if present beliefs and/or behaviors used for coping and adaptation are insufficient.

Alternative or complementary health practices and practitioners are widely used in many of the APA groups. Clinicians must determine if these practices are helpful, neutral, or maladaptive. If the practice or practitioner is helpful or neutral, these practices can be supported. Such support would indicate our respect for cultural beliefs. We might also learn other effective modalities of care. If the practice is harmful, we must work with the patient and family to help them understand how it may be counterproductive for their condition. Ultimately, the decision is between the patient and family once they are fully informed.

By drawing on the richness of the cultural support system as well as utilizing Western therapeutic techniques, practitioners and families can arrive at mutually acceptable goals, and our efforts will have a greater likelihood of achieving their intended aim of optimal cancer care.

SUMMARY

Asian Pacific Americans now constitute a significant percentage of the U.S. population. However, very little is known about this highly diverse group. Identifying issues affecting the experience of breast cancer for APAs are complicated by several factors: (1) the myth of the "model" minority; (2) the cultural diversity within the group of health beliefs and practices, and differences in levels of acculturation; and (3) the lack of ability to accurately "count" APAs in most national and other large study data bases, which restricts our ability to design culturally relevant and acceptable screening and treatment programs (Kagawa-Singer, 1992).

This chapter clearly announces a challenge to oncology researchers and practitioners to recognize Asian Pacific American women with breast cancer as an underserved population in the United States and to move forward to develop programs and practitioners who are responsive to the needs of this community and who will define and provide optimum care for these women.

References

American Cancer Society. (1995). *1995 California cancer facts and figures*; 1–31.

American Cancer Society, California Division & California State Tumor Registry. (1994). *Cancer facts and figures*. Oakland, CA: American Cancer Society.

California State Department of Health. (1993). Health Risk Survey. Unpublished data.

Centers for Disease Control. (1992a). Behavioral risk factor survey of Chinese: California, 1989. *Morbidity and Mortality Weekly Report, 41*, 266–270.

Centers for Disease Control. (1992b). Behavioral risk factor survey of Vietnamese and Hispanics: California 1989–1991. *Morbidity and Mortality Weekly Report, 41*, 69–72.

Chen, M.S., Jr. (1993). A 1993 status report on the health status of Asian Americans and Pacific Islanders: Comparison with *Healthy People 2000* objectives. *Asian American and Pacific Islander Journal of Health, 1*, 37–55.

Cheung, F. (1982). Psychological symptoms among Chinese in urban Hong Kong. *Social Science & Medicine, 16*, 1339–1344.

Chipp, S., & Green, J. (Eds.). (1980). *Asian women in transition*. University Park & London: The Pennsylvania State University Press.

Doi, T. (1985). *The anatomy of self*. Tokyo: Kodansha International.

DeVos, G., & Romannucci-Ross, L. (1982). *Ethnic identity: Cultural continuities and change*. Chicago and London: The University of Chicago Press.

Eisenberg, L.(1979). Disease and illness. *Culture, Medicine and Psychiatry 1* (9), 9–23.

Frank-Stromborg, M., & Olsen, S. J. (Eds.). (1993). *Cancer prevention in minority populations*. St. Louis: Mosby.

Fugita, S., & O'Brien, D. J. (1991). *Japanese American ethnicity: The persistence of community*. Seattle: University of Washington Press.

Geissler, E. (1994) *Pocket guide to cultural assessment*. St. Louis: Mosby-Year Book.

Gillis, D. L., Perkins, C., Snipes, K., Wright, W., & Young, J. (1994). Factors affecting regional variations in breast conserving therapy. Abstract. *California Tumor Registry*. Paper presented at the National State Tumor Registry Conference, San Diego, California.

Han, E. E. S., Kim, S. H., Lee, M. S., Miller, J. S. K., Rhee, S., Song, H., & Yu, E. Y. (1989). Korean Health Survey: A preliminary report. Los Angeles: Korean Health, Education and Information and Referral Center.

Harwood, A. (Ed.). (1981). *Ethnicity and medical care*. Cambridge, MA: Harvard University Press.

Ho, M. K. (1989). Applying family therapy theories to

Asian/Pacific Americans. *Contemporary Family Therapy, 11* (1), 61-70.

Ho, M. K. (1991). Use of ethnic-sensitive inventory to enhance practitioner skills with minorities. *Journal of Multicultural Social Work, 1* (1), 57–67.

Hubler, S. (1992). 80s failed to end economic disparity, census shows. Los Angeles Times, August 17.

Ito, K., Chung, R., & Kagawa-Singer, M. (1995). Asian/Pacific American Group, In Sheryl Rusek, Virginia Olesen, & Adele Clarke (Eds.) *Women's Health: Dynamics of Diversity*, Philadelphia: Temple University Press (in press).

Ito, K. L. (1982). NIMH final report: Health care alternative of Asian American women. Grant No. RO1MH33038.

Izard, C. (1980). Cross-cultural perspectives on emotion and emotion communication. In H. Triandis & W. Lonner (Eds.) . *Handbook of cross-cultural psychology: Basic processes*, Vol. 3 (pp. 185–221). Boston: Allyn & Bacon.

Jenkins, C., & Kagawa-Singer, M. (1994). Cancer. In N. Zane, D. Takeuchi, & K. Young (Eds.), *Confronting critical health issues of Asian and Pacific Islander Americans.* (pp. 105–147) Thousand Oaks, CA: Sage Publications.

Jenkins, C. N. H., McPhee, S. J., Bird, J.A., & Bonilla, N.-T. (1990). Cancer risks and prevention behaviors among Vietnamese refugees. *Western Journal of Medicine, 153,* 34–39.

Jones, L.A. (Ed) (1989). *Minorities and cancer*. New York: Springer.

Kagawa-Singer, M., Wellisch, D. K., & Durvasula, R. (1995). Impact of Breast Cancer on Asian- and Anglo-American women (in revision).

Kagawa-Singer, M. (1995). Resources for Asian Pacific Islanders. *Cancer Practice, 3* (6), 382–384.

Kagawa-Singer, M. (1988). Bamboo and oak: Differences in adaptation to cancer by Japanese-American and Anglo-American patients. Unpublished dissertation, UCLA School of Anthropology.

Kagawa-Singer, M. (1990). Implications for cancer nursing research. Paper presented at the 15th Annual Congress of the Oncology Nursing Society, May 15.

Kagawa-Singer, M. (1992). Paper presented at the American Psychological Association, Washington DC, September.

Kagawa-Singer, M. (1995). Socioeconomic and cultural influences on cancer in minority populations. *Seminars in Oncology Nursing, 11* (2), 109–119.

Kagawa-Singer, M., & Chung, R. C.-Y. (1994). A paradigm for culturally based care in ethnic minority populations. *Journal of Community Psychology, 22*, 310–326.

Kagawa-Singer, M., & Wellisch, D. W. (1994). Impact of breast cancer on Asian-American and Anglo-American women. (In preparation).

Kleinman, A., and Eisenberg, L., & Good, B. (1982). Culture, illness and care. *Annals of Internal Medicine, 88*, 251–258.

Lin-Fu, J. S. (1994). Asian and Pacific Islander Americans: An overview of demographic characteristics and health care issues. *Asian American and Pacific Islander Journal of Health, 1* (1), 20–36.

Lock, M. (1983). Japanese responses to social change—Making the strange familiar. *Western Journal of Medicine, 12* (139), 839–834.

Long, S., & Long, B. (1982). Curable cancer and fatal ulcers. *Social Science and Medicine, 16*, 2101–2108.

Lovejoy, N. C., Jenkins, C., Wu, T., Shankland, S., & Wilson, C. (1989). Developing a breast cancer screening program for Chinese-American women. *Oncology Nursing Forum, 16* (2,; 181–187.

Mo, B. (1992). Modesty, sexuality and breast health in Chinese-American women. In Cross-cultural Medicine—A decade later (special issue). *Western Journal of Medicine, 157*, 260–264.

National Cancer Institute, Surveillance, Epidemiology and End Results (SEER) survey, 1975 to 1984, from San Francisco/Oakland and Hawaii SEER Registries.

Ong, P. (Ed.) (1994). The State of Asian Pacific America: Economic Diversity, Issues and Policies. LEAP Asian Pacific American Public Policy Institute and UCLA Asian American Studies Center.

Peters-Golden, H. (1982). Breast cancer: Varied perceptions of social support in the illness experience. *Social Science and Medicine, 16*, 483–491.

Rosaldo, M. Z., & Lamphere, L. (Eds.). (1974). *Women, culture and society*. Stanford, CA: Stanford University Press.

Schain, W. S., Jacobs, E., & Wellisch, D. K. (1984). Psychosocial issues in breast reconstruction: Intrapsychic, interpersonal, and practical concerns. *Clinics in Plastic Surgery, 11* (2), 237–253.

Sue, S., & Morishima, J. (1982). *The mental health of Asian Americans*. San Francisco: Jossey-Bass.

Taylor, S. E., Falke, R. L., Shoptaw, S. J., & Lichtman, R. R. (1986). Social support, support groups, and the cancer patient. *Journal of Consulting and Clinical Psychology, 54* (5), 608–615.

U.S. Department of Commerce News: Census Bureau Releases 1990 census counts on specific racial groups, CB 91-215. Washington DC: Bureau of the Census, June 12, 1991.

U.S. General Accounting Office. (1990). Asian Americans, A Status report. GAO/HRD-90-36-FS. Washington DC: General Accounting Office, March.

Wellisch, D.K., et al. (1989). Psychosocial outcomes of breast cancer therapies: Lumpectomy versus mastectomy. *Psychosomatics, 30* (4), 365–373.

Wellisch, D. K., Jamison, K. R., & Pasnau, R. O. (1978). Psychosocial aspects of mastectomy: II. The man's perspective. *American Journal of Psychiatry, 135* (5), 543–546

Young, J. L., Ries, L. G., & Pollack Z. S. (1984). Cancer patient survival among ethnic groups in the U.S. *Journal of the National Cancer Institute, 43*, 341–351.

Zane, N., Takeuchi, D., & Young, K., (Eds.). (1994). *Confronting critical health issues of Asian and Pacific Islander Americans*. Thousand Oaks, CA: Sage Publications.

CHAPTER 21 | Breast Cancer Challenges in Native American Women

Jeannine M. Brant, RN, MS, AOCN

Breast cancer in Native American (NA) women presents unique challenges and opportunities for oncology nursing. Historically, little attention has been directed toward NA women with breast cancer due to the low incidence and mortality rates in this population. Unfortunately, the low incidence rates have undermined the fact that NA women have the poorest 5-year survival rate of any racial group. This chapter reviews breast cancer rates in NA women, including Indian women of the lower 48 states as well as Alaska Native women. Risk factors, barriers to early detection and treatment, and nursing implications are addressed. Because the information on NA women is limited, interviews with six NA women with breast cancer are also included.

BREAST CANCER RATES

Incidence

Cancer is the second leading cause of cancer death in NA women of the lower 48 states and the leading cause of death for Alaska Native women. Breast cancer accounts for the greatest number of cancers (18%), followed closely by cervical cancer (13%) (Burhansstipanov & Dresser, 1993).

Breast cancer incidence rates are lower among NA women when compared with other races. The rate is 21.7 in 100,000 among NA women compared with 93.3 in 100,000 among white women. Regional variability also exists. For example, Northern Plains Indian women (including Montana, South Dakota, and Wyo-

Figure 21-1   Age-Adjusted Breast Cancer Incidence Rates per 100,000 Population for Selected Tribes and IHS Areas, Females, 1982–1987

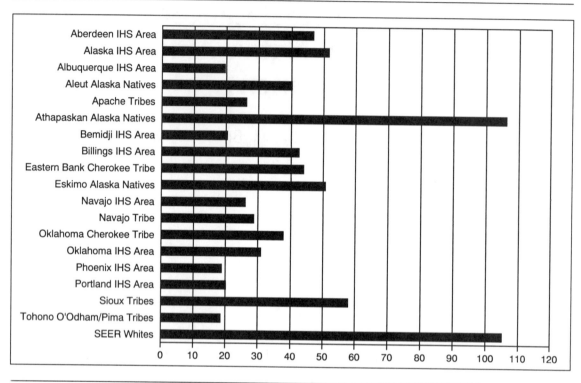

Note. From "Documentation of the Research Needs of American Indians and Alaska Natives" by L. Burhansstipanov and C. M. Dresser, 1993, National Cancer Institute: NIH Pub. No. 93–3603.

ming) have a higher incidence of breast cancer than NA women overall. Athapaskan Alaskan women have the highest incidence, which is comparable with that of white women (see Figure 21-1) (Burhansstipanov & Dresser, 1993; Frost, Taylor, & Fries, 1992; Lanier, Bulkow, & Ireland, 1989; Mahoney, Michalek, Cummings, Nasca, & Emrich, 1989a; Mahoney, Michalek, Cummings, Nasca, & Emrich, 1989b; Michalek & Mahoney, 1990; Michalek, Mahoney, Cummings, Hanley, & Snyder, 1989).

Mortality

Breast cancer mortality rates coincide with the low incidence rates among NA women of the lower 48 states (9.0 in 100,000) and Alaskan

Native women (12.8 in 100,000). The mortality rate for white women is 26.7 in 100,000 (Burhansstipanov & Dresser, 1993). These data suggest that breast cancer is not highly prevalent among NA women, however, the low incidence and mortality rates may be due to racial misclassification or inaccurate reporting by the Surveillance Epidemiologic and End Results (SEER) data (Burhansstipanov & Dresser, 1993; Frost et al., 1992).

Survival

Aside from incidence and mortality rates, NA women have the poorest breast cancer survival rates of any racial group. Native American women have a 5-year survival rate of

48.8%, African Americans 62.8%, and whites 75.7% (Burhansstipanov & Dresser, 1993). Late detection is a major factor influencing survival. Advanced disease (28 of 32, or 87.5%) was evident in one survey of women on the Crow and Northern Cheyenne reservations of Montana (Fallsdown et al., 1991). Other factors affecting survival include poor compliance with treatment, presence of concomitant disease, lack of timely access to diagnosis and treatment, and low socioeconomic status (SES) (Burhansstipanov & Dresser, 1993).

RISK FACTORS

Genetic Factors

Native Americans' ancestry originated in Asia, and the NA population shares many characteristics of Asians, including a lower incidence of breast cancer. Unlike Asian women, however, NA women have maintained a low incidence in spite of their acculturation into Western society, suggestive of distinct genetic traits (Sievers & Fisher, 1981).

In a histologic comparison of breast cancer among Southwest NA women, Hispanic women, and Anglo women (n = 45 for each group), lobular carcinoma was less common in NA women than in Anglo women. Native American women also had tumors with less differentiated nuclei or a statistically significant greater number of grade 1 tumors in comparison with both Hispanic and Anglo women. This occurred despite a less favorable stage at diagnosis among NA women (Black, Bordon, Varsa, & Herman, 1979).

Parenchymal patterns also differ among NA women. High-density parenchymal patterns are associated with a higher risk of breast cancer. NA women develop a less dense parenchymal pattern at an earlier age (21 to 40) compared with Hispanic and Anglo women (ages 41 to 50), independent of parity factors. This earlier shift correlates with the low incidence of breast cancer (Hart, Steinbock, Mettler, Pathak, & Bartow, 1989).

Environmental Factors

Despite potential genetic protective factors, breast cancer rates have increased in NAs over the past 30 years and are approaching that of the general population (Michalek & Mahoney, 1990). The increasing incidence may be attributed to a slow acculturation to Western society, including a high-fat diet and increasing obesity in NA women. Obesity is also associated with a shorter survival rate in breast cancer patients (Welty, 1991). Other factors, such as parity, age at first pregnancy, menstrual history, and history of fibrocystic changes, have not been associated with an increase in breast cancer in NA women (Hart et al., 1989; Pathak, Pike, Key, Teaf, & Bartow, 1990). More accurate SEER data may also be related to the higher incidence. Historically, SEER data did not include a category for NA people, and therefore, many NA people with cancer were classified in the "other race" or "white" category. Tumor registries now include a category for NA people.

BARRIERS TO EARLY DETECTION

Health Care

The Indian Health Service (IHS) is the governmental health care system that provides health care services to the NA people. Care is provided in IHS clinics or hospitals located on or near reservations in the 33 reservation states. The IHS may also contract care to larger referral centers for specialized needs. The IHS contract care is based on a priority rating scale for patients with the most imminent need. Those with immediate life-threatening situations, such as trauma and diabetes, are readily referred to specialists. Breast lumps may have a low priority number because of the low incidence of breast cancer in NA women (Burhansstipanov & Dresser, 1993). Many women find it difficult to understand and accept the IHS contract care system that must prioritize needs according to funding available to IHS. The funding amounts change periodically.

Mammography access may also be difficult in remote reservation areas. Most IHS clinics do not own mammography machines but rely on off-reservation facilities or mobile units, which may visit the reservation once a month. In a survey of Crow and Cheyenne women, 60% (67 of 99) had never had a mammogram (Fallsdown et al., 1991). Native American women also report that a lack of female technicians and physicians may prevent them from seeking health care.

Native American people from urban areas or nonreservation states may have to travel long distances in order to access the IHS system. There are 34 urban clinics for NA people throughout the United States, and they receive partial funding from IHS. Those who do not receive care at the IHS clinic must pay for private care. Contract care is not available to those who have been off of the reservation longer than 6 months. Urban NA women may have needs distinctly different from women living on the reservation; however, limited information is available. Several observations have been noted at the urban IHS clinic in Billings, Montana. Native American women in urban communities tend to ask more questions, and they appear to be more adept toward learning due to greater access of cable television, local American Cancer Society (ACS) units, and other health educational resources. Approximately 20% of NA urban women have seen a breast model, whereas the majority of NA women on the reservation have never seen a breast model. Urban NA women are also more comfortable with handling and palpating breast models than are NA women on the reservation. More information is needed to accurately assess the distinct needs of NA women in urban areas.

Poverty

Poverty among NA people may also interfere with early detection. Twice as many NAs than the total U.S. population live below the poverty level. The American Cancer Society (ACS) reports that the poor have a 10% to 15% lower survival rate than the general population because they often present with advanced disease at diagnosis (ACS, 1990). Twenty-five percent of homes on the reservation lack complete plumbing and 16% have no electric lights. It is also difficult to contact women for mammography screening and follow-up appointments because 56% of homes on the reservation have no phone (Department of Commerce, 1992). Many NA women in rural areas also lack transportation to health care facilities.

Education

Lower educational levels present another barrier to early detection. Approximately 65.5% of Native Americans graduate from high school and 9.3% graduate from college, compared with 77.9% and 21.5%, respectively, in the white population (Department of Commerce, 1992). In addition, NA women report that they have received minimal breast cancer education, and they are often unaware that a "painless" breast lump could potentially be cancerous. A public health nurse (PHN) shared a story regarding an NA woman with breast cancer on the Crow reservation. A family requested that the PHN visit the home because of a foul odor coming from their mother. When the nurse arrived, she observed that the family was wearing masks to lessen the odor. The nurse assessed the mother and discovered an ulcerating breast lesion. This case may have been related to a lack of education as well as other cultural factors, but serves as an example that many NA women may delay seeking health care.

Cultural Barriers

Cultural barriers may also impede the early detection of breast cancer in NA women. First, cancer is sometimes considered a "white man's disease," foreign to Indian people. Cancer was not diagnosed among NA people until governmental health care became accessible, and so some may feel that NAs never had cancer.

Many tribes have no Native word for "cancer." Second, NAs may have an overwhelming fear of cancer, such that if they talk about cancer or even think about cancer they may get the disease. This greatly interferes with cancer education and early detection. Third, fatalism about cancer (cancer = death) may also prevent women from seeking health care. In the Navajo language, *cancer* means "a sore that does not heal" (Antle, 1987). A common concern expressed is "Why find the cancer early if it will just mean I am going to die?" This perception is based on the experience that most NA women with breast cancer have died, but this is most likely due to late detection.

In addition, Indian women are highly esteemed in NA culture as the "givers of life." The woman is the caretaker of the home, and family needs may outweigh her personal need for health care. As one NA woman shared, "I know that my sister knew about that breast lump for a long time. There was just so much stress going on with her family at that time that she didn't get it checked." The woman's sister presented with advanced disease and died shortly thereafter.

BREAST CANCER TREATMENT

The literature contains very little information on NAs and cancer treatment. One survey of Crow and Cheyenne women (n = 99) asked them to rate cancer therapy in the order of importance. The results were: vitamins (85%), diet (78%), radiation therapy (77%), chemotherapy (72%), surgery (65%), and biologicals (55%) (Fallsdown et al., 1991). The major forms of treatment for breast cancer in NA women are further delineated below.

Surgery

Invasive procedures, such as a mastectomy, may be the least preferred method of treatment for NA women (Antle, 1987). This is most likely due to the fear of undergoing surgery. Some NA women may request to save

the removed breast to bury it. They believe that they will not proceed to their next life fully intact unless they bury their breast. Others believe that by burying their breast they will experience less postmastectomy pain, and the burial will also allow the woman to process her grief of losing a breast. Despite individual preference, surgery continues to be the most common treatment modality.

Chemotherapy/Radiation Therapy

Many NA women misunderstand the differences between chemotherapy and radiation therapy (RT) and link them as "one" cancer treatment. Native American women share many of the same concerns about body image changes as non-Indian women with regard to chemotherapy and RT. Hair loss may be a greater concern than suffering from other untoward side effects. It is perceived by some that the "wrong" person may use the hair for a curse against the patient.

In an interview with four Plains Indian women, one of their greatest concerns was a lack of understanding about their cancer treatment, including the difference between chemotherapy and radiation therapy, rationale for treatment, their prognosis with cancer treatment, and side effect management. English was a second language to their native tongue, and they felt that the chemotherapy/ RT education was presented too quickly to understand. In addition, some NA women wonder, "How can a treatment that makes you so sick still help you?" They may feel that the physician made them sick or caused them to lose their hair unnecessarily. This greatly affects some NA women's attitudes toward health care and the health care team. The concept of chemotherapy/RT for many NA women is that they must feel better immediately, and it may be difficult for them to wait for the delayed response. Many NA women also feel that it is disrespectful to ask the nurse or physician any additional questions about cancer treatment.

Traditional Medicine

Native American women interrelate religion with health. They consent to modern medicine to treat their breast cancer, but they consider the underlying cause of the disease (i.e., suppressed feelings) to be a spiritual matter. The goal of the traditional medicine is to establish harmony between the body, mind, and spirit. Traditional medicine seeks to explore the spirit and the mind as to the underlying cause of the disharmony and then attempts to assist the mind and spirit to achieve harmony with the body through various ceremonies. Disharmony may not actually be caused by the breast cancer itself, but it may be caused by the woman's inability to accept and cope with her illness and body changes. The woman will experience an "immediate" response from the traditional healer, which is deeply satisfying. A blending of "white medicine" with "traditional medicine" is considered the best combination for wellness in the NA woman (Locust, 1985).

NURSING IMPLICATIONS

Communicating with Native American Women

The most important thing to remember when communicating with NA women about breast cancer is that there are more than 500 recognized tribes in the United States, each with its own unique and diverse culture (Burhansstipanov & Dresser, 1993). There are also variances in each tribe, including clan affiliation, extended family membership, and each individual's degree of acculturation. Some of the more common communication patterns are listed (see Table 21-1).

Assessment

To develop an appropriate plan of care, the nurse will need to assess the woman's individual acculturation. It will be important to respect the traditional, the transitional, and the nonpracticing NA woman. Bloch's ethnic/cul-

Table 21-1 Communicating with Native American Women

1. Be yourself. Avoid trying to be a part of the NA culture. Allow the NA woman to share her culture with you.
2. Do not make any cultural assumptions.
3. Learn the client's name and ask her how she would like to be addressed (Olsen & Frank-Stromborg, 1993). Greet each person warmly and gently shake their hands.
4. Always address the patient, but acknowledge others in the room as well, especially elders and children.
5. Find the family spokesperson who has been given the informal authority to communicate with the health care team.
6. Minimize questions and allow women to communicate by storytelling. Their cancer experience will be revealed in the stories they share.
7. Listen actively as a form of respect. If possible, complete the written assessment away from the client after the information is gathered.
8. Pause and allow for silence after questions as a sign of respect for the one answering (Olsen & Frank-Stromborg, 1993).
9. Native American women may stare at the floor as a sign of attentive listening.
10. Nodding and smiling may not represent understanding or agreement (Olsen & Stromborg, 1993). Evaluate learning through return demonstration or reflection.

tural assessment tool serves as a useful guide for a comprehensive cultural, sociological, psychological, and biological/physiological assessment (Orque, Bloch, & Monroy, 1983).

Plan/Implementation

In 1989, the Billings Interhospital Oncology Project of Billings, Montana, received a grant from the National Cancer Institute (NCI) to help accrue NA subjects to clinical trials. An NA consultant was hired to accomplish the goals of the grant. During the early stages of the project, it was discovered that the NA people were reluctant to even talk about cancer. The consultant visited the reservations every week to work with PHNs, community health representatives (CHRs) who are NA lay persons with specialized health training, and the NA people. To date, she has provided more than 1,000 one-on-one contacts for cancer prevention, early detection, and referrals for cancer treatment when necessary. Cancer seminars were also presented for 3 consecutive years at the state CHR conference by oncology clinical nurse specialists. Approximately 120 CHRs attended each year, and a CHR from each reservation was assigned to cancer control in their area. In addition, the Big Sky Chapter of the Oncology Nursing Society visited each reservation to provide training to PHNs and CHRs on the early detection of cancers.

The evaluation of this program has been excellent. Mammogram use has increased from five per month to fifteen to twenty per month over the past 4 years on the Northern Cheyenne reservation. It is also significant to note that six women attended a breast cancer interview session during the writing of this chapter, and this most likely would not have occurred even 2 years prior. Unfortunately, the NCI funding is based on subject accrual to clinical trials rather than on the establishment of foundational programs for cancer prevention and early detection.

Oncology nurses have the responsibility of addressing each phase of the cancer trajectory, beginning with cancer prevention. Table 21-2 provides nursing implications for each phase, along with cultural tools available. There is a great need for the development of culturally and educationally sensitive tools for breast cancer treatment and side effect management.

Support

It is also important to understand the significant support systems of the NA woman. One survey revealed that the most prevalent sources of support for Indian women are the family (42 of 99, 42%) and God (20 of 99, 20%) (Fallsdown et al., 1991). Plains Indian women with breast cancer identified that prayer and family were their most important sources of support. Many NA women may delay surgery

and other treatment options until all decisions are discussed with the extended family (Antle, 1987). Cancer may be considered a contagious disease by some NA people. This generates additional fear of cancer, which may interfere with the patient's support system.

Support groups are another important component in breast cancer care for NA women. The groups may assist women to overcome the fear of cancer and to receive support from family, friends, and other cancer survivors. Outreach to the reservations will deliver the most success, and CHRs may need to assist patients with travel arrangements. Children are considered a blessing and are always welcome in group settings. It is important to serve food as a sign of hospitality (Cella & Yellen, 1993). One cancer support group on the Northern Cheyenne reservation is facilitated by a CHR breast cancer survivor. She prepares a full meal for those who attend the group. The Crow reservation recently began a support group as well. The facilitators, cancer patients, and families travel to a different town on the reservation each month. An average of fifteen people attend the group.

Evaluation/Follow-up

Working with NA women with breast cancer is a privilege for the oncology nurse. Unfortunately, several projects and efforts are put forth for the NA people, but the lack of follow-up has resulted in a lack of trust of "white" and professional people. The follow-up care is an integral part of building a positive, trusting relationship with the NA woman and her tribe.

FUTURE DIRECTIONS

There are numerous challenges to face for NA women with breast cancer, but along with each challenge is an opportunity to overcome barriers and challenges. The Oncology Nursing Society, in collaboration with the Multicultural Advisory Council and the Transcultural Nursing Issues Special Interest Group, has an opportunity to develop alliances and working

Table 21-2 Nursing Implications and Cultural Tools for Native American Women With Breast Cancer

Cancer Trajectory	Nursing Implications	Useful Cultural Tools
Breast cancer prevention	1. Assess regional variances in available foods, i.e., fresh vegetables are not readily available in remote areas. 2. Assess individual tribal foods for fat content/preparation methods. 3. Encourage modifying diet with consideration to available foods, traditional foods, and ACS recommendations. 4. Use culturally sensitive tools for teaching.	*National Cancer Institute:* 1. "Traditional Foods Can Be Healthy" (pamphlet) 2. "Eating Healthy the Alaska Way" (poster, table tents) 3. "Eating Healthy the American Indian Way: Why All the Talk About Fat?" (booklet) *American Cancer Society:* 1. *Better Choices* (video) *Old Man Coyote Productions:* 1. *Standing Strong Against the Cancer Enemy* (video, Brant, 1993)
Screening/ early detection	1. Assess cultural barriers that may interfere with screening. Work with PHNs, CHRs, tribal elders, and cancer survivors to overcome barriers. 2. Use round self-examination teaching models rather than breast models to practice breast self-exam. Round models may be less offensive yet provide the same tactile learning. 3. Assess individual access to mammography and screening facilities. 4. Use CHRs to help schedule, transport, and support women with the breast cancer screening process. 5. Provide ongoing education to CHRs and IHS health care professionals regarding the increasing incidence, low survival, and importance of early detection of breast cancer. 6. Use culturally sensitive tools that are available.	*American Cancer Society:* 1. "Continue the Circle: Enjoy the Gift of Health" (poster) 2. "Circle of Life" (flip chart, booklet, leaflet) 3. "What Women Should Know About Cancer" (leaflet) *Native American Women's Health Education Resource Center:* 1. "Breast Cancer" (leaflet) 2. "How to Examine Your Breasts" (poster) *University of Arizona:* 1. "Malam Nau Yahiwapo: Women's Gathering Place" (fact sheets with folder) *American Indian Health Care Association:* 1. "We are the Circle of Life: Pass on the Gift of Health" (poster) *Health Edco:* 1. "New Round Self-examination Teaching Models, Nonsexual" (Health Edco)
Breast cancer surgery	1. Draw the breast lump on a breast diagram to allow the woman to visualize the cancer. 2. Utilize word pictures to discuss breast anatomy, i.e., "a tree with branches reaching out" may represent breast ducts and lobules. 3. Explore cultural barriers if woman is reluctant to discuss lumpectomy/ mastectomy. 4. Inquire whether the woman would like to save the removed breast tissue for burial. 5. Develop individualized teaching tools as needed.	*National Cancer Institute:* 1. Breast Anatomy tablet No other specific cultural tools available concerning surgery.

Table 21-2 Continued

Cancer Trajectory	Nursing Implications	Useful Cultural Tools
Chemotherapy/ radiation therapy	1. Provide one-on-one or family teaching. 2. Explain the difference between radiation therapy and chemotherapy. 3. Give a tour of the radiation treatment center to patients and their families if applicable. 4. Use visual aids (pictures, videos, models, diagrams) to facilitate teaching. 5. Keep literacy level below 6th grade while using respect and adult education methods (applies to low-literacy NA and those who speak English as a second language). 6. Encourage return demonstration when teaching skills (i.e., vascular access device flushing) to assess learning. 7. Provide specific written instructions or information of chemotherapy/radiation schedule, drugs, and potential side effects. 8. Develop individual teaching tools as needed.	No specific cultural tools available. (All materials listed under column "Useful Cultural Tools" are referenced in Burhansstipanov & Barry, 1994 unless otherwise indicated) *American Indian Health Care Association:* 1. *Native American Women and Wellness* (video for health care providers of NA women; includes cultural differences and needs of NA women regarding cancer screening) (Burhansstipanov & Dresser, 1993).
Traditional healing ceremonies and cultural harmony	1. Allow privacy if healer or family requests. Some NAs may encourage health care professionals to participate in the ceremonies. 2. Accept the ceremony as a component of the patient's healing. 3. Encourage all health care team members to respect the culture and ceremony. 4. Avoid attempts to control the ceremony, which may result in resistance to modern medicine. 5. Work with the patient's spokesperson to accomodate large groups.	

relationships with individual tribes and reservations. Oncology nurses can share knowledge and expertise of the cancer experiences, while the NA people share their unique cultural diversity. This unique relationship will strengthen cancer care for NA people. There is also a great need to develop educationally appropriate and culturally sensitive materials that inform NA women about breast cancer surgery, chemotherapy, radiation therapy, and other treatment options. This will enable NA women to be informed about their cancer treatment plan. Finally, there is a clear need for federal grant funds to apply toward cancer program development on NA reservations. The programs must begin by encouraging NAs to talk about cancer openly, including fears associated with the word *cancer*, and educating NA people about cancer prevention and early detection. As cancer becomes more familiar to NA people, they will be able to discuss cancer openly, use cancer screening programs, and seek health care early when an abnormality is detected. Effective change will come from empowerment within the tribe itself, and the oncology nurse can be available for education, support, and encouragement during the planning and implementation process.

References

American Cancer Society. (1990). A summary of the American Cancer Society report to the nation: Cancer in the poor. *Cancer and the socioeconomically disadvantaged* (Professional Educational Publication). Atlanta: American Cancer Society.

Antle, A. (1987). Ethnic perspectives of cancer nursing: The American Indian. *Oncology Nursing Forum, 14* (3), 70–73.

Black, W. C., Bordon, G. M., Varsa, E. W., & Herman, D. (1979). Histologic comparison of mammary carcinomas among a population of Southwest American Indians, Spanish Americans, and Anglo women. *American Journal of Clinical Pathology, 71* (2), 142–145.

Brant, J. (Producer). (1993). *Standing Strong Against the Cancer Enemy* (film). Billings, MT: Old Man Coyote Productions.

Burhansstipanov, L., & Barry, K. C. (1994). *Cancer education resources for American Indians and Alaska Natives*. National Cancer Institute: NIH Pub. No. 94-3706.

Burhansstipanov, L., & Dresser, C.M. (1993). Native American Monograph No. 1: *Documentation of the research needs of American Indians and Alaska Natives*. National Cancer Institute: NIH Pub. No. 93-3603.

Cella, D. F., & Yellen, S. B. (1993). Cancer support groups: The state of the art. *Cancer Practice, 1* (1), 56–61.

Department of Commerce, Bureau of the Census. (1992). 1990 populations for the total United States by sex and race groups, for five-year age groups. General Population Characteristics from the Census Bureau tape. Washington, DC: U.S. Government Printing Office.

Fallsdown, D., Hammond, N., Kuefler, P., Marchello, B., Myers, D., Hall, S., & Weinert, C. (1991). Cancer control survey among Crow and Cheyenne Native American females who live on the Crow and Cheyenne reservations. *ASCO Proceedings , 10,* 89.

Frost, F., Taylor, V., & Fries, E. (1992). Racial misclassification of Native Americans in a surveillance, epidemiology, and end results cancer registry. *Journal of the National Cancer Institute, 84* (12), 957–962.

Hart, B. L., Steinbock, R. T., Mettler, F. A., Pathak, D. R., & Bartow, S.A. (1989). Age and race related changes in mammographic parenchymal patterns. *Cancer, 63,* 2537–2539.

Lanier, A. P., Bulkow, L. R., & Ireland, B. (1989). Cancer in Alaskan Indians, Eskimos, and Aleuts, 1969-83: Implications for etiology and control. *Public Health Reports, 104* (6), 658–664.

Locust, C. S. (1985). *American Indian beliefs concerning health and unwellness* (Native American Research and Training Center Monograph Series). Tuscon, University of Arizona.

Mahoney, M. C., Michalek, A. M., Cummings, K. M., Nasca, P. C., & Emrich, L. J. (1989a). Cancer mortality in a northeastern Native American population. *Cancer, 64,* 187–190.

Mahoney, M. C., Michalek, A. M., Cummings, K. M., Nasca, P. C., & Emrich, L. J. (1989b). Cancer surveillance in a northeastern Native American population. *Cancer, 64,* 191–195.

Michalek, A. M., & Mahoney, M. C. (1990). Cancer in Native populations: Lessons to be learned. *Journal of Cancer Education, 5,* 243–249.

Michalek, A. M., Mahoney, M. C., Cummings, K. M., Hanley, J., & Snyder, R. (1989). Mortality patterns among a Native American population in New York state. *New York State Journal of Medicine, 89,* 557–561.

Olsen, S. J., & Frank-Stromborg, M. (1993). Cancer prevention and early detection in ethnically diverse populations. *Seminars in Oncology Nursing, 9* (3), 198–209.

Orque, M., Bloch, B., & Monroy, L. (1983). *Ethnic nursing care: A multicultural approach*. St. Louis: Mosby.

Pathak, D. R., Pike, M. C., Key, C. R., Teaf, S. R., & Bartow, S. A. (1991). Parity factors and prevalence of fibrocystic breast change in a forensic autopsy series. *British Journal of Cancer, 63* (6), 1005–1009.

Sievers, M. L., Fisher, J. R. (1981). Diseases of North American Indians. In H. Rothschild (Ed.), *Biocultural aspects of disease*. New York: Academic.

Welty, T.K. (1991). Health implications of obesity in American Indians and Alaska Natives. *American Journal of Clinical Nutrition, 53,* 1616–1620.

PART 8 | Activism, Health Policy, and Research

CHAPTER 22 | Breast Cancer Advocacy

Judith Hirshfield-Bartek, RN, MS, OCN

In 1960, the incidence of breast cancer in American women was 1 in 20. Today 12% of the female population, or 1 in 8 women, will develop breast cancer by the age of 84, and 35% will die of their disease (Harris, et al., 1992). The incidence of breast cancer continues to rise with little change in mortality, despite the development of new treatments. Furthermore, medical researchers know little about what causes breast cancer, let alone how to prevent it, or how to cure it. These discouraging facts have united women across the country who have come to realize that federal research funding agencies of this country need to focus more attention on finding the causes, prevention, and ultimately a cure for breast cancer.

Nurses are the largest providers of health care in the United States. As care providers, we are given many opportunities to empower our patients with the information they need to personally fight this disease, and to teach them how to become activists if they so desire. This chapter reviews information about why and

how breast cancer has become a political issue in the United States, discusses nursing advocacy, and suggests avenues for empowering women to become activists about women's health issues.

BREAST CANCER: A SENSE OF URGENCY

Breast cancer is a major public health problem in the United States (Harris, et al., 1992). In 1995, it is projected that over 182,000 women will have been diagnosed with breast cancer (1 every 3 minutes), and 46,000 women will die of this disease (1 every 11 minutes) (American Cancer Society, 1995). Breast cancer is the number-one cancer diagnosed in women and the leading cause of death among American women between the ages of 40 and 55 years. (National Center for Health Statistics, 1990). Over 1.6 million women have survived breast cancer, and another 1 million are predicted to be diagnosed with the disease by the year 2000 (Liotta, 1992).

The incidence, survival, and mortality rates for breast cancer vary among ethnic groups and by age. For example, Caucasian women have a 20% higher incidence of breast cancer than African American women. However, mortality rates for breast cancer among Caucasians are about 16% lower. For all women, breast cancer mortality increased 2.7% from 1973 to 1990, but for African American women, there was over a 17% increase in mortality (Hankey, Brinton, Kessler, & Abrams, 1992). This statistic is compounded by the fact that many women, particularly those in rural settings, do not have equal access to health care services. As a result, detection of breast cancer for undeserved and underinsured women often occurs when the disease is more advanced.

While the mortality rates from breast cancer for women less than 65 years of age have decreased by 5.9%, the rates have increased by 14.7% for women over the age of 65 (Broder, 1993). While many of these statistics about breast cancer are familiar to us as nurses, these startling facts have only recently come to the public's attention.

- The Northeast corridor from Maine to the Mid-Atlantic states has the highest incidence of breast cancer and there are no clues as to why this is happening (NIH 1993a).
- 800,000 women years are lost annually from breast cancer deaths (20 years lost each death x 46,000) (Davis, 1992).
- In 1990, the dollar value of medical care for the nation's breast cancer patients was estimated at over $6 billion. Federal funding for breast cancer research equals only 6.7% of that cost (Brown & Fintor, 1994).
- Since 1960 almost 1 million women have died from breast cancer, more than twice the number of Americans that died in WWI, WWII, the Vietnam War, and the Persian Gulf Wars combined (President's Commission on Veteran's Pension 1956, U.S. Department of Defense, 1992).
- During a 31-month period between 1990 and 1993, the U.S. government spent more on military research than all the monies spent on medical research since the turn of the century (Harkin, personal communication, October 1993).

Health care providers teach women the detection methods that are presently available. Unfortunately, by the time a breast mass is visualized on mammography or palpated by an individual, it has most likely micrometastasized. As women become more educated about breast disease, they realize that there needs to be more than just the "early" detection methods presently available. Women are seeking a more activist role in combating this disease. They also feel a sense of urgency and the need for change in public policy and research priorities at the national level.

BIRTH OF THE BREAST CANCER ADVOCACY MOVEMENT

Despite the increased attention to breast cancer in the political arena over the last few years, the breast cancer movement actually began in the early 1970s. This happened when several prominent women publicly discussed their breast cancers. Shirley Temple Black, former First Lady Betty Ford, and Happy Rockefeller shared their breast cancer experiences with the nation, and thus increased public awareness about the importance of mammography and breast self-examination.

At the same time, Rose Kushner, a journalist, began to publicly question the accepted and commonly practiced one-step biopsy to mastectomy procedure. Kushner had a vision to educate women about breast cancer. She was instrumental in establishing many organizations and programs, including Y-Me, a national breast cancer support group hot line established in 1978, National Breast Cancer

Awareness Week in 1984 (now a month long), and the National Alliance of Breast Cancer Organizations (NABCO) in 1986.

PUBLIC ATTENTION

More recently, the media has focused public attention on the magnitude of breast cancer. Major newspapers and women's journals have published breast cancer issues, including the topics of prevention, environmetal influences, politics, and the need for better early detection methods. The increased level of public information also brings confusion and highlights the fact that little is known about breast cancer. The public has become confused by the conflicting reports they read. For example, the National Cancer Institute's (NCI's) 1994 change in screening mammography guidelines left many women and providers questioning the benefits of mammography for women under age 50, and when a woman should have a baseline mammogram. Conflicting reports in medical and lay literature leave the public wondering about the role of dietary fat or hormone replacement therapy in the development of breast cancer. What is the validity of risk factors for breast cancer, such as age of first pregnancy or age at menarche or menopause? (See Table 22-1).

The anxiety and fear experienced by women with breast cancer were escalated by the barrage of events occurring in early 1994. The National Surgical Adjuvant Breast and Bowel Project (NSABP) and NCI admitted to scientific misconduct among some investigators who were accruing subjects for the partial mastectomy plus radiation therapy versus mastectomy clinical trials. Despite re-analysis of the data and reassurance from the NCI that other research studies supported the results of the NSABP study, many women felt betrayed by the medical establishment. As a result, women throughout the country living with breast cancer worry that the local treatment choice they made could have been based on false information (Visco, 1994).

Women have begun to take charge, seek answers, and ask questions about detection and treatment. They are demanding an active role in the decision-making process. Activists insist that research into the causes of breast cancer be adequately funded. Some activists believe that breast cancer has been ignored because it is a woman's disease and suggest that breast cancer may be the feminist issue of the 1990s (Ferraro, 1993).

In June 1990, a General Accounting Office report revealed that the National Institutes of Health (NIH) was not implementing its policy of including women in clinical trials (Howes & Bass, 1991). This report ignited a fire and, for the first time, the public realized that women's health issues have not been a priority in the research world. The activists contend that something needed to change.

DEVELOPMENT OF THE NATIONAL BREAST CANCER COALITION

Early in 1991, several women joined together to discuss the possibility of a national coalition of breast cancer activists. Amy Langer of NABCO, Susan Love, MD, then director at the Faulkner Breast Center in Boston, and Susan Hester, founder of the Mary Helen Mautner Project for Lesbians with Cancer, met in Washington, D.C., to discuss the development of a national strategy that would unite and mobilize American women against breast cancer. They were angered and dissatisfied by the status quo and felt that women's health issues and breast cancer were not receiving a fair allocation of research dollars in proportion to the magnitude of the problem. Their vision was that women, their families, and anyone who had been touched by breast cancer would join together and create change. Women slowly realized that breast cancer was not just an issue for those living with it, nor is it just a woman's problem. Rather, breast cancer affects all of us.

Women, inspired by the AIDS activists of the 1980s, began to use support groups as a

Table 22-1   Established and Probable Risk Factors for Breast Cancer

Risk Factor	Comparison Category	Typical Risk Category	Relative Risk	Study
Family history of breast cancer	No 1st-degree relatives affected	Mother affected before the age of 60	2.0	Nurses' Health Study[a]
		Mother affected after the age of 60	1.4	Nurses' Health Study[a]
		Two 1st-degree relatives affected	4–6	Gail et al. (1989)
Age at menarche	16 yr	11 yr	1.3	Kampert et al. (1988)
		12 yr	1.3	
		13 yr	1.3	
		14 yr	1.3	
		15 yr	1.1	
Age at birth of 1st child	Before 20 yr	20–24 yr	1.3	White (1987)
		25–29 yr	1.6	
		≥30 yr	1.9	
		Nulliparous	1.9	
Age at menopause	45–54 yr	After 55 yr	1.5	Trichopoulos et al. (1972)
		Before 45 yr	0.7	
		Oophorectomy before 35 yr	0.4	
Benign breast disease	No biopsy or aspiration	Any benign disease	1.5	Willett et al. (1987)
		Proliferation only	2.0	Dupont and Page (1985)
		Atypical hyperplasia	4.0	Dupont and Page (1985)
Radiation	No special exposure	Atomic bomb (100 rad)	3.0	Boice and Monson (1977)
		Repeated fluoroscopy	1.5–2.0	McGregor et al. (1989)
Obesity	10th percentile	90th percentile:		Tretli (1989)
		Age, 30–49 yr	0.8	
		Age, ≥ 50 yr	1.2	
Height	10th percentile	90th percentile:		Tretli (1989)
		Age, 30–49 yr	1.3	
		Age, ≥ 50 yr	1.4	
Oral contraceptive use	Never used	Current use[b]	1.5	Romieu et al. (1989)
		Past use[b]	1.0	
Postmenopausal estrogen-replacement therapy	Never used	Current use all ages	1.4	Colditz et al. (1990)
		Age, <55 yr	1.2	
		Age, 50–59 yr	1.5	
		Age, ≥60 yr	2.1	
		Past use	1.0	
Alcohol use	Nondrinker	1 drink/day	1.4	Longnecker et al. (1988)
		2 drinks/day	1.7	
		3 drinks/day	2.0	

[a]Unpublished prospective data were obtained from Graham Colditz (personal communication).

[b]Relative risks may be higher for women given a diagnosis of breast cancer before the age of 40.

Note. From "Breast Cancer" by J. R. Harris, M. Lippmann, et al., 1992, *New England Journal of Medicine, 327* (5), p. 321.

means to activate a national political advocacy movement. Today, the National Breast Cancer Coalition (NBCC) has grown from a grassroots advocacy effort to more than 250 member organizations, including the American Cancer Society, Y-Me National Organization for Breast Cancer Information and Support, National Alliance of Breast Cancer Organizations, National Women's Health Network, and the Oncology Nursing Society. NABCO represents millions of women, health care professionals, patients, their families, and friends. The mission of the NBCC is to eradicate breast cancer through focusing national attention on the disease and by involving individuals who are advocates for action, advances, and change.

The first major action of the NBCC occurred in September 1991 with 175,000 letters to President Bush and Congress. This number represented the number of women expected to be diagnosed with breast cancer in 1991. The letters called for more attention to breast cancer at the national level. Actually, over 675,000 letters were sent and, for the first time, attracted attention to the urgency of the problem. However, Congressional members seemed to know very little about breast cancer, and believed that mammography was enough to address women's concerns. Congresswomen Patricia Schroeder (D-Colorado) summed up the congressional consensus: "They don't fund what they don't fear, and they don't fear breast cancer." The activists were challenged to educate Congress about breast cancer.

The process began a long hard journey. Governmental funding for breast cancer research is appropriated by Congress. It is a political reality that it is difficult, at best, for committed volunteers to compete with well-paid professional lobbyists. Volunteers, primarily women with breast cancer, walked the halls of Congress only to realize that professional lobbyists had already successfully lobbied the allocation of tax dollars in other directions. Over the past few years, the momentum has changed. Activists succeeded in moving breast cancer from a medical condition to a political issue.

Initially, Congress questioned how much money was actually needed for breast cancer research. In February 1992, the NBCC held open hearings and invited researchers to present their vision for the future of breast cancer research. This was the first time that scientists and activists had come together to discuss breast cancer funding issues. From these hearings, NBCC compiled a "wish list," requesting over $300 million annually to fund breast cancer research into cause, prevention, environmental influences, rehabilitation, psychosocial issues, improved detection, and treatment. This wish list gave the NBCC necessary data to approach Congress with a plan for funding appropriations and spending priorities. The NBCC requested an additional $300 million for fiscal year 1993 to bring the breast cancer budget up to $439 million. Initially, Congress indicated that the request was excessive. NCI officials believed that enough money was being allocated for breast cancer research. However, because 1992 was an election year, Congressional members were highly motivated to support women's health issues. They became keenly interested in learning more about breast cancer.

Senator Tom Harkin, (D-Iowa), whose family members had breast cancer, supported the NBCC mission. Harkin proposed that Congress support an amendment to transfer 1% of the military research budget to the NIH for the express purpose of funding women's health research. However, during the Bush Administration (1989–1993), an agreement between Congress and the President known as the "Fire Wall Agreement" meant that Congress could not tranfer monies from one domestic budget to another. Harkin's Tranfer Amendent was vetoed. Senator Harkin pushed on. After reviewing details of the Department of Defense (DoD) budget, he discovered a line item for "Breast Cancer Programs" that already existed. He went back to Congress and proposed the transfer of 1% of the military research budget to the already existing breast cancer program within the DoD. After much debate, the Harkin Transfer Amendment passed and became a major victory for women. Between 1993 and 1994, the Department of Defense Breast Cancer Research Program received 2,500 applications for breast cancer-related research, and over 950 were awarded funding.

The second major action taken by the NBCC took place in 1993. The strategy was to collect 2.6 million signatures. This number represented the 1.6 million women living with breast cancer and the 1 million who have the disease but don't know it. In October 1993, the NBCC delivered over 2.6 million signatures to President Clinton asking for a national strategy against breast cancer. During the White House ceremony President Clinton stated "...[breast cancer] is not only tearing the heart out of so many families, but also has left us again with no excuse for why we would spend so much money picking up the pieces of broken lives when we could spend a little bit of money trying to save them." Secretary of Health and Human Services Donna Shalala offered the Administration's commitment to plan a national strategy, calling for a coordinated effort between the Administration, Congress, and the scientific community. The first step in this process began in December 1993 when experts joined activists to begin planning a National Strategy (NIH, 1993b).

Clearly, progress has occurred since women voiced their concerns about the need for more breast cancer research. As activists have been recognized for their accomplishments, they have become concerned about additional areas related to women's health. Access to health care has become a major part of the NBCC agenda. Equal access to the health care system for diagnosis, treatment, and clinical trials must be addressed. The impact of changes in the health care industry due to managed care programs, rationing of services, and health care reform is particularly important for the millions of underserved and uninsured women in the United States.

Another area of great concern is the exploding field of human genetics. With the discovery of the BRCA1 susceptibility gene, legal safeguards must be in place that protect women from insurance and employment discrimination. It is crucial that the activists be involved in the Ethical, Legal, and Social Implications (ELSI) Task Force within the National Center for Human Genome Research and the Breast Cancer Hereditary Susceptibility Working Group of the National Action Plan to address these concerns before widespread public testing is made available. These and other issues make it even more important that informed consumers participate in the process and be actively involved in health care delivery decisions.

EMPOWERMENT THROUGH POLITICAL ACTIVISM

Some women surviving breast cancer believe that the only cure for breast cancer is political action. Most of the women who have become involved were amateurs at activism; however, the energy that drives them is hope and anger.

Involvement as an activist helps women with breast cancer feel supported at a time when their lives may seem out of control. One NBCC member stated, "When I was first diagnosed with breast cancer I was scared . . . but when I started working with the Coalition, I began to have hope . . . hope for the future." (Osimo, 1993). Another woman who was nearing the end of her battle against breast cancer wanted to feel she could contribute toward lobbying efforts. Homebound, she was asked to count and bundle petitions from Massachusetts, which would be delivered to President Clinton. Her daughter explained that this activity gave her mother a feeling of dignity and worth even when everything else was falling apart.

Women who have breast cancer are motivated to become activists for change not out of concern for themselves, but because of the knowledge that their daughters, the next generation, may be faced with an even greater threat of developing this disease. Artist Hollis Sigler expressed her feelings about her own breast cancer in an exhibition at the National Museum for Women in the Arts entitled "Walking with the Ghosts of My Grandmother." Many of her paintings captured the empowerment women feel through activism.

TEACHING WOMEN ABOUT ACTIVISM

What can we do to teach women about activism? In reality, activism is about exercising rights as American citizens. The Constitution makes this possible. Oncology nurses can teach women to become activists. Nurses should view this role as a new and unique dimension of patient advocacy. As nurses, we look at many issues that affect patient care, and help patients acquire the knowledge they need to make decisions. The power women achieve when they learn how to become activists is immeasureable. They are empowered when they feel their efforts may change the future. For many women, activism is a healing experience.

There is no one "typical" breast cancer activist. Activism crosses lifespans because breast cancer is an "equal opportunity" disease cutting across socioeconomic, educational, and racial lines.

Nurses might consider developing an action network within their locale. An action network links individuals with information and provides a way to contact their congressperson. Developing such an action network can be both enjoyable and challenging. Often it involves breaking the barriers that hold individuals back from calling a state representative or member of Congress. People often don't realize how important their voices can be. Nurses can encourage others to exercise their constitutional rights. Following a few easy steps can help accomplish this goal.

- The NBCC national office is a good number to keep handy. Staff members can give you the name of the State Coordinator. They can become the contact person and can provide you with up-to-date information about NBCC activities and pending national and state legislation.

- Select an area on the nursing unit or ambulatory care center to post information about local and national activities. Include brochures about legislative alerts and what action needs to be taken. For example, if people are asked to call or write their legislator about a particular issue, it's helpful to have specific information available. Post the name of a contact person who can answer questions.
- Make sure information is made available for feedback of the action and suggestions for the next action. People want to know that their efforts were worthwhile. This encourages them to act on a legislative alert in the future.
- Network with other health care services, especially if they are breast centers or women's health centers, to see if other health care professionals are interested in information on political advocacy.
- Work with grassroots organizations to develop a statewide telephone chain that can be activated within 24 hours. The NBCC can provide a list of members within one's state. Discuss the possibility of a call-in "Hot Line" that will bring up-to-date local information to individuals.
- Obtain a copy of the *US Congress Handbook*, which is published annually. The address is Box 566, McLean, VA 22101, Phone: (800) 229-3572. This book includes information about all members of Congress and the committees on which they serve.
- Contact local newspapers and television stations, particularly if there is a local event planned around breast cancer. Encourage the media to run stories about women's health issues.
- Use this resource list:
  National Breast Cancer Coalition (202) 296-7477
  National Alliance of Breast Cancer Organizations (212) 719-0154

Y-Me National Organization for Breast Cancer Information and Support
(800) 221-2141
National Women's Health Network
(202) 347-1140
White House Comment Line
(202) 456-1111
Washington Congressional Switchboard for Phone Numbers of Congress
(202) 224-3121

CONCLUSION

Women across the United States are tired of the status quo and finally realize that a change in public policy about women's health issues is needed. Grassroots advocacy groups such as the NBCC have gained momentum in the political arena as a voice for change. Professional nurses can encourage and help women, their friends, and families become involved as activists and view this as an important dimension to our role as patient advocates. As Margaret Meade observed, "Never doubt that a small group of thoughtful, committed citizens can change the world. Indeed it's the only thing that ever does."

ACKNOWLEDGMENT

To all the courageous women with breast cancer who have taught me about life, living, and speaking out.

References

American Cancer Society. (1995). *Facts and figures 1995.* Atlanta: American Cancer Society, Inc.

Avery, B. (1994). President National Black Women's Health Project, Statement at Mass Leadership Summit: The Challenge of Breast Cancer. Boston, May.

Boice, J.D., Jr., Monson, R.R. (1977). Breast cancer in women after repeated fluoroscopic examinations of the chest. *Journal of the National Cancer Institute, 59,* 799–811.

Broder, S. (1993). *1995 Budget estimate National Cancer Institute,* pp. 22–23, 133 NCI, September.

Brown, M., & Fintor, L. (1994).The economic burden of cancer. In P. Greenwald, B. Kramer, & D. Weed (Eds.), *Cancer prevention and control.* Marcel-Dekker.

Colditz, G. A., Stampfer, M. J., Willett, W. C., Hennekens, C. H., Rosner, B., & Speizer, F. E. (1990). Prospective study of estrogen replacement therapy and risk of breast cancer in postmenopausal women. *Journal of the American Medical Association, 264,* 2648–2653.

Davis, D. L. (1992). *Testimony Before the National Breast Cancer Coalition.* Washington, DC: Marcel-Dekker. February.

Dupont, W. D., & Page, D. (1985). Risk factors for breast cancer in women with proliferative breast disease. *New England Journal of Medicine, 312,* 146–151.

Ferraro, S. (1993). The anguished politics of breast cancer, *New York Times Magazine, 15,* 25.

Gail, M. H., Brinton, L. A., Byar, D. P., et al. (1989). Projecting individualized probabilities of developing breast cancer for white females who are being examined annually. *Journal of the National Cancer Institute, 81,* 1870–1886.

Hankey, B., Brinton, L., Kessler, L., & Abrams, J., (1992). *SEER Cancer Statistics Review 1973–90.* NIH NCI Section IV Breast, pp. 1–24.

Harkin, T. (1993). Personal communication, October.

Harris, J. R., Lippmann, M. et al. (1992). Breast cancer. *New England Journal of Medicine, 327,* 319–328.

Healy, B. (1991). Statement before the House Committee on Government Operation Subcommittee on Human Resources and Intergovernmental Relations, Dec. 11.

Howes, J., & Bass, M., (1991). Women's health research prescription for life, *Annual Report: Society for the Advancement of Women's Research.* Washington, DC.

Institute of Medicine. (1993). *Strategies for managing the breast cancer research program.* Washington, DC: National Academy Press.

Kampert, J. B., Whittemore, A. S., Paffenbarger, & R. S., Jr. (1988). Combined effect of childbearing, menstrual events, and body size on age-specific breast cancer risk. *American Journal of Epidemiology, 128,* 962–979.

Liotta, L. (1992). *Testimony Before President's Cancer Panel on Breast Cancer.* Bethesda, Maryland. May.

Longnecker, M. P., Berlin, J. A., Orza, M. J., & Chalmers, T. C. (1988). A meta-analysis of alcohol consumption in relation to risk of breast cancer. *Journal of the American Medical Association, 260,* 652–656.

Love, S. (1992). Proceedings—Opportunities for research on women's health. Hunt Valley. National Institutes of Health. Maryland Sept 1-4 ,1991 NIH Publication no. 92-3459 Sept 1992. p186.

McGregor, H., Land, C. E., Choi, K., et al., (1989). Breast cancer incidence among atomic bomb survivors, Hiroshima and Nagasaki, 1950–69. *Journal of the National Cancer Institute, 81,* 1313–1321.

Miller, B., Feuer, E., & Hankey, B. (1994). The significance of the rising incidence in the United States. In *Important advances in oncology.* V. DeVita, S. Hellman, & S. Rosenberg, (Eds.). Philadelphia: J.B. Lippincott Company, P. 193.

National Center for Health Statistics. (1990). Vital statistics of the U.S., 1987. Vol. 2. Mortality, Part A. Washington DC: U.S. Government Printing Office, DHHS Publication No. (PHS) 90–1101.

National Institutes of Health. (1993a). Breast cancer in the northeastern and middle Atlantic United States. *NIH Guide, 22* (2) pg. 1, Publication No. 93–39.

National Institutes of Health. (1993b). Proceedings: Secretary's conference to establish a national action plan on breast cancer. December 14-15.

National Institutes of Health. (1993c). *National Cancer Institute Breast Cancer Research and Programs.* U.S. Department of Health and Human Services, May, pg. 24.

Osimo, C. (1993). Breast cancer survivor, Personal communication.

President's Cancer Panel Special Commission on Breast Cancer. (1993). Breast cancer: A national strategy. A report to the nation. National Institutes of Health, *NCI,* October.

President's Commission on Veteran's Pension. (1956). Veteran's benefits in the U.S. Vol. 1.

Romieu, I., Willett, W. C., Colditz, G. A. et al. (1989). Prospective study of oral contraceptive use and the risk of breast cancer in women. *Journal of the National Cancer Institute, 81,* 1313–1321.

Tretli, S. (1989). Height and weight in relation to breast cancer morbidity and mortality: A prospective study of 570,000 women in Norway. *International Journal of Cancer, 44,* 23–30.

Trichopoulos, D., MacMahon, B., & Cole, P. (1972). Menopause and breast cancer risk. *Journal of the National Cancer Institute, 48,* 605–613.

U.S. Department of Defense. (1992). Statistical abstract of the U.S. 112th ed.

Visco, F., (1994). President, National Breast Cancer Coalition, Testimony before Energy and Commerce Subcommittee on Oversight and Investigations of NSABP Fraud, April 13.

White, E. (1987). Projected changes in breast cancer incidence due to the trend toward delayed childbearing. *American Journal of Public Health, 77,* 495–497.

Willett, W. C., Stampfer, M. J., Colditz, G. A., Rosner, B. A., Hennekens, C. H., & Speitzer, F. E. (1987). Dietary fat and the risk of breast cancer. *New England Journal of Medicine, 316,* 22–28.

CHAPTER 23 | Health Policy and Breast Cancer

Deborah K. Mayer, RN, MSN, AOCN, FAAN

Health care policy has a major effect on breast cancer care and research. Understanding what health policy is and how it is formulated and implemented is an important first step in influencing it. Nurses can influence health policy development in a variety of ways, from involvement in local issues affecting cancer to conducting research to political activism. This chapter reviews public health policy formulation, uses screening mammography as an example of how health policy influences breast cancer care and research, and, finally, identifies ways in which nurses can influence health policy.

HEALTH POLICY FORMULATION

Public health policy formulation is "the way in which issues are raised on the public agenda, the process by which laws are passed committing resources to programs that affect people; the development of withdrawal rules and regulations that interpret laws; the pro-

cess of program development; and the evaluation of the usefulness of the program" (Abdellah, 1991, p.4). Current federal government health policies affect health care providers because federal programs pay for care of the poor, elderly, and disabled; support training of health care providers; fund research; and provide capital support for health care facilities (Abdellah, p.7).

According to Davis (1988), health policy processes include identifying values and issues that guide policy direction, while policy making includes analysis of various data about the problem and the possible solutions. Resultant public policy becomes official through law and regulations. The effects of the policy should be evaluated on a variety of levels of impact (e.g., social and economic) and revised as needed. Screening mammography is just one example of the many breast cancer specific complex health policy issues.

Policy analysis is political argument and vice versa. "Ideas are a medium of exchange and a mode of influence even more powerful than money and votes and guns" (Stone, 1988, p. 306). "Shared meanings motivate people to action and meld individual striving into collective action. Ideas are at the center of all political conflict. Policy making, in turn, is a constant struggle over the criteria for classification, the boundaries of categories, and the definition of ideals that guide the way people behave" (Stone, p. 7). Policy making is an active, ever-evolving process influenced by and affecting many groups and individuals. Our values are influenced by social and economic issues, which, in turn, influence political processes, which develop our social and health care policies. For example, oncology nurses have witnessed and been a part of the political arguments surrounding health care and breast cancer.

Resource allocation is a political activity because it reflects the struggle over ideas, principles, and priorities (National Cancer Advisory Board, 1994). Resource allocation in health care and cancer has been an explicit reflection of implicit values. Take for example, one's own ideas and values about the myriad of ways to allocate cancer-related resources: How would one go about allocation—by disease type? incidence? mortality? gender? age? race or ethnic group? type of treatment? Health policy attempts to address these issues. However, the debates, both public and private, help shape not only the definition of the problem, but also possible solutions as well.

ANATOMY OF A HEALTH POLICY ISSUE: SCREENING MAMMOGRAPHY

Breast cancer screening with routine mammography has been the focus of much heated debate about health policy resource, development, and implementation (DeBor, 1993; Horsch & Willson, 1993). A brief review of screening mammography reveals how health policy influences breast cancer issues. Since

the first breast radiography was made in 1901, imaging techniques have developed dramatically (Feig, 1993). Two landmark studies, the Health Insurance Plan of Greater New York (HIP) and the Breast Cancer Detection Demonstration Project (BCDDP), conducted in the late 1960s and early 1970s, established screening mammography as a valid means for detecting breast cancer at an earlier stage. Detecting smaller tumors in the absence of lymph node involvement correlates with a higher survival rate (Feig, 1993). It was therefore concluded that widespread use of screening mammography should contribute to the overall reduction of breast cancer mortality. Based on this premise, why have we not seen an anticipated reduction in overall mortality from breast cancer? What are the health policy issues and how have these issues affected the debate and controversies over screening mammography?

Many clinical studies have been conducted on screening mammography, which has led to the general acceptance of a 30% mortality reduction if mammography is used on a regular basis for women over 50 years of age (a relatively arbitrary year chosen to represent a cutoff between pre- and postmenopausal women). The survival data for women under the age of 50 remain more controversial because a similar endpoint of mortality reduction has yet to be realized. The first recommended guidelines for screening mammography were established during the 1977 National Cancer Institute Breast Cancer Consensus Development Conference.

In 1987, the American College of Radiology hosted meetings with eleven other organizations to promote uniform guidelines on this topic. These guidelines included annual screening for women over 50 years of age. Although imperfect, screening mammography is currently the best technology available for reducing breast cancer mortality (Love, 1994).

Why is it that annual mammograms for women over age 50 are still not routinely used? It appears that having guidelines issued by health professionals is not enough to influence health policy or clinical practice (Hamwi, 1990). Other factors influencing a woman's decision to obtain a mammogram include insurance coverage, access, and mammogram quality issues. These factors are discussed below.

Insurance coverage has not been routinely provided for screening mammography, making cost a significant barrier. Biennial coverage of screening mammography only began for Medicare recipients in 1991. By 1992, 42 states had legislation requiring some form of private health insurance coverage for screening mam-

also
ven-
ncer
for
de-
am-
this

gra-
igh
be-
her
nan
of
Ef-
een
of
io-
nd
for
to
Re-
nit-
to
ey,
&
or,
ed
te
es

Third, the *quality of mammography* varies widely throughout the country in both image and radiation dose. The effectiveness of screen-

ing mammography will be altered if adequate quality cannot be assured (Hendrick, 1993). As a result of studies documenting problems with consistent-quality mammograms, the American College of Radiology (ACR) established a voluntary Mammography Accreditation Program (MAP) in 1987. This program, paid for by the mammography unit seeking certification, consists of a site survey questionnaire, an assessment of clinical images, and image quality and measurement of radiation dose during the procedure. As of January 1993, 75% to 80% of mammography sites have been or are in the process of becoming accredited by the MAP (Hendrick, 1993).

Legislative acts that dealt with screening mammography also addressed some of these quality assurance issues (e.g., any place providing Medicare-funded mammography had to meet certain criteria); however, it wasn't until 1992 that the Mammography Quality Standards Act (MQSA) was passed. The MQSA, instituted in 1994, superseded other legislation and is mandatory for all screening and diagnostic mammography units or sites regardless of funding sources or populations studied. Unfortunately, funding has not been provided to institute this piece of legislation.

In summary, technology is available that, theoretically, can reduce breast cancer mortality if uniformly applied across the United States. Tangible reductions in mortality should become apparent within 5 to 10 years if good-quality mammography is routinely administered. For that goal to become a reality, a complex array of factors, including beliefs, attitudes, perceptions of women, and physician-patient interactions as they relate to mammography need to be understood (White et al., 1993). Most of these factors will require some form of health policy research and policy development to identify the best strategies to increase utilization. A 1993 national strategic plan for early detection and control of breast and cervical cancers has been developed as a joint effort of the CDC, FDA, and NCI to begin addressing some of these issues. From this brief review of screening mammography within a health policy context, it is apparent that much more research is needed.

HEALTH POLICY AND NURSING

Nurses can contribute to health policy formulation in many ways, affecting individuals at the local, regional, or national level. Contributions include conducting research, participating at the local level in health policy issues, and promoting political activism.

Research is one of the major ways in which nursing can shape public and health care policy (Hinshaw, 1988; Nagelkerk & Henry, 1991). Nurses have contributed to our knowledge about breast cancer, which in turn, has contributed to health policy development. The chapter by Coleman in this book outlines the many research studies on breast cancer conducted by nurses.

Becoming involved at the local level includes documenting the effects of policy on women with breast cancer and being aware of other practices available for advocating for a change in services. Another way to be involved is identifying the variations in insurance reimbursement for other treatments, for example, bone marrow transplantation (Peters & Rogers, 1994). Support for breast cancer advocacy through involvement in the many breast cancer advocacy and activist groups is another way in which nurses can affect health policy (President's Cancer Panel Special Commission on Breast Cancer, 1993). Participation on committees or boards can help shape the debate.

Third, becoming involved in the political process and showing support for activism is another way in which nurses can greatly influence health policy (Gray, Doan, & Church, 1991; Wachter, 1992). Unfortunately, many nurses underestimate their personal influence as constitutents and underuse their tremendous clinical expertise in relationship to health policy. In an earlier chapter, Hirshfield-Bartek outlines ways in which nurses can become involved with legislative issues affecting breast cancer health policy.

CONCLUSION

The public debate about breast cancer is an ongoing way to explore and define society's values regarding breast cancer and health care. Nurses must continually articulate their values in society. Nursing's values, as documented in the American Nurses Association Social Policy Statement (1980), include:

- belief in the individual's right to health care;
- belief in humanistic health care;
- belief in the individual's responsibility for his or her own health care;
- belief in the provision of health care by the best qualified practitioner.

Davis (1988) recommends implementing a values-policy model within nursing by presenting a unified nursing front, by serving as advocates for the underprivileged, by demonstrating cost-effect services, and by developing innovative and humanistic nursing approaches that are responsive to a competitive health care system.

References

Abdellah, F. (1991). Nursing's role in the future: The case for health policy decision making. Sigma Theta Tau Monograph Series #91. Indianapolis, IN: Center Nursing Press of Sigma Theta Tau International.

American Nurses Association. (1980). A social policy statement. Kansas City, MO: The association.

Davis, G. (1988). Nursing values and health care policy. *Nursing Outlook, 36,* 289–292.

DeBor, M. (1993). What do women do now? *Cancer, 72,* 1486–1489.

Feig, S. (1993). Mammographic screening: An historical perspective. *Seminars in Roentgenology, 28,*193–203.

Gray, R., Doan, B., & Church, K. (1991). Empowerment issues in cancer. *Health Values, 15,* 22–28.

Hamwi, D. (1990). Screening mammography: Increasing the effort toward breast cancer detection. *Nurse Practitioner, 16,* 27–32.

Hendrick, R. (1993). Mammography quality assurance: Current issues. *Cancer, 72* (Suppl 4), 1466–1474.

Hinshaw, A. (1988). Using research to shape health policy. *Nursing Outlook, 36,* 21–24.

Horsch, K., & Willson, K. (1993). Legislative issues related to breast cancer. *Cancer, 72,* 1483–1485.

Hurley, S., Jolley, D., Livingston, P., Reading, D., Cockburn, J., & Flint-Richter, D. (1992). Effectiveness, costs, and cost-effectiveness of recruitment strategies for a mammographic screening program to detect breast cancer. *Journal of the National Cancer Institute, 84,* 855–863.

Love, S. (1994). Truth behind mammogram dispute. *LA Times,* March 16.

Nagelkerk, J., & Henry, B. (1991). Leadership through policy research. *Journal of Nursing Administration, 21,* 20–24.

National Cancer Advisory Board. (1994). Report to Congress on the Evaluation of the National Cancer Program. Bethesda, MD.

National Strategic Plan for the Early Detection and Control of Breast and Cervical Cancers. (1993). US Department of Health and Human Services: CDC, FDA, and NCI.

Peters, W., & Rogers, M. (1994). Variation in approval by insurance companies of coverage for autologous bone marrow transplantation for breast cancer. *New England Journal of Medicine, 330,* 473–477.

President's Cancer Panel Special Commission on Breast Cancer. (1993). Breast cancer: A national strategy: A report to the nation. Bethesda, MD: National Institutes of Health.

Romans, M. C. (1993). Utlization of mammography: Social and behavioral trends. *Cancer, 72* (Suppl 4), 1475–1477.

Stone, D. (1988). *Policy paradox and political reason.* Boston: Scott, Foresman & Co.

Wachter, R. (1992). AIDS, activism and the politics of health. *New England Journal of Medicine, 326,* 128–133.

White, E., Urban, N., & Taylor, V. (1993). Mammography utilization, public health impact, and cost effectiveness in the United States. *Annual Review of Public Health, 14,* 605–633.

CHAPTER 24 | Breast Cancer Research
History and Opportunities

Elizabeth Ann Coleman, PhD, RNP, AOCN
Karen Hassey Dow, PhD, RN, FAAN

In recent years, breast cancer researchers have made advances in biology, epidemiology, diagnosis, and treatment. One of the most significant findings in the area of biology was the identification of the breast cancer gene, which may be responsible for 5% of all breast cancers (Hall et al., 1990). In addition, researchers have identified new prognostic markers to aid in the treatment of the disease (Chen et al., 1991; Clark, Dressler, Owens, Pounds, Oldaker, & McGuire, 1989; Slamon, Clark, Wong, Levin, Ullrich, & McGuire, 1987; Folkman, 1990; Steeg, et al., 1988; Tandom, Clark, Chamness, Chirgwin, & McGuire, 1990).

Significant epidemiologic research findings include the mounting evidence to support mass breast cancer screening with mammography for women age 50 and older (Fletcher, Black, Harris, Rimer, & Shapiro, 1993) and the apparent lack of evidence to support mammographic screening for women age 40 to 49 years (Elwood, Cox, & Richardson, 1993). There is also a suggestive association between organochlorine insecticides in the environment and the food chain and an increase in breast cancer risk (Hunter & Kelsey, 1993); and statistics that indicate lower survival rates for African American women than for Caucasian women (Coates et al., 1992; Howard et al., 1992).

Study results pertinent to diagnosis and treatment include findings that the type of surgical treatment for breast cancer varies by geographical region (Coleman, Kessler, Wun, & Feuer, 1992; Nattinger, Gottlieb, Veum, Yahnke, & Goodwin, 1992); the advantage of combining radiation therapy with breast-conserving surgery for the treatment of intraductal breast cancer (Fisher et al., 1993); and the use of bone marrow transplantation in the treatment of breast cancer (Peters et al., 1993).

Research investigations are ongoing in evaluating hormonal (Pike, Bernstein, & Spicer, 1993) and dietary risk factors (Howe, Friedenreich, Jain, & Miller, 1991; Mills, Beeson, Phillips, & Fraser, 1989); breast implants and the risk of systemic diseases (Coleman, Lennon, Rudki, Depuy, & Baker, 1994; Gabriel, O'Fallon, Kurland, Beard, Woods, & Melton, 1994); and the development of chemopreventive agents (Nayfield, Karp, Ford, Dorr, & Kramer, 1991).

A REVIEW OF BREAST CANCER STUDIES CONDUCTED BY NURSES: 1970s TO 1990s

Methods

Two methods were used for reviewing breast cancer studies conducted by nurses during the last 20 years. A literature search was conducted using Medline, CINAHL, Health, AIDSline, and Cancerlit data bases as well as the Sigma Theta Tau electronic library. To include as wide a network of articles as possible in the literature searches, breast neoplasms were referenced by cancer nursing or nursing research journals. Second, interviews were conducted with personnel from the National Institute for Nursing Research (NINR), the National Cancer Institute (NCI), and the Oncology Nursing Society. When interviews with the various agency personnel or professional organization members indicated the need, articles from journals other than nursing were also included in this review. Otherwise, a search among journals other than nursing was not conducted because it would have been nearly impossible to identify all nursing authors.

Results

The review of *Oncology Nursing Forum* (n=31), *Cancer Nursing* (n=20), *Nursing Research* (n=18), *Research in Nursing and Health* (n=8), *Western Journal of Nursing Research* (n=3), *Image* (n=2), *Journal of Public Health Nursing* (n=2), *Applied Nursing Research* (n=1), *Journal of Advanced Nursing* (n=1), *Journal of Holistic Nursing* (n=1), and *Journal of Nursing Quality Assurance* (n=1) yielded a total of 88 articles. A review of ten articles from journals in fields other than nursing were also included because nurses had a significant role in conducting and reporting on the research results.

The studies were grouped into six areas: prevention, risk factors, screening/early detection, diagnosis, treatment, and rehabilitation.

Prevention. None of the studies addressed the prevention of breast cancer.

Risk Factors. Two studies dealt with the laterality of breast cancer and the association of handedness (Kramer, Albrecht, & Miller, 1985; London & Albrecht, 1991) and season of birth (Albrecht & London, 1990).

Screening. The overwhelming majority of studies focused on early detection, and nearly all of the studies addressed breast self-examination (BSE) practices. Most often, nurse researchers used the Health Belief Model in descriptive correlational studies (Champion, 1992; Champion, 1991; Champion, 1990; Glenn & Moore, 1990; Wyper, 1990; Champion, 1988; Rutledge & Davis, 1988; Champion, 1987; Rutledge, 1987; Massey, 1986; Champion, 1985; Hallal, 1982; Hirshfield-Bartek, 1982; Schlueter, 1982; Trotta, 1980; Stillman, 1977). One study sought to refine an instrument to measure the Health Belief Model using the context of breast cancer and BSE (Champion, 1993), and another researcher developed a questionnaire to measure beliefs and attitudes about BSE (Lauver & Angerame, 1988).

The review included studies of BSE among African American women (Nemcek, 1989), rural populations (Gray, 1990), women older than 35 years versus women younger than 35 (Turnbull, 1978), women age 80 years and older (Lierman, Kasprzyk, & Benoliel, 1991; Williams, 1988), and Hispanic women (Longman, Saint-Germain, & Modiano, 1992). A few studies focused on the nurse's role in BSE: the ability of nurses to detect nodules in silicone breast models (Haughey, Marshall, Mettlin, Nemoto, Kroldart, & Swanson, 1984) and the nurses' knowledge of BSE and personal practices in teaching the elderly to perform BSE (Ludwick, 1992). One study used husbands as health educators (Rose et al., 1980), and another discussed health teaching in the workplace (Brailey, 1986).

One study correlated reported practices and proficiency of BSE with stage of breast cancer at diagnosis (Haughey, Marshall Nemoto, Kroldart, Mettlin, & Swanson, 1988). Two researchers produced a performance scoring tool for BSE research and a check list for teaching BSE and evaluating BSE performance in clinical practice (Coleman & Pennypacker, 1991a, 1991b).

A few studies examined the predictors of more than the one component of breast cancer screening, such as BSE and mammography (Champion, 1991; Coleman, Feuer, & the NCI Breast Cancer Screening Consortium, 1992; Kurtz, Given, Given, & Kurtz, 1993; Wehrwein & Eddy, 1993). Only one reported study focused on mammography and the nurse's influence on patient behavior (Mandelblatt et al., 1993), even though research has demonstrated a reduction of up to 30% in mortality among women older than 50 years with a screening mammogram. The one study by Mandelblatt et al. demonstrated a significant increase in mammography use among women seen by nurse practitioners compared with the mammography use among women followed in a physician-reminder system.

A few intervention studies addressed the need to reduce the barriers to breast cancer screening, especially among the elderly and medically underserved populations (Ansell, Lacey, Whitman, Chen, & Phillips, 1994; Coleman, Lord, Bowie, & Worley, 1993; Fintor, Coleman, Debor, Gibson, & Sutton, 1994). Some studies investigated the effectiveness of different BSE educational methods (Coleman, Riley, Fields, & Prior, 1991; Edwards, 1980; Kuhns-Hastings, Brakey, & Marshall, 1993; Lauver, 1989).

Diagnosis.   Two studies focused on anxiety and critical thinking during breast biopsy and care-seeking behaviors for breast lumps (Lierman, 1988; Scott, 1983). One study investigated the relationship between commitments, uncertainty about the cancer situation, threat of recurrence, and control of the cancer situation and the coping strategies that the women used (Hilton, 1989). Another study examined how care-seeking behaviors varied by racial differences (Lauver, 1992).

Two studies, using Roy's Adaptation Model, developed a framework for studying functional status after diagnosis of breast cancer

(Tulman, Fawcett, & McEvoy, 1991; Tulman & Fawcett, 1990). Two other researchers studied the adjustment of patients and their husbands to the initial impact of breast cancer on their lives (Northouse & Swain, 1987).

Treatment.   Three studies looked at informational needs, decision-making behaviors, choice for breast-conserving surgery over mastectomy, and psychosocial needs of women choosing breastconserving surgery (Cawley, Kostic, & Cappello, 1990; Pierce, 1993; Ward, Heidrich, & Wolberg, 1989). One study resulted in an instrument that tests a woman's knowledge of surgical treatment options for early-stage breast cancer (Ward & Griffin, 1990). Cimprich (1992) studied attentional fatigue following breast cancer surgery and subsequently tested interventions to restore attention in cancer patients (Cimprich, 1993).

Studies of symptom management during treatment included pain in advanced cancer (Arathuzik, 1991a; Arathuzik, 1991b), management of hypercalcemia (Meriney, 1990), the effectiveness of scalp hypothermia in preventing cyclophosphamide-induced alopecia (Parker, 1987), and correlates of fatigue (Blesch et al., 1991). Several researchers focused on self-care patterns during cancer treatment (Dodd, 1988; Dodd, 1984).

Other studies focused on information seeking during chemotherapy (Hopkins, 1986), self-care activities while receiving chemotherapy (Nail, Jones, Greene, Shipper, & Jensen, 1991), the professional support and information received by a group of 100 patients in Finland (Suominen, 1992), and issues affecting Indian women with breast cancer (David, Roul, & Kuruvilla, 1988). Patients' reactions to completing treatment (Ward, Viergutz, Tormey, deMuth, & Paulen, 1992), demands of illness among younger women (Loveys & Klaich, 1991), symptom distress (Ehlke, 1988), and hopelessness (Brandt, 1987) were the foci of other studies.

Rehabilitation.   Several studies spanning the period from 1978 to 1990 focused on the issue of weight gain during adjuvant chemotherapy. These included early descriptions of weight gain (Dixon, Moritz, & Baker 1978; Foltz, 1985; Knobf, Mullen, Xistris, & Moritz, 1983), factors affecting weight gain (DeGeorge, Gray, Fetting, & Rolls, 1990), and food intake of women (Grindel, Cahill, & Walker, 1989).

Another group of researchers sought to determine the effects of aerobic interval training in improving the functional capacity of breast cancer patients on adjuvant chemotherapy (MacVicar, Winningham, & Nickel, 1989; Winningham, MacVicar, Bondoc, Anderson, & Minton, 1989), decreasing reports of nausea (Winningham & MacVicar, 1988), and improving the quality of life (Young-McCaughan & Sexton, 1991). Nelson (1991) studied perceived health, self-esteem, health habits, and perceived benefits and barriers to exercise in women who have and who have not experienced stage I breast cancer.

Other researchers discussed a wide range of topics, including threat of recurrence (Hilton, 1989); spiritual well-being (Mickley, Soeken, & Belcher 1992); health within illness (Moch, 1990); self-transcendence and emotional well-being (Coward, 1991); demands of illness, social support, and psychological adjustment (Heidrich & Ward, 1989); longitudinal adjustment to breast cancer (Krouse & Krouse, 1982); and life change loss and stress and breast cancer (Simmons, 1984). One study developed a quality of life instrument that would account for individual values as well as satisfaction (Ferrans, 1990).

Another study measured the relationships among social support, attitudes toward mastectomy, and self-esteem in women post-mastectomy (Feather & Wainstock, 1989a, 1989b). One study dealt with social support and adjustment of women cured of breast cancer and their perceived quality of life (Woods & Earp, 1978).

Several researchers described the care needs of home-based cancer patients and their caregivers with quantitative methods (Longman, Atwood, Sherman, Benedict, & Shang, 1992). Other researchers used qualita-

tive methods to describe the impact of breast cancer on patients and their husbands (Wilson & Morse, 1991; Northouse, 1988; Northouse, 1989a, 1989b), and how children cope with their mother's breast cancer (Issel, Ersek, & Lewis, 1990). Another study described the mental health (depression), symptoms, and functional status of breast cancer patients, and the mental health (depression) and reaction to care of their caregivers (Given & Given, 1992).

Two researchers tested the addition of coaching by a caring partner to support groups on enhancing the adaptation to breast cancer (Samarel & Fawcett, 1992); others studying social support for women during chronic illness found that women perceived more support from their partners than from any other sources (Primomo, Yates, & Woods, 1990).

GAPS IN RESEARCH KNOWLEDGE

While we have learned a great deal about breast cancer in both the basic and applied sciences over the past 20 years, there are significant areas where there are gaps in research knowledge. For example, in the area of cancer biology, there is a need to address the natural history of premalignant disease; the differences in breast cancer biology among pre- and postmenopausal women; and the contribution of changes in the structure or regulation of oncogenes, tumor suppressor genes, and other important cellular genes to the development and biologic behavior of breast cancer.

Epidemiologic research has yielded several risk factors for breast cancer. Yet, these known factors account for only a small part of the diagnosed breast cancers, and 70% of women with breast cancer have no known risk factors. There is a great need for epidemiologic studies that look for other risk factors and that use better methods to identify the women at high risk. More work should address understanding the role of exogenous hormones, diet, and environmental factors in breast cancer etiology.

In the area of screening and early detection, there is need for studies in the following areas:

In the United States, there is a need for population-based prospective studies that address the difference in the biology of screen-detected and non–screened-detected cases; the difference in the clinical management and outcome between screen-detected and non–screened-detected cases; genetic differences among women with breast cancer detected through screening and those with breast cancer not detected through screening; significant variability in the predictive value of screening mammography; the effect of screening on shift-in-stage distribution and on mortality in the population within target age groups; and coverage and compliance with screening programs. We need studies on the effectiveness of BSE and physical examination of the breast as well as mammography. Linking screening facilities with pathology laboratories with quality-controlled, population-based cancer registries would also facilitate research.

There is a need for studies that improve treatment, and, in the area of rehabilitation, better reconstructive methods, especially in light of questionable problems with breast implants and the number of women having mastectomies, are also needed. Furthermore, studies on quality of life issues and reproductive issues for younger women are paramount. Finally, as cost becomes more important, studies are needed to consider the cost effectiveness of interventions in any of these areas of breast cancer research.

NURSES' ROLES IN FUTURE BREAST CANCER RESEARCH

The following discussion offers some suggested areas in which nurses could take a significant role. We will consider each of the following areas as in the review of the literature: prevention, risk factors, screening/early detection, diagnosis, treatment, and rehabilitation.

In the area of prevention, nurses could conduct intervention studies on established risk factors that a woman can modify or eliminate. For example, evaluating postmenopausal obesity fits this description. Further,

since the NCI, in collaboration with the National Heart, Lung, and Blood Institute, is proceeding with the Breast Cancer Prevention Trial using the chemotherapeutic agent tamoxifen, nurses could evaluate women's adherence to tamoxifen.

Once geneticists clone the breast cancer gene and biologists establish a laboratory test to identify women at high risk for breast cancer because they have the gene, nurses could study and test interventions in counseling, teaching, and supporting these women.

In the realm of screening and early detection, nurses could consider conducting the following studies: the effectiveness of screening by mammography for women younger than 50 years of age, and the effectiveness of screening by physical breast examination and BSE for women of all ages. The psychosocial concerns of women undergoing additional tests for a positive finding on a screening test (whether mammogram, physical breast examination, or BSE) are also needed, as well as ways to improve the health care professional's adherence to teaching breast cancer screening guidelines.

Patterns of care and symptom management studies will help women with breast cancer undergoing treatment. Nurses need to include women with advanced disease as well as those with early-stage breast cancer. Nurses have increasingly studied rehabilitation and cost issues, and this important endeavor needs to continue.

AVAILABILITY OF RESEARCH DOLLARS

Agencies are distributing more funds for breast cancer research. For example, the Department of Defense Army Medical Research and Development Command allocated $210 million to award in research grants in 1994 for breast cancer research, and the NCI received increased funding for breast cancer research. The NINR supports studies to improve women's knowledge and behavior concerning breast cancer prevention and detection, and research that leads to effective nursing interventions to support and enhance treatment of women with breast cancer.

From a listing of current breast cancer research projects, prepared by the Research Analysis and Evaluation Branch at the NCI, nurses are currently working in at least four projects. At least two nurse researchers have received academic awards from the NCI Division of Cancer Prevention and Control to conduct research in breast cancer, and at least three nurses have received funding from the NINR for breast cancer studies. A search for principal investigators in the Cancer Control Protocol Index in the Division of Cancer Prevention and Control at the NCI revealed one protocol on breast cancer with a nurse investigator in 1993.

Although agencies are allocating more funding for breast cancer research, more nurses are competing for research support. To increase the quality and quantity of nursing's role in breast cancer research, nurses will need to develop stronger collaborative working relationships with each other and with researchers in other disciplines. Nurse researchers have made and can continue to make significant contributions in breast cancer research in biology, diagnosis and treatment, and epidemiology, as well as the body of nursing knowledge.

References

Albrecht, S. A., & London, W. P. (1990). Season of birth and laterality of breast cancer. *Nursing Research, 39* (2), 118–120.

Ansell, D., Lacey, L., Whitman, S., Chen, E., & Phillips, C. (1994). A nurse-delivered intervention to reduce barriers to breast and cervical cancer screening in Chicago inner city clinics. *Public Health Reports—Hyattsville, 109* (1), 104–111.

Arathuzik, D. (1991a). Pain experience for metastatic breast cancer patients. Unraveling the mystery. *Cancer Nursing, 14* (1), 41–48.

Arathuzik, D. (1991b). The appraisal of pain and coping in cancer patients. *Western Journal of Nursing Research, 13* (6), 714–731.

Blesch, K. S., Paice, J. A., Wickham, R., Harte, N., Schnoor, D. K., Purl, S., Rehwalt, M., Kopp, P. L., Manson, S., Coveny, S. B., et al. (1991). Correlates of fatigue in people with breast or lung cancer. *Oncology Nursing Forum, 18* (1), 81–87.

Brailey, L. J. (1986). Effects of health teaching in the workplace on women's knowledge, beliefs, and practices regarding breast self-examination. *Research in Nursing and Health, 9* (3), 223–231.

Brandt, B. T. (1987). The relationship between hopelessness and selected variables in women receiving chemotherapy for breast cancer. *Oncology Nursing Forum, 14* (2), 35–39.

Cawley, M., Kostic, J., & Cappello, C. (1990). Informational and psychosocial needs of women choosing conservative surgery/primary radiation for early stage breast cancer. *Cancer Nursing, 13* (2), 90–94.

Champion, V. L. (1985). Use of the health belief model in determining frequency of breast self-examination. *Research in Nursing and Health, 8* (4), 373–379.

Champion, V. L. (1987). The relationship of breast self-examination to health belief model variables. *Research in Nursing and Health, 10* (6), 375–382.

Champion, V. L. (1988). Attitudinal variables related to intention, frequency and proficiency of breast self-examination in women 35 and over. *Research in Nursing and Health, 11* (5), 283–291.

Champion, V. L. (1990). Breast self-examination in women 35 and older: A prospective study. *Journal of Behavioral Medicine, 13* (6), 523–538.

Champion, V. L. (1991). The relationship of selected variables to breast cancer detection behaviors in women 35 and older. *Oncology Nursing Forum, 18* (4), 733–739.

Champion, V. L. (1992). Relationship of age to factors influencing breast self-examination practice. *Health Care for Women International, 13* (1), 1–9.

Champion, V. L. (1993). Instrument refinement for breast cancer screening behaviors. *Nursing Research, 42* (3), 139-143.

Chen, L., Neubauer, A., Kurisu, W., Waldman, F., Ljung, B., Goodson, W., III, Goldman, E., Moore, D., II, Balazs, M., Liu, E., et al. (1991). Loss of heterozygosity on the short arm of chromosome 17 is associated with high proliferative capacity and DNA aneuploidy in primary breast cancer. *Proceedings of the National Academy of Sciences, 88,* 3847–3851.

Cimprich, B. (1992). Attentional fatigue following breast cancer surgery. *Research in Nursing and Health, 15* (3), 199–207.

Cimprich, B. (1993). Development of an intervention to restore attention in cancer patients. *Cancer Nursing, 16* (2), 83–92.

Clark, G., Dressler, L., Owens, M., Pounds, G., Oldaker, T., & McGuire, W. (1989). Prediction of relapse or survival in patients with node negative breast cancer by DNA flow cytometry. *New England Journal of Medicine, 320,* 627–633.

Coates, R., Bransfield, D., Wesley, M., Hankey, B., Eley, W., Greenberg, R., Flanders, D., Hunter, C., Edwards, B., Forman, M., Chen, V., Reynolds, P., Boyd, P., Austin, D., Muss, H., Blacklow, R., & the Black/White Cancer

Survival Study Group. (1992). Differences between black and white women with breast cancer in time from symptom recognition to medical consultation. *Journal of the National Cancer Institute, 84*, 938–950.

Coleman, E. A., Feuer, E. J., & the NCI Breast Cancer Screening Consortium. (1992). Breast cancer screening among women from 65 to 74 years of age in 1987-88 and 1991. *Annals of Internal Medicine, 117* (11), 961–966.

Coleman, E. A., Kessler, L. G., Wun, L. M., Feuer, E. J. (1992). Trends in the surgical treatment of ductal carcinoma in situ of the breast. *American Journal of Surgery, 164* (1), 74–76.

Coleman, E. A., Lemon, S., Rudik, J., Depuy, S., & Baker, B.K. (1994). Rheumatic disease among 1167 women reporting local implant and systemic problems after breast implant surgery. *Journal of Women's Health, 3* (3), 165–177.

Coleman, E. A., Lord, J. E., Bowie, M., & Worley, M. J. (1993). A statewide breast cancer screening project. *Cancer Nursing, 16* (5), 347–353.

Coleman, E. A., & Pennypacker, H. (1991a). Evaluating breast self-examination performance. *Journal of Nursing Quality Assurance, 5* (3), 65–69.

Coleman, E. A., & Pennypacker, H. (1991b). Measuring breast self-examination proficiency. A scoring system developed from a paired comparison study. *Cancer Nursing, 14* (4), 211–217.

Coleman, E. A., Riley, M. B., Fields, F., & Prior, B. (1991). Efficacy of breast self-examination teaching methods among older women. *Oncology Nursing Forum, 18* (3), 561–566.

Coward, D. D. (1991). Self-transcendence and emotional well-being in women with advanced breast cancer. *Oncology Nursing Forum, 18* (5), 857–863.

Crooks, C. E., & Jones, S. D. (1989). Educating women about the importance of breast screenings: The nurse's role. *Cancer Nursing, 12* (3), 161–164.

David, A. J., Roul, R. K., & Kuruvilla, J. (1988). Lessons of self-help for Indian women with breast cancer. *Cancer Nursing, 11* (5), 283–287.

DeGeorge, D., Gray, J. J., Fetting, J. H., & Rolls, B. J. (1990). Weight gain in patients with breast cancer receiving adjuvant treatment as a function of restraint, disinhibition, and hunger. *Oncology Nursing Forum, 17* (suppl 3), 23–28.

Dixon, J. K., Moritz, D. A., & Baker, F. L. (1978). Breast cancer and weight gain: an unexpected finding. *Oncology Nursing Forum, 5* (3), 5–7.

Dodd, M. J. (1984). Self-care for patients with breast cancer to prevent side effects of chemotherapy: A concern for public health nursing. *Public Health Nursing, 1* (4), 202–209.

Dodd, M. J. (1988). Patterns of self-care in patients with breast cancer. *Western Journal of Nursing Research, 10* (1), 7–20.

Edwards, V. (1980). Changing breast self-examination behavior. *Nursing Research, 29* (5), 301–306.

Ehlke, G. (1988). Symptom distress in breast cancer patients receiving chemotherapy in the outpatient setting. *Oncology Nursing Forum, 15* (3), 343–346.

Elwood, J. M., Cox, B., & Richardson, A. K. (1993). The effectiveness of breast cancer screening by mammography in younger women. *The Online Journal of Current Clinical Trials [serial online]*, 25 Feb 1993 (Doc No 32).

Feather, B. L., & Wainstock, J. M. (1989a). Perceptions of postmastectomy patients. Part I. The relationships between social support and network providers. *Cancer Nursing, 12*(5), 293–300.

Feather, B. L., & Wainstock, J. M. (1989b). Perceptions of postmastectomy patients. Part II. Social support and attitudes towards mastectomy. *Cancer Nursing, 12* (5), 301–309.

Ferrans, C. E. (1990). Development of a quality of life index for patients with cancer. *Oncology Nursing Forum, 17* (Suppl 3), 15–19.

Fintor, L., Coleman, E. A., DeBor, M., Gibson, J., & Sutton, S. (1994). Promoting breast cancer screening to the public: Results from a community-based intervention model. In *Proceedings of the 2nd High Tatras International Health Symposium: Health and Quality of Life in Changing Europe in the Year 2000.* New York: Symposium International.

Fisher, B., Costantino, J., Redmond, C., Fisher, E., Margolese, R., Dimitrov, N., Wolmark, N., Wickerham, D. L., Deutsch, M., Ore, L., et al. (1993). Lumpectomy compared with lumpectomy and radiation therapy for the treatment of intraductal breast cancer. *New England Journal of Medicine, 328* (22), 1581–1586.

Fletcher, S. W., Black, W., Harris, R., Rimer, B. K., & Shapiro, S. (1993). Report of the International Workshop on Screening for Breast Cancer. *Journal of the National Cancer Institute, 85* (20), 1644–1656.

Folkman, J. (1990). What is the evidence that tumors are angiogenesis dependent? *Journal of the National Cancer Institute, 84*, 4–6.

Foltz, A. T. (1985). Weight gain among stage II breast cancer patients: A study of five factors: Activity, depression, intake, serum estradiol, and metabolic rate. *Oncology Nursing Forum, 12* (3), 21–26.

Gabriel, S. E., O'Fallon, W. M., Kurland, L. T., Beard, C. M., Woods, J. E., & Melton, L. J. (1994). Risk of connective-tissue diseases and other disorders after breast implantation. *The New England Journal of Medicine, 330* (24), 1697–1749.

Given, B., & Given, C. W. (1992). Patient and family caregiver reaction to new and recurrent breast cancer. *Journal of the American Medical Womens Association, 47* (5), 201–206.

Glenn, B. L., & Moore, L. A. (1990). Relationship of self-concept, health locus of control, and perceived cancer treatment options to the practice of breast self-examination. *Cancer Nursing, 13* (6), 361–365.

Gray, M. E. (1990). Factors related to practice of breast self-examination in rural women. *Cancer Nursing, 13* (2), 100–107.

Grindel, C. G., Cahill, C. A., & Walker, M. (1989). Food intake of women with breast cancer during their first six month of chemotherapy. *Oncology Nursing Forum, 16* (3), 401–407.

Hall, J., Lee, M., Newman, B., Morrow, J., Anderson, L., Huey, B., & King, M. C. (1990). Linkage of early-onset familial breast cancer to chromosome 17q21. *Science, 250,* 1684–1689.

Hallal, J. C. (1982). The relationship of health beliefs, health locus of control, and self concept to the practice of breast self-examination in adult women. *Nursing Research, 31* (3), 137–142.

Haughey, B. P., Marshall, J. R., Mettlin, C., Nemoto, T., Kroldart, K., & Swanson, M. (1984). Nurses' ability to detect nodules in silicone breast models. *Oncology Nursing Forum, 11* (1), 37–42.

Haughey, B. P., Marshall, J. R., Nemoto, T., Kroldart, K., Mettlin, C., & Swanson, M. (1988). Breast self-examination: Reported practices, proficiency, and stage of disease at diagnosis. *Oncology Nursing Forum, 15* (3), 315–319.

Heidrich, S. M., & Ward, S. E. (1992). The role of the self in adjustment to cancer in elderly women. *Oncology Nursing Forum, 19* (10), 1491–1496.

Hilton, B. A. (1989). The relationship of uncertainty, control, commitment, and threat of recurrence to coping strategies used by women diagnosed with breast cancer. *Journal of Behavioral Medicine, 12* (1), 39–54.

Hirshfield-Bartek, J. (1982). Health beliefs and their influence on breast self-examination practices in women with breast cancer. *Oncology Nursing Forum, 9* (3), 77–81.

Hopkins, M. B. (1986). Information-seeking and adaptational outcomes in women receiving chemotherapy for breast cancer. *Cancer Nursing, 9* (5), 256–262.

Howard, J., Hankey, B., Greenberg, R., Austin, D., Correa, P., Chen, V., & Durako, S. (1992). A collaborative study of differences in the survival rates of black patients and white patients with cancer. *Cancer, 69,* 2349–2359.

Howe, G., Friedenreich, C., Jain, M., & Miller, A. (1991). A cohort study of fat intake and risk of breast cancer. *Journal of the National Cancer Institute, 83,* 336–340.

Hunter, D., & Kelsey, L. (1993). Pesticide residues and breast cancer: The harvest of a silent spring? *Journal of the National Cancer Institute, 85* (8), 598–599.

Issel, L. M., Ersek, M., & Lewis, F. M. (1990). How children cope with mother's breast cancer. *Oncology Nursing Forum, 17* (Suppl 3), 5–12.

Knobf, M. K., Mullen, J. C., Xistris, D., & Moritz, D. A. (1983). Weight gain in women with breast cancer receiving adjuvant chemotherapy. *Oncology Nursing Forum, 10* (2), 28–33.

Kramer, M. A., Albrecht, S., & Miller, R. A. (1985). Handedness and the laterality of breast cancer in women. *Nursing Research, 34* (6), 333–337.

Krouse, H. J., & Krouse, J. H. (1982). Cancer as crisis: The critical elements of adjustment. *Nursing Research, 31* (2), 96–101.

Kuhns-Hastings, J., Brakey, M. R., & Marshall, I. A. (1993). Effectiveness of a comprehensive breast cancer-screening class for women residing in rural areas. *Applied Nursing Research, 6* (2), 71–79.

Kurtz, M. E., Given, B., Given, C. W., & Kurtz, J. C. (1993). Relationships of barriers and facilitators to breast self-examination, mammography, and clinical breast self-examination in a worksite population. *Cancer Nursing, 16*(4), 251–259.

Lauver, D. (1989). Instructional information and breast self-examination practice. *Research in Nursing and Health, 12* (1), 11–19.

Lauver, D., & Angerame, M. (1988). Development of a questionnaire to measure beliefs and attitudes about breast self-examination. *Cancer Nursing, 11* (1), 51–57

Lauver, D. (1992). Psychosocial variables, race, and intention to seek care for breast cancer symptoms. *Nursing Research, 41* (4), 236–241.

Lierman, L. M. (1988). Discovery of breast changes. Women's responses and nursing implications. *Cancer Nursing, 11* (6), 352–361.

Lierman, L. M., Kasprzyk, D., & Benoliel, J. Q. (1991). Understanding adherence to breast self-examination in older women. *Western Journal of Nursing Research, 13* (1), 46–61.

London, W. P., & Albrecht, S. A. (1991). Breast cancer and cerebral laterality. *Perceptual & Motor Skills, 72* (1), 112–114.

Longman, A. J., Atwood, J. R., Sherman, J. B., Benedict, J., & Shang, T. (1992). Care needs of home-based cancer patients and their caregivers: Quantitative findings. *Cancer Nursing, 15* (3), 182–190.

Longman, A. J., Saint-Germain, M. A., & Modiano, M. (1992). Use of breast cancer screening by older Hispanic women. *Public Health Nursing, 9* (2), 118–124.

Loveys, B. J., & Klaich, K. (1991). Breast cancer: Demands of illness. *Oncology Nursing Forum, 18* (1), 75–80.

Ludwick, R. (1992). Registered nurses' knowledge and practices of teaching and performing breast exams among elderly women. *Cancer Nursing, 15* (1), 161–167.

MacVicar, M. G., Winningham, M. L., & Nickel, J. L. (1989). Effects of aerobic interval training on cancer patients' functional capacity. *Nursing Research, 38* (6), 348–351.

Mandelblatt, J., Traxler, M., Lakin, P., Thomas, L., Chauhan, P., Matseoane, S., & Kanetsky, P. (1993). A nurse practitioner intervention to increase breast and cervical cancer screening for poor, elderly black women. The Harlem Study Team. *Journal of General Internal Medicine, 8* (4), 173–178.

Massey, V. (1986). Perceived susceptibility to breast cancer and practice of breast self-examination. *Nursing Research, 35* (3), 183–185.

Meriney, D. K. (1990). Application of Orem's conceptual framework to patients with hypercalcemia related to breast cancer. *Cancer Nursing, 13* (5), 316–323.

Mickley, J. R., Soeken, K., & Belcher, A. (1992). Spiritual well-being, religiousness, and hope among women with breast cancer. *Image: Journal of Nursing Scholarship, 24* (4), 267–272.

Mills, P., Beeson, W., Phillips, R., & Fraser, G. (1989). Dietary habits and breast cancer incidence among Seventh-Day Adventists. *Cancer, 64,* 582–590.

Moch, S. D. (1990). Health within the experience of breast cancer. *Journal of Advanced Nursing, 15* (12), 1426–1435.

Nail, L. M., Jones, L. S., Greene, D., Schipper, D. L., & Jensen, R. (1991). Use and perceived efficacy of self-care activities in patients receiving chemotherapy. *Oncology Nursing Forum, 18* (5), 883–887.

Nattinger, A., Gottlieb, M., Veum, J., Yahnke, D., & Goodwin, J. (1992). Geographic variation in the use of breast-conserving treatment for breast cancer. *New England Journal of Medicine, 326,* 1102–1107.

Nayfield, S., Karp, J., Ford, L., Dorr, F., & Kramer, B. (1991). Potential role of tamoxifen in prevention of breast cancer. *Journal of the National Cancer Institute, 83,* 1450–1459.

Nelson, J. P. (1991). Perceived health, self-esteem, health habits, and perceived benefits and barriers to exercise in women who have and who have not experienced stage I breast cancer. *Oncology Nursing Forum, 18* (7), 1191–1197.

Nemcek, M. A. (1989). Factors influencing black women's breast self-examination practice. *Cancer Nursing, 12* (6), 339–343.

Northouse, L. L. (1988). Social support in patients' and husbands' adjustment to breast cancer. *Nursing Research, 37* (2), 91–95.

Northouse, L. L. (1989a). A longitudinal study of the adjustment of patients and husbands to breast cancer. *Oncology Nursing Forum, 16* (4), 511–516.

Northouse, L. L. (1989b). The impact of breast cancer on patients and husbands. *Cancer Nursing, 12* (5), 276–284.

Northouse, L. L., & Swain, M. A. (1987). Adjustment of patients and husbands to the initial impact of breast cancer. *Nursing Research, 36* (4), 221–225.

Parker, R. (1987). The effectiveness of scalp hypothermia in preventing cyclophosphamide-induced alopecia. *Oncology Nursing Forum, 14* (6), 49–53

Peters, W. P., Ross, M., Vredenburgh, J. J., Meisenberg, B., Marks, L. B., Winer, E., Kurtzberg, J., Bast, R. C. Jr., Jones, R., Shpall, E., Wu, K., Rosner, G., Gilbert, C., Mathias, B., Coniglio, D., Petros, W., Henderson, I. C., Norton, L., Weiss, R. B., Budman, D., & Hurd, D. (1993). High-dose chemotherapy and autologous bone marrow support as consolidation after standard-dose adjuvant therapy for high-risk primary breast cancer. *Journal of Clinical Oncology, 11* (6), 1132–1143.

Pierce, P. F. (1993). Deciding on breast cancer treatment: A description of decision behavior. *Nursing Research, 42* (1), 22–28.

Pike, M., Bernstein, L., & Spicer, D. (1993). The relationship of exogenous hormones to breast cancer risk. In J. E. Niederhuber (Ed.). *Current therapy in oncology.* St. Louis: Mosby.

Primomo, J., Yates, B. C., & Woods, N. F. (1990). Social support for women during chronic illness: The relationship among sources and types to adjustment. *Research in Nursing and Health, 13* (3), 153–161.

Rose, M. A., Fore, V., Rachide, M., Cummings, H., Creech, D., Price, D., & Elesha, M. (1980). Husbands as health educators for their wives: A pilot study in breast cancer education. *Oncology Nursing Forum, 7* (3), 18–20.

Rutledge, D. N. (1987). Factors related to women's practice of breast self-examination. *Nursing Research, 36* (2), 117–121.

Rutledge, D. N., & Davis, G. T. (1988). Breast self-examination compliance and the health belief model. *Oncology Nursing Forum, 15* (2), 175–179.

Samarel, N., & Fawcett, J. (1992). Enhancing adaptation to breast cancer: The addition of coaching to support groups. *Oncology Nursing Forum, 19* (4), 591–596.

Schlueter, L. A. (1982). Knowledge and beliefs about breast cancer and breast self-examination among athletic and nonathletic women. *Nursing Research, 31* (6), 348–353.

Scott, D. W. (1983). Anxiety, critical thinking, and information processing during and after breast biopsy. *Nursing Research, 32* (1), 24–28.

Simmons, C. C. (1984). The relationship between life change losses and stress levels for females with breast cancer. *Oncology Nursing Forum, 11* (2), 37–41.

Slamon, D., Clark, G., Wong, S., Levin, W., Ullrich, A., McGuire, W. (1987). Human breast cancer: Correlation of relapse and survival with amplification of the HER-2/neu oncogene. *Science, 235,* 177–182.

Steeg, P., Bevilacqua, G., Kopper, L., Thorgeirsson, U., Talmadge, J., Liotta, L., & Sobel, M. (1988). Evidence for a novel gene associated with low tumor metastatic potential. *Journal of the National Cancer Institute, 80,* 200–204.

Stillman, M. J. (1977). Women's health beliefs about breast cancer and breast self-examination. *Nursing Research, 26*(2), 121–127.

Suominen, T. (1992). Breast cancer patients' opportunities to participate in their care. *Cancer Nursing, 15* (1), 68–72.

Tandom, A., Clark, G., Chamness, G., Chirgwin, J., & McGuire, W. (1990). Cathepsin D and prognosis in breast cancer. *New England Journal of Medicine, 322,* 297–302.

Trotta, P. (1980). Breast self-examination: Factors influencing compliance. *Oncology Nursing Forum, (3),* 13–17.

Tulman, L., & Fawcett, J. (1990). A framework for studying functional status after diagnosis of breast cancer. *Cancer Nursing, 13* (2), 95–99.

Tulman, L., Fawcett, J., & McEvoy, M. D. (1991). Development of the inventory of functional status-cancer. *Cancer Nursing, 14*(5), 254–260.

Turnbull, E. M. (1978). Effect of basic preventive health practices and mass media on the practice of breast self-examination. *Nursing Research, 27* (2), 98-102.

Ward, S., & Griffin, J. (1990). Developing a test of knowledge of surgical options for breast cancer. *Cancer Nursing, 13* (3), 191–196.

Ward, S., Heidrich, S., & Wolberg, W. (1989). Factors women take into account when deciding upon type of surgery for breast cancer. *Cancer Nursing, 12* (6), 344–351.

Ward, S. E., Viergutz, G., Tormey, D., deMuth, J., & Paulen, A. (1992). Patients' reactions to completion of adjuvant breast cancer therapy. *Nursing Research, 41* (6), 362–366.

Wehrwein, T. C., & Eddy, M. E. (1993). Breast health promotion: Behaviors of midlife women. *Journal of Holistic Nursing, 11* (3), 223–236.

Williams, R. D. (1988). Factors affecting the practice of breast self-examination in older women. *Oncology Nursing Forum, 15* (5), 611–616.

Wilson, S., & Morse, J. M. (1991). Living with a wife undergoing chemotherapy. *Image: Journal of Nursing Scholarship, 23* (2), 78–84.

Winningham, M. L., & MacVicar, M. G. (1988). The effect of aerobic exercise on patient reports of nausea. *Oncology Nursing Forum, 15* (4), 447–450.

Winningham, M. L., MacVicar, M. G., Bondoc, M., Anderson, J. I., & Minton, J. P. (1989). Effect of aerobic exercise on body weight and composition in patients with breast cancer on adjuvant chemotherapy. *Oncology Nursing Forum, 16* (5), 683–689.

Woods, N. F., & Earp, J. A. (1978). Women with cured breast cancer—a study of mastectomy patients in North Carolina. *Nursing Research, 27* (5), 279–285.

Wyper, M. A. (1990). Breast self-examination and the health belief model: Variations on a theme. *Research in Nursing and Health, 13* (6), 421–428.

Young-McCaughan, S., & Sexton, D. L. (1991). A retrospective investigation of the relationship between aerobic exercise and quality of life in women with breast cancer. *Oncology Nursing Forum, 18* (4), 751–757.

Index